Mastering The World Of Herbs

A Know How – How To
Reference Guide To Herbs, Essential Oils,
And All Things Natural

To Mary,
To the wise woman in you. I hope it will bring you joy & happiness
Leilah 6/21/14

Leilah

Mastering The World Of Herbs
Copyright ©2002 By The Herb Start, Inc.

Published and distributed in the United States by:
The Herb Start, Inc.
PO BOX 673
Pine, AZ 85544

Cover and back page designed by Natalie Hajdu-Voakes
Leilah's cover photo by Studio No. 5, Scottsdale, AZ
Leilah's back cover photo by Lawrence Duncan
Saguaro and Ocotillo illustration by Lawrence Duncan

All rights reserved. No part of this book may be reproduced by any mechanical, photoraphic, or electronic process, or in the form of a phonographic recording, nor may it be stored in a retrieval system, transmitted, or otherwise be copied for public or private use - other than for "fair use" without prior written permisson of the publisher.

The author of this book does not diagnose or prescribe treatments for diseases or injuries. Although the information in this book is drawn from many traditional herbal sources, the author is mindful that each person is unique and complex. For this reason, the reader is advised to consult a qualified health care professional regarding the use of herbs.

ISBN-13: 978-1494477431
ISBN-10: 1494477432

1st printing, 2002
2nd printing November 2008
3rd printing, January 2014

To my daughter Natalie,
Thank you for your loving, wise, and passionate support of my life's work as an herbalist and for your essential and greatly appreciated help with this book, and the many more hours you have lovingly worked by my side. You are my inspiration. I am honored to be passing the torch on to you, the next generation, so that this knowledge will exist forever. Working with you is a gift I treasure. I love you so much.

To my husband Lawrence,
Thank you for sharing your ancestoral wisdom and knowledge.
You have taught me both patience, and the wisdom that all good things happen in their own time.
I love you and the life we share.

Table Of Contents

Chapter Title	Pages	Chapter Title	Pages
24-Hour Energy Flow in the Body	1	Dosing	69
Additives, Preservatives & Other Ingredients	2-8	Ear Coning	70-73
Algeas and Lichens	9-12	Essential Oils & Attar Oils	74-112
Astrology and Herbs	13-17	Exfoliants	113-116
Ayurvedic Herbs	18-31	Gifts from the Honeybee	117-118
Castor Oil Packs	32	Henna & Mendhi	119-120
Cell Salts	33-35	Herb List	121-190
Chakras and Herbs	36-39	First Aid for Radiation Protection	191
Chinese Patent Formulas	40-53	Herbal Safety Guide	192-199
Clays and Muds	54-58	Hot Peppers & Spicy Recipes	200-203
Desert Medicinal Plants	59-64	Hydrosols	204-213
Different Forms of Herbal Medicine	65-68	Incense	214-220

Chapter Title	Pages
Infused Oils	221-226
Minerals	227-229
Moxibustion	230
Mushrooms & Fungi	231-232
Neti Pot	233-234
Plant Constituents Solvent Guide	235
Natural Preservatives	236
Salts	237-240
Sweeteners	241-244
Vegetable, Nut & Seed Carrier Oils	245-258
Vegetable, Nut & Seed Butters	259-261
Waxes	262-264
Index	266-275

Endorsements

As a practicing and experienced herbalist, I absolutely love Leilah's book. Mastering the Word of Herbs is the first reference guide I go to when I have health questions. Her stories and side notes are incredibly entertaining and truly unique. A must have on your shelf and in your practice.

Natalie Hajdu-Voakes – Herbalist, Herbal Teacher, Reiki II Practitioner,
Spectro- Chrome Therapist, Vegan, and owner of the Herb Stop, Pine, AZ

This is the book I've been waiting for. Leilah's wisdom is a gift to a generation of health seekers. Finally, it's the complete resource I need to keep handy for my own use and the guide I'm eager to pass on. As a caretaker for many with special health considerations and an advocate for the benefit of this wisdom, this book is an essential key in gaining access to this vast knowledge. Clearly organized and written in a personal, professional tone that is to be trusted and honored, this is a book to be kept open, referred to and applied as we seek a more whole, healthy and sustainable way of living.

Sam – Artistic Director, Detour Company Theatre, Phoenix, AZ

This is an easy to read encyclopedia of herbs, oils and natural remedies. A tool box for the prevention and cure of ailments and an endless supply of beauty tips. This book belongs next to your favorite cookbook. You'll want to use it often.

Rebekah Belanger – Certified Pilates and Dance instructor, Tuscon, AZ

"Mastering The World Of Herbs" is the most comprehensive reference guide for natural and herbal medicine to date. It takes complex botanical and medical information and puts it in everyday langage that is easy to understand and accessible to all. I use this guide on a weekly basis to brush up my knowledge on western, ayurvedic and Chinese herbal medicine.

Steven D. Hajdu, M.D., Lausanne, Switzerland

This extensive study of practical everyday use of our immense world of herbs is outlined for us by the author, one who is genuine and creative. She is concerned and cares about guiding us into a healthier life. When we realize the benefits our world of herbs have to offer, then we will recive the gift of healing.

Suzanne B. Blaauw, Caretaker, Herbalist, Payson, AZ

In a quest to achieve my own physical goals I realize there is an importance in seeking knowledge that keeps me healthy and strong from a natural whole body perspective. As a novice in using reference guides, and as one who has no time to persue this body of knowledge, Leilah's book is an important key to gaining quick, dependable and useable answers without having to wade through complicated material.

Paul Voakes, Firefighter, Bodybuilder, Payson, AZ

I find this book provides alternative, practical and essential theories for using a wholistic approach to curing ailments and conditions shared in the animal world. The knowledge it contains is timeless, but its application and the vast range of materials it covers makes it a book for a daily use.

Timothy A. Patterson, DVM, CVA, VCP, Payson, AZ

The World of Herbs not only belongs to two-footed creatures. As a horse-trainer, I see the application of the natural healing therapies and the use of Leilah's knowledge that works for the many animals I deal with.

Kandy Christensen, Horse Trainer, Herbalist, Payson, AZ

The wisdom of Mother Earth is sacred. Leilah, in her book, honors the spiritual wisdom Nature holds for us all. Gently, and with great respect, Leilah shares the secrets and a rich body of knowledge that has been guarded and handed down for many generations. She offers it to her readers now through a strong conviction that we can no longer ignore the timeless Truth that Nature holds the key to providing healing for a broken world.

Spotted Eagle, Native American Healing & Counseling, Azeé Bee Nahaghá of Diné Nation, Arizona

As a professional homeopath and spiritual teacher of some 30-odd years, it is easy for me to see a truly gifted, intuitive, talented healer when I see one, and Leilah is just that. It would be easy to go on and on about her genuine gifts, qualifications and accomplishements, but the truth to me is much simpler than that: Leilah is a gift to humanity and a blessing for us all. Leilah has just written the book which healers of generations past - of all disciplines - could only dream about, and now we have the opportunity to own. She is a fine, intelligent and hard-working individual and her book cannot help but be a reflection of those attributes.

Sati L. Tripp - Professional Homeopath, Spiritualist and
mother of five grown children, with two grandkids and another on the way.
Pine, AZ

I believe that every person needs to take the responsability to improve their own health and without knowledge we can not make appropriate judejements. Thank you for an informational book that will help us make the much needed changes

Judy J. Scofield RN, AZ

Leilah's Introduction And Acknowledgements

I started writing this book many, many years before putting words onto paper. As a child and growing up, I carried knowledge gained from my grandmother in Switzerland. I continued to explore remedies, cures and solutions through my formal education and work as an herbalist. Finally I was gifted knowledge gained from my husband who shared with me the natural healing wisdom found in his Native American tradition. This complex body of knowledge began to find its way onto slips of paper, note cards and the like. I continually shared this knowledge through phone calls, store visits and random encounters with eager, expectant and hopeful seekers longing for answers. Finally it became clear to me that it was time to write, to weave together this body of knowledge so it could make a difference in the lives of people everywhere. I always wanted to have a book, one complete book, where I could have at my fingertips complete access to the world of herbs and all things natural. This book is written for the novice, as well as for the experienced herbalist, medical healers and those who are simply curious. It provides easy access to the fascinating and life-enhancing gifts nature so abundantly offers each of us.

Many people contributed to the creation of this book. No list can truly hold every name but to this group I am most appreciative. I am thankful for Natalie, and Spotted Eagle for their patience, practical knowledge and never failing support. I am grateful to my proof reader Cindy as well as to my many customers, clients, and students, from whom I learned so much. I am thankful for my teachers in Switzerland at the Apothekenhelferinnen Schule, for Dr. Dorothy Marshall at Canadian College of Natural Healing, and for Sam. I am forever indebted to my grand-mother Marie who saved my life through the use of herbs when I was just a child. Finally, in all that I teach, share and offer here, I appreciate and honor the natural world who is the supreme teacher of all.

x

24-HOUR ENERGY FLOW IN THE BODY

Every 24 hours the circulation of energy (Chi) flows through the entire body in a specific pattern, so that each 2-hour period, one organ is dominant. For example, the peak energy for the heart occurs between 11am and 1 pm. If there is an excess of energy, it may become apparent at this time. Twelve hours from the peak time is a low energy point, for the heart it is 11 pm to 1 am. If symptoms occur from a weak heart, it may manifest during this time.

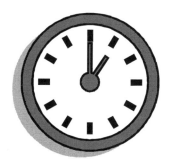

Peak	Organ	Low
11 pm – 1 am	GALLBLADDER	11 am – 1 pm
1 am – 3 am	LIVER	1 pm – 3 pm
3 am – 5 am	LUNGS	3 pm – 5 pm
5 am – 7 am	LARGE INTESTINE	5 pm – 7 pm
7 am – 9 am	STOMACH	7 pm – 9 pm
9 am – 11 am	SPLEEN	9 pm – 11 pm
11 am – 1 pm	HEART	11 pm – 1 am
1 pm – 3 pm	SMALL INTESTINE	1 am – 3 am
3 pm – 5 pm	BLADDER	3 am – 5 am
5 pm – 7 pm	KIDNEYS	5 am – 7 am
7 pm – 9 pm	PERICARDIUM	7 am – 9 am
9 pm – 11 pm	THREE HEATER	9 am – 11 am

ADDITIVES AND OTHER INGREDIENTS

Acacia Gum, Gum Arabic
(Acacia senegal)
Gum acacia is a sap that is tapped from the acacia Senegal tree. These trees grow exclusively south of the Sahara desert, the so-called "Gum Belt". The first recorded uses of gum arabic are more than 4000 years old; the Egyptians used it for the conservation of mummies. Today, gum arabic is being used for a wide array of applications in the food, beverage, and pharmaceutical industries. It is also used in cosmetics as a thickener, emulsifier and stabilizer for creams and lotions, in hair styling gels and sprays. Add a small amount of gum arabic to increase viscosity to your creams and lotions, and also to give the skin a smooth feel and protective coating.

Aloe Vera Gel
(Aloe barbadensis)
Aloe vera relieves sunburn and the symptoms associated with adverse skin conditions, such as dry skin, psoriasis and eczema. Aloe vera is a skin soother and moisturizer. Research has shown that aloe vera penetrates human skin almost four times faster than water. When combined with other healing agents, aloe vera helps these substances penetrate the skin more effectively, carrying them to the deeper layers of the skin. Aloe vera has anti-inflammatory and pain-relieving properties. Aloe vera can reduce the negative effects radiation has on the skin, accelerates tissue repair and normal cell growth. Internally, aloe vera has the capability to heal the whole digestive tract. Here is an excellent remedy some people have used to heal ulcers is: Mix one drop of 3% hydrogen peroxide into one ounce of aloe vera, drink before bed for two days. Thereafter, every night before bed take one ounce of aloe vera juice only, for about two weeks.

Apple Cider Vinegar
(Acetic acid)
Apple cider vinegar has been used for over 10,000 years and the benefits are endless. The word "vinegar" comes from *vin aigre*, French for "sour wine", but other ingredients can be used to make vinegar. Apple cider vinegar is made from the juice of fresh apples. Apple cider vinegar is rich in enzymes and potassium. It is a natural antibiotic, germ fighter, fights E.Coli and other bacteria. Helps control and normalize weight, improves digestions and assimilation, improves immune system, helps soothe dry throats, and removes body toxins. Take one to two teaspoons of raw, organic apple cider vinegar, add a sweeter like honey, maple syrup, or molasses and add it to 8 oz of distilled water. Take it two to three times daily and see an increase in

energy, soft skin, and decreased muscle and joint stiffness. Because of apple cider vinegar's antiseptic properties, it can be used topically to treat dozens of common conditions, including, sunburn, bruises and cuts, aches and pains, body odor, ear infections, yeast infections, dandruff, hair loss, and to restore ph levels to skin and hair. Apple cider is also helpful for animals. It is great for maintaining a healthy, shiny coat. It also works as a repellant for fleas, ticks and other insects because they don't like the acidic environment of the skin. Apple cider vinegar also alleviates hot spots, constant wound licking and skin allergies.

Hair Rinse for Shiny and Manageable Hair

Hair rinses are conditioning treatments that soften the hair, encourage shine and body, and make hair more manageable. Rinses can also help bring out the natural highlights in hair.

<u>Method 1</u> – To make a vinegar rinse, make a vinegar extract by macerating one ounce of herbs in one to two cups of apple cider vinegar. Cover and set in a dark place for one week. Strain and combine with an equal amount of water (distilled or rain water) and pour onto hair as a final rinse.

<u>Method 2</u> – To make an infusion, warm selected herbs in vinegar, one ounce of herbs to one cup of vinegar and one cup of water, steep for 30 minutes. Cool to desired temperature. Strain and pour over hair as a final rinse.

Suggested herbs for hair rinses:

Herb	Properties
Sage	astringent and refreshing
Chamomile	healthful and highlighting
Nettles	tonic and strengthening
Rosemary	conditioning and stimulating
Lemon Grass	cleansing and astringent

Arrowroot
(Maranta arudinacea)

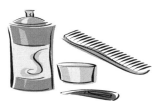

Arrowroot is made from the root of the maranta arudinacea plant. It is a thickening agent with excellent absorbent properties, and can be added to pastes and facial masques. Arrowroot can also be used as a main ingredient in body powders, giving a smooth, silky feeling to the skin and helping to absorb moisture. In cooking, arrowroot thickens at lower temperature and is virtually odorless. Use same amount as you would cornstarch and 1/3 less when substituting wheat flour. It makes a clear sauce instead of cloudy, excellent when preparing fruit sauces.

Foot Powder (for smelly feet)

1 oz arrowroot
8 drops peppermint essential oil
8 drops tea tree essential oil
4 drops sage essential oil
Mix ingredients thoroughly and store in a shaker

Baking Soda
(Sodium bicarbonate)

Did you know that baking soda helps alkalize the body? Baking soda is excellent for any acidic condition in the body. Baking soda is known to destroy any virus lingering in the body, because when the body is in a slight alkaline state, virus cannot survive. The most effective way I have found to do this is to add one *level* teaspoon of baking soda to one cup of hot distilled water. Drink this mix as hot as you are able to tolerate. Do this three to four times a day. The next day, I find I am free of any viruses. Baking soda can also be added to baths for itchy skin, and other skin problems, and as a gentle abrasive and cleaning agent in toothpowder. Leaves your teeth white and clean.

Borax
(Sodium borate)

Borax is the gentlest soap. It is an emulsifier, natural preservative and buffering agent for moisturizers, scrubs and bath salts. Borax increases cleaning power, softens water, disinfects, loosen dirt and stains, and removes odors. Where does borax come from? During rainy seasons the water runoffs from adjacent mineral-rich mountains accumulate in nearby lakes. The runoff is rich in the element boron and becomes highly concentrated when it evaporates during dry seasons. Eventually the concentration is so great that crystals of borax and other boron minerals form.

Camphor crystals
(Cinnamomum camphora)

Camphor is a resin colleted from the cinnamon camphora tree and has been used externally for upper respiratory problems, asthma, nasal congestion, sinus headaches, rheumatic pain and gout. In ayurveda, camphor is known to increase Prana (breathing), opens up the senses and brings clarity to the mind. Fill a small jar with camphor crystals, and keep it tightly sealed. To relieve congestion, headaches, and to awaken perception, open the small jar and breathe in the aroma forcefully.

Fizzy Bath Salts and Bomb

Mix 1 cup of baking soda with ½ cup of citric acid in a large bowl. Scoop out ½ cup in a smaller bowl. Add coloring and scent, and mix well. Slowly incorporate back into large bowl. Remove 1/3 cup of the mixture, spritz lightly with witch hazel, so that the mixture will "clump" together. Pack the mixture inside a mold. Release onto a cardboard and repeat.

Mineral Bath

1 cup borax	1 tbsp clay
1 cup epsom salt	20 drops essential oils
1 cup sea salt	20 drops essences

Mix thoroughly and store in a glass jar. Add 2 tbsp. per bath. You may add a little milk, cream or oils if you have dry skin.

Citric Acid
(Citric acid)
Derived from citrus fruits, citric acid is an acidifier and antioxidant used in foods. Citric acid is used in cosmetics to adjust the pH level and prevent the cosmetics from becoming too alkaline.

Cornstarch
(Zea mays
Cornstarch is made from corn and is used in body powders and milk baths to add silkiness and to soothe the skin. To prevent diaper rash in babies, cornstarch is a safer alternative than talc. Cornstarch can also be used in the same way as arrowroot as a thickening agent when mixed with water or other liquids.

Guar Gum
(Cyamopsis tetragonoloba)
Guar gum is derived from the guar plant, and is a natural thickener, emulsifier and stabilizer. Guar gum is useful because it has the ability to thicken without heat.

Glycerin, Vegetable
(Vegetable Glycerin, USP)
Glycerin is a substance that occurs naturally in vegetables fats. It is a colorless, odorless, sweet and syrupy liquid. Use it in creams, lotions, bath salts, soap making, herb tinctures (glycerites) and cough syrups. Vegetable glycerin's humectant properties are useful in moisturizing and soothing dry and parched skin. However, it is very sticky, if more than 20 % is added to cosmetic. Add vegetable glycerin to an alcohol menstrum when extracting tannin-rich herbs to help liberate their medicinal properties while neutralizing the tannins. The menstrum should be 10 % vegetable glycerin to 90% brandy or vodka. To make a non-alcohol herb tincture (glycerite) I use 70 % vegetable glycerin to 30 % water.

> **Baby Powder**
> - 1 cup cornstarch
> - 10 drops mandarin essential oil
> - 5 drops lavender essential oil
>
> Mix ingredients well and store in a shaker.

A Tasty Glycerite

Place your herbs into a jar, add enough brandy to cover, and macerate for one to three months. Strain out the solids, and squeeze all the liquid through cheesecloth. Measure the volume of extract, and then add the same amount of vegetable glycerin. Place this liquid into a crock-pot and simmer down to half of the original amount of liquid. Add two to ten percent of something tasty, such as maple syrup, honey, molasses, vanilla, fruit concentrate, flavored vinegar, natural flavors, essential oils, etc. Here you have the concentration and benefits of an alcohol extract, but without the alcohol. And best of all, it tastes good!

Lanolin, Anhydrous
(Lanolin)
Lanolin is considered a wax (chemically it is not a fat) and is obtained from the wool of sheep. It has a heavy and thick feel. When it is added to cosmetics, it provides a protective and moisturizing barrier. Lanolin absorbs and holds water in the skin, preventing water loss, which gives the skin a soft and smooth feeling. Lanolin can be used as a bees wax substitute in making cosmetics to emulsify and bind creams, lotions, salves, etc. Lanolin is excellent for dry, rough and cracking skin. Lanolin can possibly retard the development of fine wrinkles of aging.

Lecithin
(Lecithin)
Lecithin is naturally derived from egg yokes, sunflowers, soybeans or corn. It is being used as a moisturizer, restorative and nutrient for the skin and hair. It has the ability to penetrate the epidermis and carrying nutrients deep into the cells. You can use lecithin as a thickening agent in creams and lotions. Taken internally, lecithin helps with oil absorption into the body, deep into the organs. If you are unable to assimilate dietary oils or are lacking oils in your body, your skin and hair may be dry and your joints may feel stiff. Lecithin is high in vitamin B and B complex, the stress vitamin.

Menthol crystals
(Mentha piperita)
Menthol crystals are clear and colorless crystals obtained from steam distilled peppermint oil. Menthol acts as an analgesic by numbing the nerves after it cools. It can be added to arthritis ointments and sports rubs. As an inhalant, it can help clear up congested respiratory passages. Camphor is specific for upper respiratory problems, where as menthol is more for lower respiratory situations.

Pumice
(Pumex)
Pumice is a light, porous volcanic rock that forms during explosive eruptions. Pumice stone is good for removing dead skin. For an effective scrubbing effect, add pumice stone powder to foot scrubs and soaps.

Silk Amino Acid
(Silk amino acids)
Silk amino acid is essentially 100 % pure natural silk protein, carefully processed to retain its original physical structure, and chemical composition. Silk amino acid is very unique, as it has the ability to hold and release moisture depending on the temperature and humidity of the surroundings. Available in powdered and liquid hydrolyzed form, it is used in cosmetics and

soaps because of the silky feel. To give a cream or lotion a truly special feel, use silk amino acid at 1-5%. In soaps, use it at 4-10% to achieve a silky lather. Mix into the water phase of your formulations. Silk amino acid has been used by a number of leading cosmetic manufactures in the U.S., Europe and Japan.

Stearic Acid
(Stearic acid)
Stearic acid is derived from soybean and is a white waxy natural fatty acid. Stearic acid is a major ingredient in soap making and lubricants, because it helps to bind and thicken creams.

Tragacanth Gum
(Astragalus gummifer)
Tragacanth gum is native to the arid regions of Iran, Asia Minor, and Greece. Tragacanth gum is an emollient, demulcent, and thickener for lotions and creams. The name *"tragacanth"* comes from the appearance of the exuded gum, which tends to form ribbons similar in appearance to a goat horn (from the Greek *"tragos"* meaning goat and *"akantha"* meaning horn).

Whey
Whey is what remains after the cream and casein (protein) have been removed from milk when making cheese. One tablespoon of dried whey is made from almost two quarts of regular liquid whey. Whey contains the highest amount of sodium, known as the "youth maintainer" because naturally occurring sodium is considered to bring youthfulness to the body's tissues. Sodium is essential for healthy capillaries and arteries. It is required for maintaining flexibility and mobility in the joints. Without proper sodium the joints would stiffen and calcify prematurely, and the lining of the stomach would not secrete the necessary enzymes for healthy digestion. Sodium is a blood builder and a great neutralizer. It aids digestion, counteracts acidosis, halts intestinal fermentation and purifies the blood. It holds calcium in solution to maintain the suppleness of youth in the joints. Whey is a wonderful culture to feed the friendly bacteria that live in the intestinal tract. To encourage this germ life use it regularly and especially after using antibiotics. When whey is ingested in the evening, one wakes up in the morning highly energized both physically and mentally. Whey is one of the best youth foods available to us. When we lack sodium, the first organ to show disorder is the stomach and this disorder gradually spreads throughout the body.

Witch Hazel
(Hamamelis virginiana)
Witch hazel is extracted from the witch hazel shrub. Traditionally, it has been used as a natural astringent, toner, cleanser, and anti-inflammatory. It is excellent in reducing fevers (especially for infants and children) when applied to extremities.

Xanthan Gum

(Xanthan)

Xanthan gum is a natural thickener derived from fermented corn sugar, often used to thicken and stabilize salad dressings and soups. It can thicken and add volume to lotions, creams and gels. A tiny amount thickens a very large amount of water.

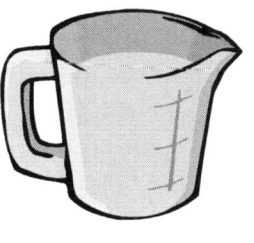

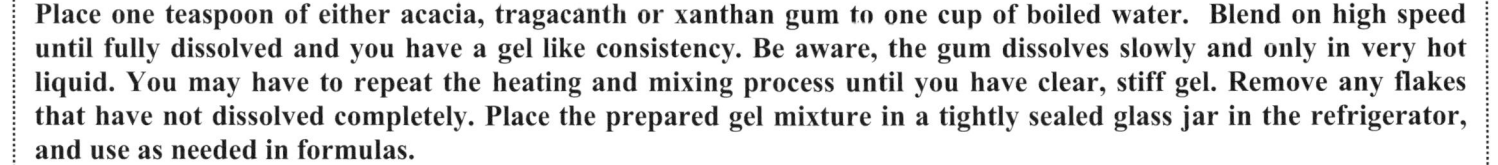

How to Prepare Acacia, Tragacanth and Xanthan Gum Gel

Place one teaspoon of either acacia, tragacanth or xanthan gum to one cup of boiled water. Blend on high speed until fully dissolved and you have a gel like consistency. Be aware, the gum dissolves slowly and only in very hot liquid. You may have to repeat the heating and mixing process until you have clear, stiff gel. Remove any flakes that have not dissolved completely. Place the prepared gel mixture in a tightly sealed glass jar in the refrigerator, and use as needed in formulas.

ALGAES & LICHENS

Since the time of recorded history algaes and lichens have been utilized by many cultures in various parts of the world. Algaes and lichens are one of nature's richest sources of micro-nutrients, minerals, and trace minerals. They contain approximately 25% protein and 2% fat and are low in calories. Algaes are differentiated according to their predominant colorations and divided into blue-green, green, red and brown algaes.

Algaes and lichens are yummy and tasty! Crush, chop, snip or crumble any mix of dry sea greens you like into soups and sauces, pizzas, casseroles, rice and salads. Roast them into anything you cook. If you add sea veggies, no other salt is needed. This is an advantage for people on a low salt diet. Store them in a moisture proof container and they will keep indefinitely.

Algaes and lichens are also great to add to a bath. It takes approximately forty-five minutes to balance the acid-alkaline system, encourage liver activity, cellulite release and fat metabolism. To get the most from a seaweed treatment, dry brush cellulite skin areas before your seaweed bath. Or, indulge in a body wrap to exfoliate dead skin, open up pores for waste elimination and increase blood flow to affected areas. Skin tone, color, and better circulation are almost immediately noticeable.

Dulse

Dulse can be added to potoatoes, eggs, vegetables, rice, casseroles and chowders. Dulse is great sprinkled on salads, pizza, (like anchovies), or in omelettes or scrambled eggs, (like bacon). Because dulse is so delicate and fragile in texture, it becomes mushy when cooked. Use it raw, sprinkled as flakes on cooked food, or steamed for a moment, or cooked in scrambled eggs and omelettes.

Kelp

Kelp can be used to replace chicken or beef stock. Simmer with liquid, at least 10 minutes and remove if desired, or leave it in for a richer broth. Add dry kelp to any pickle recipe for a sea treat. Kelp contains natural glutamates, which enhance flavors and tenderize high protein foods like beans. Kelp in the kitchen reduces or eliminates the need for salt.

Agar Agar

Agar agar is also called kanten, a vegetable gelatin derived from seaweeds, excellent for vegans, as it is a replacement for animal derived gelatin. It is not necessary to boil il to make it thick. Add it to fruit pies, jellies, jams and soups. Soak two tablespoons of agar agar in three cups of liquid for about 45 minutes before adding to your ingredients. If it is not as thick as you like it, just remember that it thickens when it cools. Agar agar is an excellent soluble fiber, and is excellent in cases of constipation. Remember to drink a lot of water when you use it for this purpose.

Arame
(Eisenia bycyclis)

Arame has been used to help reduce breast and uterine fibroids, and to normalize menopausal symptoms. Arame promotes soft, wrinkle-free skin, shiny hair and prevents hair loss.

Bladderwrack
(Fucus vesiculosus)

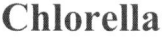

Bladderwrack is a brown algae species common in colder waters of the North Atlantic. Bladderwrack is the best remedy for obesity. Where obesity is associated with thyroid trouble, this herb may be very helpful in reducing excess weight. Good for all glandular afflictions, goiter, and scrofula. Has an excellent effect on the kidneys. It also has a reputation to help with rheumatism and rheumatoid arthritis, both used internally and as an external application upon inflamed joints. Bladderwrack is packed with vitamin K - an excellent adrenal stimulant.

Chlorella
(Chlorella pyrenoidosa)

Chlorella is a single-celled, blue-green algae, which thrives in fresh water. It has survived throughout its two-billion-year history on this planet, because its tough outer shell protects its genetic integrity. Chlorella is rich in protein, vitamins and minerals, and can promote cell reproduction, reduce cholesterol and increase hemoglobin levels. Since chlorella is such a broad-spectrum plant, it can help support and repair organs and tissues that have been injured by a variety of causes. Numerous research projects in the USA and Europe have indicated that chlorella can also aid the body in breaking down persistent hydrocarbon and toxic metals such as DDT, PCB, mercury, cadmium and lead as well as strengthening the immune system response. The fibrous materials in chlorella can also improve digestion and promote the growth of beneficial bacteria in the intestinal tract. Other research programs have indicated that regular use of chlorella can help guard against heart disease, reduce high blood pressure and lower serum cholesterol levels.

Dulse
(Palmaria palmata)
Dulse is a reddish algae that grows on exposed shores, known in Ireland as Creathnach. It is a supremely balanced nutrient rich in iron, protein, and vitamin A. Dulse has 300 times more iodine and 50 times more iron than wheat. Tests on dulse have shown positive activity against herpes virus. It has purifying, nourishing and toning effects on the body. Dulse does not induce thirst!

Kelp
(Laminaria digitata)
Kelp is a dark brown algae, common on some coasts of Britain, Ireland, Iceland and the western Atlantic. Kelp is especially high in iodine and potassium, and has shown to be most useful in the treatment of under-active thyroid function and for alkalizing blood chemistry. Extensive research done on this remarkable seaweed has shown to have anti-tumor properties (Japanese researchers have claimed kelp has "conclusively been proven to prevent breast cancer"). Kelp has antibiotic, antioxidant and anti-bacterial properties. Kelp has the ability to protect against environmental toxins, increase circulation and help lower cholesterol, among many other benefits.

Kombu
(Laminaria digitata)
Kombu is a traditional Japanese delicacy with great nutritional and healing value. It is a decongestant for excess mucous, and helps lower blood pressure. Kombu is rich in iodine, carotenes, vitamins B, C, D and E, as well as other minerals, such as calcium, magnesium, potassium, silica, iron and zinc. It also contains the powerful skin healing nutrient germanium. Kombu is a high-protein seaweed. Add a strip of kombu to your bean pot to reduce gas.

Icelandic Moss
(Cetraria islandica)
Icelandic moss is not a seaweed, but a foliaceous lichen. It is found on barren stony ground throughout all northern countries and mountainous areas. Icelandic moss is rich in mucilage and its demulcent action is of value in the treatment of gastritis, gastric ulcer, hiatal hernia, reflux oesophagitis, vomiting and dyspepsia. In addition, its nutritive qualities contribute to the treatment of malnourishment, debility, and anorexia. Icelandic moss is often used in the treatment of respiratory catarrh and bronchitis, especially in constantly recurring acute irritation in the elderly. It generally soothes the mucous membranes. It is useful for coughs and hoarseness.

Irish Moss
(Chondrus crispus)
Irish moss is cartilaginous, dark purplish-red algae, frequently iridescent under water, gathered in the Maritime Provinces of Canada. It is a source of carrageenan, which is an ingredient used to make (thicken) soups, jellies, etc. In Ireland, it is a remedy for respiratory disorders. Irish moss is full of electrolyte minerals - calcium, magnesium, sodium and potassium. Its mucilaginous compounds help to detoxify, boost metabolism and strengthen hair, skin and nails. Traditionally used for a low sex drive.

Nori
(Porphyra laver)
Nori is a red sea weed with a sweet, meaty taste when dried. It contains protein, higher than any other sea plant. Nori's fiber makes it a perfect sushi wrapper.

Sea Palm, a.k.a. American Arame
(Postelsia palmaeformis)
Sea palm looks like a miniature palm tree and grows only on the Pacific Coast of North America, on top of rocks in areas of intense wave action, where it receives nutrients and oxygen. It is an annual plant. When it reaches maturity, spores are produced that slime off of the sharply attenuated blades during low tide, where they then settle and multiply. Has a sweet, salty taste.

Spirulina
(Arthrospira plantensis)
Spirulina is a single-celled, blue-green algae, which thrives in warm, alkaline fresh water. It is one of nature's most concentrated sources of vegetarian nutrition. Acre for acre, spirulina yields 20 times more protein than soybeans, 400 times more protein than beef. It is a complete protein, with all 22 amino acids, the entire vitamin B-complex, including B-12 (one teaspoon supplies 2 ½ times the RDA), carotenes, minerals, and essential fatty acids. Digestibility is high, for both immediate and long-range energy. Spirulina is also well known for its ability to curb appetite.

Wakame
(Undaria pinnatifida)
Wakame is high in protein and calcium. It is widely used for hair growth and luster, and for healthy skin tone.

HERBS AND ASTROLOGY

♈ Aries
♂ *(Mars)*

The first house of the Zodiac is ruled by Aries and governs the head and face. Mars is the planetary ruler. Mars herbs are fiery and move obstructions in the body. The herbs of Mars are: all-spice, anemones, asafetida, barberry, basil, bearberry, blessed thistle, bloodroot, cactus, carrot, cashews, cayenne, chili powder, chives, coriander, cubeb, cumin, curry, damiana, dragon's blood, fireweed, galangal, garlic, gentian, ginger, grains of paradise, hawthorn, high john the conqueror, hops, horseradish, leeks, mustard, nettles, onion, paprika, pennyroyal, peppers, peppermint, pine, poke, prickly ash, radish, rue, shallot, snapdragon, tarragon, thistles, tobacco, uva ursi, vitex, woodruff, wormwood, yucca.

♉ Taurus
♀ *(Venus)*

The second house of the Zodiac is ruled by Taurus and governs the neck and throat. Venus is the planetary ruler. Venus/Taurus herbs are sweet, gentle and cleansing. The herbs of Venus/Taurus are: alder, alfalfa, alkanet, apple blossom, apricot, balm of gilead, birch, blackberry, burdock, cardamom, catnip, cherry, cocoa, coltsfoot, columbines, cornflowers, cowslip, crocus, daisies, dittany of crete, elder, feverfew, figwort, foxglove, geranium, goldenrod, gooseberry, groundsel, heather, hibiscus, indian paint brush, iris, lady's mantle, lemon balm, licorice, motherwort, mugwort, oats, orchid, passionflower, pea, peach, pear, periwinkle, plantain, plum, primrose, raspberry, rhubarb, rose, rose geranium, sagebrush, spearmint, spikenard, strawberries, sugarcane, thyme, tomato, valerian, vanilla, vervain, vetivert, verbena, violets, willow, yarrow.

♊ Gemini
☿ *(Mercury)*

The third house of the Zodiac is ruled by Gemini and governs the arms and shoulders, the power of breath and the nervous system, including the brain. Mercury is the planetary ruler. Mercury/Gemini herbs are calming nervines, and respiratory tonics. The herbs of Mercury/Gemini are: almond, aspen, bergamot, brazil nut, caraway, celery, dill, elecampane, fennel, fenugreek, filbert, flax, horehound, lavender, lemongrass, lemon verbena, lily of the valley, mace, mandrake, marjoram, mulberry, papyrus, parsley, pecan, peppermint, pistachio, pomegranate, summer savory, senna.

♋ Cancer
☽ *(Moon)*

The fourth house of the Zodiac is ruled by Cancer and governs the stomach, uterus and mammary glands. The Moon is the planetary ruler. Moon herbs work with the subconscious mind, and are for emotions and instincts. They bring a higher degree of sensibility and help us flow with the rhythm of life. The Moon herbs are: aloe, bladderwrack, buchu, cabbage, calamus, camphor, chickweed, club moss, coconut, cucumber, dulse, eucalyptus, gardenia, grape, irish moss, jasmine, lemon, lettuce, lily, loosestrife, lotus, mallow, mesquite, myrrh, papaya, poppy, purslane, sandalwood, turnip, willow, wintergreen.

♌ Leo
☉ *(Sun)*

The fifth house of the Zodiac is ruled by Leo and governs the upper spine, heart and arterial circulation, as well as the eyes. The Sun is the planetary ruler. Sun herbs strengthen the heart and eyes, equalize circulation, and relieve spasmodic afflictions. They are good for those who have trouble with their self-image. Sun herbs build self-confidence and motivate to complete one's goals. The Sun herbs are: angelica, gum arabic, ash, bay, benzoin, carnation, cashew, cedar, celandine, centaury, chamomile, chicory, chrysanthemum, cinnamon, copal, eyebright, frankincense, ginseng, goldenseal, juniper, lime, lovage, marigold, mastic, mistletoe, oak, olive, orange, peony, pineapple, rice, rosemary, saffron, st. john's wort, sesame, sunflower, tangerine, tea, tormentil, walnut, witch hazel.

♍ Virgo
☿ *(Mercury)*

The sixth house of the Zodiac is ruled by Virgo and governs the liver, solar plexus and the intestines. Mercury is the planetary ruler. The herbs of Virgo/Mercury nourish the liver and bring it back to normal activity, soothe the nervous system, allay fear and heal the intestinal tract. The herbs of Mercury are: almond, aspen, bergamot, brazil nut, caraway, celery, dill, elecampane, fennel, fenugreek, filbert, flax, horehound, lavender, lemongrass, lemon verbena, lily of the valley, mace, mandrake, marjoram, mulberry, papyrus, parsley, pecan, peppermint, pistachio, pomegranate, summer savory, senna.

♎ Libra
♀ *(Venus)*

The seventh house of the Zodiac is ruled by Libra and governs the kidneys, small of back and endocrine system. Venus is the planetary ruler. Venus herbs are gentle and cleansing. The herbs of Venus/Libra are: alder, alfalfa, alkanet, apple blossom, apricot, balm of gilead, birch, blackberry, burdock, cardamom, catnip, cherry, cocoa, coltsfoot, columbines, cornflowers, cowslip, crocus, daisies, dittany of crete, elder, feverfew, figwort, foxglove, geranium, goldenrod, gooseberry, groundsel, heather, hibiscus, indian paint brush, iris, lady's mantle, lemon balm, licorice, motherwort, mugwort, oats, orchid, passionflower, pea, peach, pear, periwinkle, plantain, plum, primrose, raspberry, rhubarb, rose, rose geranium, sagebrush, spearmint, spikenard, strawberries, sugarcane, thyme, tomato, valerian, vanilla, vervain, vetivert, verbena, violets, willow, yarrow.

♏ Scorpio
♇ *(Pluto)*

The eight house of the Zodiac is ruled by Scorpio and governs the reproductive organs and genitals. Pluto is the planetary ruler. Pluto herbs affect the glandular system, sexual drive and desire to procreate. The herbs of Pluto are: blessed thistle, leek, horseradish, wormwood, and sarsaparilla. All these herbs have antiseptic properties, which stimulate the glandular system so it can throw off the poisonous wastes that may otherwise accumulate in the bladder and reproductive organs causing serious inflammatory disorders.

♐ Sagittarius
♃ *(Jupiter)*

The ninth house of the Zodiac is ruled by Jupiter and governs the hips, thighs, liver and lower spine. Jupiter is the planetary ruler. Jupiter herbs cool the blood, reduce fever and heal. The herbs of Jupiter are: agrimony, anise, borage, chestnut, cinquefoil, clove, dandelion, endive, fig, honeysuckle, horse chestnut, hyssop, linden, liverwort, maple, meadowsweet, nutmeg, sage, sarsaparilla, sassafras, star anise, wood betony, yellow dock.

♑ Capricorn
♄ *(Saturn)*

The tenth house of the Zodiac is ruled by Capricorn and governs the knees, bone structure and skin. Saturn is the planetary ruler. Saturn herbs govern the skeletal structure, ligaments, teeth, and possibly the gallbladder. The herbs of Saturn are: amaranth, beech, beet, belladonna, bistort, boneset, buckthorn, comfrey, cypress, datura, elm, hemp, horsetail, kava kava, lady's slipper, lobelia, mimosa, morning glory, mullein, pansy, patchouli, poplar, quince, skullcap, skunk cabbage, slippery elm, solomon's seal, tamarisk, tamarind.

♒ Aquarius
♅ *(Uranus)*

The eleventh house of the Zodiac is ruled by Aquarius and governs the calves, ankles (organs of locomotion) and the bloodstream. Uranus is the planetary ruler. Uranus herbs govern the nervous system, many areas of the brain, and nerve impulses. Restriction in any form is irritating to the Aquarian; yet paradoxical as it may seem, inwardly they crave discipline. Choose herbs and flower essences that bring inspiration, as well as an ability to follow one's feelings in trying new endeavors, or when one's thinking is stuck. The herbs for Aquarius are: valerian and lady's slipper, nervines, herbs for emotional stress, anxiety and insomnia. These are also excellent for muscle cramps, nervous system, pain, spasms, and ulcers.

♓ Pisces
♆ *(Neptune)*

The twelfth house of the Zodiac is ruled by Pisces and governs the feet and toes. Neptune is the planetary ruler. Neptune herbs work with the kidneys and urinary system, which pass fluids within the body. They also rule the spinal canal and the parathyroid. Choose herbs and flower essences that open the mind to a greater sense of vision, as well as the ability to dream, both when asleep and awake. Neptune herbs have been used to enhance astral travel, but may only be used as a key to learning. The herb for Pisces is Irish moss, as it aids in the formation of stools and good for many intestinal disorders. Also used in skin lotions. It contains iron and iodine in the only form in which these can be assimilated by the body. If used persistently, irish moss relieves every Pisces complaint. Wild lettuce, lobelia, lotus, mescal, mugwort, opium, willow, and the flower essence of yerba mansa.

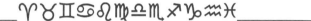

Fire signs – Aries, Leo, Sagittarius
These may suffer from strong, hard, acute illnesses, fevers, inflammation, injuries, sudden occurrences – strong and rapid recoveries.

Earth signs – Taurus, Virgo, Capricorn
These may suffer from deep-rooted ailments that take years to develop – chronic issues – deep depressions – recuperation powerful but slow.

Air Signs – Gemini, Libra, Aquarius
These may suffer from mental stress – nervous exhaustion, respiratory difficulties – poor circulation – recuperative powers unpredictable.

Water signs – Cancer, Scorpio, Pisces
These may suffer from peculiar illnesses with difficult diagnosis – lingering issues – melancholia – from fears, not letting go. They can direct their own recovery.

AYURVEDIC MEDICINE

Ayurvedic Medicine is an ancient healing system. Some experts say that it is over 5000 years old and perhaps older than the Chinese Healing System. Ayurveda is a Sanskrit word and means "The Science of Life". Ayurvedic doctors say that knowing how to live your life in balance and harmony with nature you will have eternal youth. If you are in search of a healthy and long life, it is important to find out where you are in relation to nature. The following chart can help you discover your dosha.

Constitution	Vata		Pitta		Kapha	
Body frame	Thin	☐	Moderate	☐	Large	☐
Body weight	Low	☐	Moderate	☐	Heavy	☐
Skin	Dry, rough	☐	Soft, oily	☐	Thick, oily	☐
Hair	Dry, kinky	☐	Soft, oily	☐	Thick, oily, wavy	☐
Appetite	Variable, low	☐	Good, excessive	☐	Slow but steady	☐
Disease Tendency	Nervous, pain	☐	Heat, infection, inflammation	☐	Water, mucous	☐
Disease Resistance	Poor, weak, low immunity	☐	Moderate, infections, bleeding	☐	Good, strong immunity	☐
Healing Tendency	Quick, low dosages	☐	Moderate	☐	Slow, higher dosages	☐
Physical Activity	Very active	☐	Moderate	☐	Lethargic	☐
Nature	Adaptable, quick, indecisive	☐	Penetrating, critical, intelligent	☐	Slow, steady, dull	☐
Sexual nature	Strong desire but low energy	☐	Moderate, passionate	☐	Low desire, devoted	☐
Sensitivities	Noise	☐	Bright lights	☐	Strong odors	☐
Memory	Understands quickly, forgets	☐	Clear, sharp	☐	Slow, never forgets	☐
Mind	Restless, active	☐	Aggressive, intelligent	☐	Calm, slow	☐
Emotion	Fear, insecure, anxiety	☐	Aggressive, irrational, jealous	☐	Greedy, attached	☐
Dreams	Flying, running	☐	Fiery, passionate	☐	Watery, romantic	☐
Sleep	Interrupted	☐	Little but sound	☐	Prolonged	☐
Speech	Fast, uninterrupted	☐	Sharp, clear, cutting	☐	Slow, monotone	☐
Spending Habits	Spends quickly	☐	Spends methodically	☐	Spends slowly	☐
Voice	Low, weak, talkative	☐	High, sharp, clear, argumentative	☐	Deep, slow, silent	☐

Vata ☐   Pitta ☐   Kapha ☐

Doshas (Trouble or Humor)

There are three basic life forces, doshas, which regulate the physiological and biochemical activities of the body.

Vata	Air	Wind	Life
Pitta	Fire	Sun	Light
Kapha	Water	Rain	Love

Vata - that which moves things, motivation, mental

Pitta - that which digests things, chemical and metabolic transformation, understanding

Kapha - that which holds things together, emotional support

Vata is dry, cold, light, mobile, subtle, hard, rough, changeable and clear. It is the most powerful doshas, being the life force itself, the strongest to create disease. It governs all movement, and carries both pitta and kapha.

Pitta is hot, light, fluid, subtle, sharp, malodorous, soft and clear. It governs heat, temperature and all chemical reactions.

Kapha is cold, wet, heavy, slow, dull, static, smooth, dense and cloudy. It maintains substance, weight and coherence in the body.

Actions

Vata (air) is the most important, of the three doshas. It governs the other two. Disturbances in vata tend to have more severe implications than the other two humors, and often affect the mind as well as the entire physical body.

Pitta (fire) governs digestion, heat, visual perception, hunger, thirst, luster, complexion, understanding, intelligence, courage and softness of the body. It represents all aspects of light and warmth in the body and mind.

Kapha (water) gives stability, lubrication, and holding together of the joints, and such qualities as patience. It gives emotional stability to the other two doshas.

Aggravated

When aggravated the humors give rise to various symptoms and diseases.

Vata in excess causes emaciation, debility, tremors, constipation, insomnia, sensory disorientation, incoherent speech, dizziness, confusion and depression. The life force and the mind lose their connection with the body, causing decay and loss of coordination.

Pitta in excess causes yellow color of stool, urine, eyes and skin, thirst, burning sensation and difficulty sleeping. Burning up.

Kapha in excess causes a decrease in digestive fire, lethargy, heaviness, white color, chills, cough, difficulty breathing and excessive sleeping. Hypo activity, excess tissue accumulation.

Sites of the doshas

Vata is located in the colon, thighs, hips, ears, bones, and skin.

Pitta is located in the small intestine, stomach, sweat, blood, lymph, and eyes.

Kapha is located in the chest, throat, head, pancreas, fat, nose and tongue.

The Dhatus

The dhatus are the 7 body tissues: plasma and lymph, hemoglobin, muscle tissues, adipose tissues, bone tissues, marrow and nerves, and reproductive system. The dhatus transform into each other with the aid of nutrient plasma that arises from the digestive process. Thirteen channels of circulation transport the nutrient plasma, the doshas, to the organs, tissues and system to maintain them. For the organism to function well, these channels must remain open so that the process of circulation is unimpeded. Faulty circulation leads to an accumulation of substances in the channels, adverse metabolic reactions and other effects, which result in illness.

The Malas

The malas are the substances used by the body and excreted in modified form as waste products.

The Six Tastes

All foods and herbs are classified as hot or cold and by their six tastes (sweet, sour, salty, pungent, bitter and astringent), which indicate its molecular composition, properties and therapeutic action. In general, substances with attributes opposite to those of the doshas are used in ayurvedic medicine. Vata people should avoid cold, pungent, bitter, light, rough substances, and take hot, heavy, smooth, sweet and sour substances. Pitta people should avoid hot, acrid, sour, salty, sharp smooth substances and take cool, bitter, astringent and soft substances. Kapha people should avoid cold, bitter, sweet, soft substances and take hot, acrid, pungent, astringent, sour, salty, light and rough substances.

Tastes	Energy	Wet/Dry	Heavy/Light	Elements
Sweet	Cooling	Wet	Heavy	Earth/Water
Salty	Heating	Wet	Heavy	Water/Fire
Sour	Heating	Wet	Light	Earth/Fire
Astringent	Cooling	Dry	Heavy	Earth/Air
Pungent	Heating	Dry	Light	Air/Fire
Bitter	Cooling	Dry	Light	Air/Ether

Ayurvedic Herbs

Ajowan *(Wild Caraway)*
Carum copticum
Ajowan is an appetite stimulant that is commonly used in India as a carminative to alleviate gas and indigestion.

Amalaki, Amla *(The Nurse)*
Emblica officinalis
A traditional rejuvenative used to cleanse and nourish the bodily tissues. Balancing for all doshas, especially pitta. High in Vitamin C. Each berry contains approximately 3000 mg of vitamin C. In ayurveda it is used for AIDS, anemia, biliousness, colitis, constipation, diabetes, gout, premature gray, balding hair, liver weakness, hepatitis, mental disorders, osteoporosis, spleen weakness, and vertigo. It regulates blood sugar, increases red blood cell count, a heart tonic, strengthens teeth, stops gum bleeding, stops stomach and colon inflammation, aids eyesight, treats lung inflammations, and soothes painful urination. The spiritual qualities of amalaki are pure in quality, it gives love, longevity, and good fortune. For mothers who behave angrily towards their children, it calms and balances their emotions. In Sanskrit, amalaki has another name, *dhatri,* meaning "mother".

Arjuna
Terminalia arjuna
A famous cardiac tonic used in India for a variety of heart conditions.

Asafoetida *(Hing)*
Ferula asafoetida
Also known as hing, and devil's dung, this pungent and heating resin is especially calming for vata. It helps correct the flow of vata in the GI tract, promoting healthy digestion. It is effective in breaking up impacted fecal matter. Similar in flavor to garlic, asafoetida cleanses the intestinal flora, destroys worms and dispels gas. It has a grounding but dulling effect upon the mind.

Ashwagandha *(Vitality of the horse)*
Withania somnifera

Ashwagandha, "which has the smell of a horse, as it gives the vitality and sexual energy of a horse". A well-known rejuvenative tonic used in ayurveda for stress-induced fatigue, nervous exhaustion and general debility. Strengthens and nourishes both mind and body. Also known as "Indian Ginseng". It is one of the best herbs for the mind upon which it is nurturing and clarifying. It is calming and promotes deep, dreamless sleep. Ashwagandha is good for weak pregnant women; it stabilizes the fetus.

Bala *(Strength giving)*
Sida cordifolia

Literally meaning "strength", bala is a rejuvenative and aphrodisiac that strengthens all tissues and is especially useful for the heart, lungs and nervous system.

Bhringaraj *(Ruler of the hair)*
Eclipta Alba

Known in India for its abilities to promote hair growth and help prevent premature graying. It is actually a preventative for the aging process, rejuvenating bones, teeth, hair, eyesight, hearing and memory. Bhringaraj is also used in ayurveda to calm the mind from excessive activity and promotes sound sleep, as well as for a variety of pitta-related imbalances (heat and inflammation). It combines the properties of dandelion leaf and gotu kola. Externally, it draws out poisons and reduces inflammation.

Bibhitaki
Terminalia belerica

Bibhitaki is a rejuvenative herb and used to cleanse and nourish the bodily tissues. It is useful for all doshas, especially kapha.

Boswellia
Boswellia serrata

Boswellia has traditionally been used to reduce pain and inflammation of the joints.

Brahmi/Gotu Kola *(Divine creative energy)*
Centella asiatica

A calming, rejuvenating herb that is believed to revitalize the nerves and brain, strengthen memory and intelligence, and improve concentration. In Sri Lanka, gotu kola is a favorite food for elephants.

Calamus
See Vacha

Cardamom
Elettaria cardamomum
Cardamom is a household spice that is commonly used to support digestion without increasing pitta. Cardamom has expectorant, anti-mucoid, and diaphoretic properties. It is a great breath freshener. Green cardamom is better for kidneys, white is better for the lungs.

Cinnamon
Cinnamomum cassia
This warming spice reduces vata and kapha and is traditionally used in cold formulas and for strengthening digestion. Cinnamon has thermogenic properties used in weight loss formulas. Recent studies have shown that cinnamon reduces blood sugar levels in Type II diabetics. Cinnamon increases glucose metabolism, triggering insulin release, which also affects cholesterol metabolism.

Coriander
Coriandrum sativum
Coriander is a household spice that is traditionally used to improve digestion and absorption without aggravating pitta.

Cumin
Cuminum cyminum
Cumin is a common cooking spice known for supporting digestion, which controls vata and kapha without aggravating pitta.

Fennel
Foeniculum vulgare
Fennel is a common spice that is traditionally used to improve digestion and absorption without increasing pitta. The seeds are also chewed after meals to freshen the breath and alleviate gas.

Ginger
Zingiber officinalis
Ginger is considered in ayurveda to be a general panacea that is especially useful for digestive and respiratory complaints. Also dispels nausea, motion sickness and acts as a diaphoretic.

> ## Pickled Ginger
>
> To make pickled ginger (pink ginger) commonly served in Japanese dishes, slice young ginger very thin, dip it in lemon juice and season with celtic salt. The lemon juice turns the ginger root pink.

Gokshura *(Shape of the Cow's hoof)*
Tribulus terrestris
Gokshura is a rejuvenating herb and used by ayurvedic practitioners to support proper function of the urinary tract and prostate. It increases sperm production. Gokshura is also being used for back pain, lumbago, nerve pain, and gout. It increases testosterone without raising estrogen.

Gotu Kola
See Brahmi

Guggulu
Commiphora mukul
Guggal is famous in ayurveda for its rejuvenating and detoxifying actions. It is used to remove impurities from the tissues and to assist the normal function of the joints and nervous system. For hyper cholesterol and arthritis it is the best herb (resin). Interestingly, it disinfects secretions (e.g., sweat, mucus, urination).
Caution: Do not take guggulu while experiencing acute kidney infections and rashes; avoid eating sour foods, exhaustion, sun exposure, alcohol, and anger, when taking this herb.

Gymnema
(see Shardunika)

Haritaki
Terminalia chebula
Haritaki is a traditional rejuvenative herb used to cleanse and nourish the body's tissues. It is balancing for all doshas, especially vata. Haritaki is one of the three herbs in triphala. If you take triphala on a daily basis for one year without let up, you will have rebuilt your whole digestive system.

Jatamansi
Nardostachys jatamansi
Jatamansi is calming to the nerves and it is said to strengthen the mind. Its sedative properties increase awareness, whereas its cousin, valerian, dulls the mind. Jatamansi is also known as "nard". Nard oil was applied to Jesus' feet. Jatamansi has also been used for heart palpitations, nervous headaches, respiratory and digestive diseases. It removes impurities from the blood.

Manjista
Rubia cordifolia
Manjista is considered in ayurveda to be one of the best herbs for detoxifying the blood. It is also used externally for pitta-related skin inflammation.

Neem
Azadirachta indica
Neem is a bitter herb that reduces pitta and kapha. It is known to purify the blood, detoxify the liver, and alleviate skin irritations and itching. Neem has powerful anti-fungal and anti-bacterial properties. I knew a lady who had skin tags all over her neck. After taking neem for about 2 weeks all her skin tags fell off. Another person told me after taking neem for one month she did no longer need her reading glasses. Neem can be used on your house plants or in your garden as an effective non-toxic pesticide.

Pippali
Piper longum
Pippali is a member of the pepper family. This pungent rejuvenative herb stimulates the respiratory and digestive systems.

Shardunika *(Killer of sweetness)*
Gymnema sylvestre
Shardunika has been used to maintain healthy blood glucose levels, stimulate the production of insulin and reduce cravings for sweets.

Shatavari *(Hundred husbands)*
Asparagus racemosus
Sweet, bitter and cooling, this herb nourishes the body and mind and reduces pitta. Shatavari is also considered one of the best ayurvedic rejuvenatives for women. It supplies female hormones, increases fertility, and is excellent for strengthening the female reproductive organs. In my first herb store a woman came in to discuss her difficulties with numerous failed

pregnancies. She did not have a problem conceiving, but by her third month of pregnancy she miscarried. I told her about shatavari and she began taking three capsules, three times a day. Her next pregnancy was a success, she had a full term pregnancy and easy childbirth. I have seen shatavari work this way on numerous occasions. Shatavari can also be taken for sexual debility, vaginal dryness and overall dryness in the body. Shatavari increases quantity and quality of breast milk. Because of its nourishing properties it can be used for male impotence and low sperm count. Boosts the immune system – good for AIDS, Epstein Barr, cancer - strengthens one from and for chemotherapy. Externally, it is an emollient used for stiff joints, and for neck and muscle spasms.

Turmeric
Curcuma longa

Turmeric is a traditional Indian cooking spice that stimulates and improves digestion and also purifies the blood. It is believed to act as a natural antibiotic, and at the same time improve intestinal flora. Good for all inflammatory conditions, turmeric is a metabolism regulator, assists in protein digestion, and known to be excellent for arthritis. It is a valuable anti-oxidant. Externally, turmeric can be mixed with honey or aloe vera and applied on acne and insect bites.

Vacha/Calamus *(Speaking)*
Acornus calamus

Vacha has been used in ayurveda for thousands of years, vacha is a rejuvenative for the brain and the nervous system. It promotes cerebral circulation, increases sensitivity, sharpens memory, and enhances awareness. It is the best herb for nasal administration, for nasal congestion, as it revitalizes prana (life-force). Transmutes sexual energy and feeds kundalini (spiritual life-force).

Vidari Kanda
Ipomoea digitata

Vidari kanda is a sweet, nutritive tonic to rejuvenate vata and pitta. It is used for general debility and weakness, and as an aphrodisiac.

Ayurvedic Formula For Weight Gain

This is a great formula for anyone who needs to gain weight. Some people have gained as much as 25 lbs in one month. Measure one teaspoon each of ashwagandha and shatavari, ½ tsp each of cinnamon, coriander, cumin, turmeric, and ¼ teaspoon of ginger. Pour one cup of the purest milk you can get into a blender (no soy milk, please), add a little honey, and blend at high speed for 30 seconds. You will notice that the volume of milk has doubled. Add the first herb to the honey milk and blend for 30 seconds, add the second herb, blend for 30 seconds, and continue this process, until you have added all the herbs. This process may sound trivial, but it is an ancient ayurvedic secret! Now sit down and drink this delicious herbal honey milk slowly. It is important to actually "chew" this liquid. Saliva contains enzymes and other digestive ingredients and prepares foods and drinks for the next step in the digestive processes, facilitated digestion.

Ghee (Clarified Butter)

Ghee (Clarified Butter)
According to ayurveda, clarified butter is the best form of fat for the body, and taken with herbs, it transports their nutrients and energies to all seven-tissue layers. Ghee promotes longevity. It is good for memory and digestion. It improves intelligence, vision, and voice. It is nourishing to the liver, kidneys and the brain. Ghee also reduces the desire for eating animal products. Ghee increases flexibility. When special herbs like ashwagandha are made into medicated ghee, they remove harmful cholesterol from the body.

How to prepare Ghee (Clarified Butter)
Heat one pound of raw and unsalted butter on a medium fire for 15 minutes. As it starts boiling, broth will rise to the surface. Do not remove this foam for it contains medicinal properties. Turn the fire to low. The butter will turn to a golden yellow color. When a drop or two of water placed in the ghee produces a crackling sound, the ghee is ready. Let it cool slightly and then pour it through a strainer into a container. Ghee may be stored without refrigeration.

Sesame Seed Oil

Occasionally, I rub my feet with warm sesame seed oil before bedtime, for its sedative, nourishing, and rejuvenating properties. According to ayurveda, sesame seed oil is the best of all oils, and heals all diseases. The oil can be used internally as well for dryness in the body (especially the bowels), and nervous exhaustion. Sesame seed oil calms the nerves, relieves anxiety, good to use for muscle tension, stiff back, problems with voice and vision, growth of hair, nails, teeth and bones, and to improve the function of the immune system. (Suggestion: 1 tablespoon a day in the evening).

Black Sesame Seed Oil

The oil from black sesame seeds contains high amounts of solar energy. Its high calcium content is easier to absorb than from white sesame seed oil. It is also the best oil for head massages, to prevent graying of hair and to restore it to its natural color, for migraines, tinnitus, blurry vision, and dizziness.

Facial Cleanser

Combine the juice of one lemon and one tbsp wheat germ oil. Add flour and mix into a paste, the consistency of yogurt. Apply to face and leave on for a few minutes, then wash off.

Face Glow Mask

Mix turmeric powder with whipping cream and honey (optional) to make a paste, the consistency of yoghurt. With a brush apply to face, neck and décolleté. Leave it on for 20 minutes. Rinse off, and apply vedic nourishing cream.

Vedic Nourishing Cream

In a crockpot heat 2 tbsp sesame seed oil, 2 tablespoon coconut oil, and 1 tbsp mustard seed oil. Add 3-4 tbsp of beeswax to the oils and warm it all up until the beeswax has completed melted. Let it cool a little, and then add 1 tbsp almond oil, 1 tbsp wheat germ oil, ½ tsp sandalwood essential oil, and ½ tsp rose oil. Store in a glass jar.

Traditional Ayurvedic Formulas

Chyavanprash

Nutritive jam for pitta

This formula promotes rejuvenation and proper function of the immune system. It is a combination of over 20 herbs, this calming blend is formulated to promote healthy digestion without aggravating pitta, and to strengthen the body against the effects of a stressful lifestyle. This formula is suitable for all doshas as a mental rejuvenative to enhance memory and intelligence.

Chyavanprash

Nutritive jam for vata and kapha

This formula promotes rejuvenation and proper functioning of the immune system. It is a traditional recipe containing over 40 herbs, including ashwagandha, pippali and saffron, which nourish the tissues and balances vata and kapha. This energizing formula has a slight heating quality that enkindles the digestive fire and stimulates metabolism.

Curry

The original intent for making Indian curry was to combine spices in a balanced way to promote digestion and optimal absorption. Indian curry's three primary spices are: cumin, which is heating and carminative; coriander, which is cooling and mild; and turmeric, which is pleasantly bitter, liver detoxifying, blood moving and digestive. Turmeric was also added for its golden color in food. In addition, various local regions add different spices according to climate and geography, e.g., cayenne, black pepper, and ginger, in cold weather areas. Curries have been used by people for over four thousand years. Curry preparations include: masalas, spice blends that usually lack turmeric. According to Ayurvedic medicine, a balanced curry blend can greatly enhance general health and well-being.

Curry Potatoes

1 lb potatoes cut into pieces	1 tsp curry powder
1 head cauliflower, chopped into florets	½ tsp whole cumin
1 tbsp olive oil	¼ tsp black pepper

Boil potatoes for 5 minutes, add cauliflower and boil another 5 minutes. Drain. Add oil and spices to a wok. Cook 1-2 minutes, add potatoes and cauliflower. Stir well. Cook 5 minutes.

Dashamula
This formula literally means "ten roots" and is used to pacify vata and kapha. It is commonly prepared as a tea for basti (herbal enemas).

Lavanbhaska
This formula includes five types of salt, pippali, trikatu, coriander, clove and other spices. It is used to pacify vata and stimulate agni (digestive enzymes).

Sitopaladi
This formula contains rock candy, banslochan, pippali, cardamom and cinnamon. It is being used for colds, congestion and bronchial conditions.

Trikatu
This formula contains ginger, black pepper, and pippali. It is a pungent recipe to enkindle digestive fire and to promote healthy absorption and assimilation. Trikatu supports fat metabolism and reduces ama (undigested food) and kapha.

Triphala
This formula contains amalaki, bibhitaki and haritaki. It cleanses the entire GI tract, supporting digestion and gently maintaining regularity. Considered in ayurveda to be a general panacea for all doshas, it is also used to support weight management, improve the complexion and strengthen the urinary tract.

Triphala/Guggula
Triphala/guggula can be taken for cholesterol, arthritis, high blood pressure and heart conditions associated with cholesterol, enlargement of the prostate gland, obesity, blood disorders, constipation, skin problems, and sores that are difficult to heal. Triphala guggula is a remedy against ama (undigested food, toxins), an accumulation of cholesterol, thickened mucus and other materials associated with the aging process, which inhibits the natural rejuvenative processes.

CASTOR OIL PACK

Castor oil, applied topically, can greatly reduce pain, swelling due to sprains, bruises and fractures. The emollient properties of castor oil make it excellent for soothing chapped lips and dry skin. Warmed castor oil dropped in the ear can lessen pain of ear infections. Castor oil packs are thought to help with conditions such as:

- Arthritis
- Colitis and other disturbances of the colon and intestines
- Kidney, liver and gallbladder problems
- Disturbances of the lymphatic system
- Helps soothe the nervous system.
  And much, much more. . . . .

Castor oil has shown to be effective in preventing the growth of numerous species of viruses, bacterias, yeast, and mold. This explains the high degree of success in the topical use of the oil for treating skin inflammation, warts and ringworm. Castor oil applications increase the flow of lymph throughout the body, which speeds up detoxification at the cellular level and reduces swollen lymph nodes. The end result is an improvement in organ function and a lessening of fatigue and depression.

Here is how to prepare and use a castor oil pack:

1. Fold a white or off white piece of cloth (unbleached cotton or wool) 3 times, large enough to cover the desired area
2. Saturate with castor oil.
3. Apply to body and cover with plastic sheet to keep oil from staining clothes and linen.
4. Place heating pad over plastic and cover with towel. Continue for at least 1 ½ hour.
5. Remove cloth and store in refrigerator (or under your bed). Can be reused many times
6. Wash body area to remove oil. (Apply baking soda first before washing oil off).

Castor oil packs can be used 1-3 times a day for acute ailments and 1-3 times a week for chronic ailments. This castor oil pack is yours; please do not share it with anyone!

Gorgeous Long Eye Lashes

For long eye lashes try this: Clean off eye make-up every night before retiring, then apply castor oil to your eyelashes and watch them transform.

CELL SALTS/TISSUE SALTS

Dr. W. H. Schuessler, M.D., of Oldenburg, Germany, was a key researcher investigating the many roles of minerals in the human body. He studied the work of another great 19th century thinker, Virchow, who in 1858, announced that the body is a collection of cells and medical treatment should be directed toward healing the individual cell. By 1873 Dr. Schuessler was analyzing blood from humans as well as the ashes after death. He discovered 12 mineral compounds and he called them "cell salts" or "tissue salts".

Dr. Schuessler stated that if an imbalance were to occur, sickness might follow. Each one of the 12 salts has a certain duty, and a deficiency in any one will produce certain symptoms.

Cell/Tissue Salts and Astrology

Sign	Cell Salt
ARIES	Kali Phosphoricum (Kali Phos)
TAURUS	Natrum Sulphuricum (Nat Sulph)
GEMINI	Kali Muriaticum (Kali Mur)
CANCER	Calcium Fluoride (Calc Fluor)
LEO	Magnesium Phosphate (Mag Phos)
VIRGO	Kali Sulphuricum (Kali Sulph)
LIBRA	Natrum Phosphoricum (Nat Phos)
SCORPIO	Calcium Sulphate (Calc Sulph)
SAGITTARIUS	Silica Oxide (Silica)
CAPRICORN	Calcium Phosphate (Calc Phos)
AQUARIUS	Natrum Muriaticum (Nat Mur)
PISCES	Ferrum Phosphate (Ferr Phos)

Individual Cell/Tissue Salts

Individual cell/tissue salts are meticulously extracted from living plants in an alcohol process. Manufacturers pulverize the natural mineral substances and blend them with milk sugar to make them more palatable. By placing the tablets under the tongue, cell/tissue salts are absorbed directly into to bloodstream.

Calcium Fluoride (Calc Fluor)
Necessary for retaining proper elasticity of tissues. May be of help in treating varicose veins, hemorrhoids, cracked skin, muscle strain, backache and torn ligaments.

Calcium Phosphate (Calc Phos)
Beneficial where digestion and nutrient assimilation are a problem. It may also be of assistance in treating osteoporosis, osteomalacia, bone disease, menstrual cramps and convalescence.

Calcium Sulphate (Calc Sulph)
It is a constituent of connective tissues, mucous membranes and the skin. It is a powerful blood purifier and may assist in cleaning the body of unwanted toxic accumulations.

Ferrum Phosphate (Ferr Phos)
It has the ability to carry oxygen to all cells of the body for use in the conversion to energy. It may also be helpful for the proper absorption of iron. Use it for sudden onsets of ailments.

Kali Muriaticum (Kali Mur)
It is helpful in relieving mucus congestion during colds and sinusitis. It may also be of help in treating a sore throat, tonsillitis, thrush and swollen glands.

Kali Phosphoricum (Kali Phos)
It is helpful in nerve related illnesses. It may also be of use in cases of insomnia.

Kali Sulphuricum (Kali Sulph)
It is helpful in respiratory and circulatory functions.

Magnesium Phosphate (Mag Phos)
It is helpful where cramping is a problem such as cramps due to sports, menstruation, chest cramps, leg and feet cramps.

Natrum Muriaticum (Nat Mur)
It is often referred to as the water salt. It is a regulator of water in the cells and may be of help in conditions where there is too little or too much water anywhere in the body.

Natrum Phosphoricum (Nat Phos)
It is helpful in maintaining the alkalinity of the blood.

Natrum Sulphuricum (Nat Sulph)
It is helpful in balancing the body's overall water content. It may also be of assistance in cases of mild fluid retention.

Silica Oxide (Silica)
It assists in the purification of waste. It may also be useful in relieving constipation.

The Twelve Cell/Tissue Salts

A balanced combination of the 12 cell/tissue salts gives an overall protection against any deficiencies. They are basically electrolytes the body requires to facilitate bioelectric and biochemical functions. Well-nourished cells provide us with the building blocks of health, chemically, energetically and beyond.

> **Before entering the sweat lodge, the Lakota medicine woman gave each of us a dose of the twelve-cell/tissue salts.**

THE SEVEN CHAKRAS

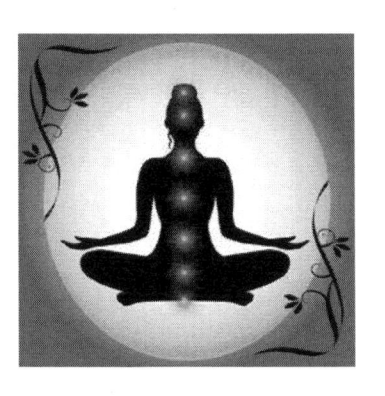

The word chakra is an ancient Sanskrit word meaning whirling vortex (or wheel) of light. Chakras are energy centers through which energy is taken in, dispersed, and released. Each center represents a psychological and spiritual quality. They are responsible for the brightness or dimness of the energy field surrounding your body. The endocrine glands are located in the same areas as the chakras. Chakras can be open, closed, or any of the various stages in between. These are the basics of someone's personality, which changes from moment to moment, in response to a situation. For example, someone with a closed third chakra (personal power) would be terrified of making a public speech. You can understand what condition your chakras are by turning your attention to the area of the body. Green tourmaline balances the the entire chakric system, as well as the endocrine glands.

THE FIRST CHAKRA

The first chakra is located at the base of the spine, is associated with survival. Its element is earth.

Organs: Circulatory, urinary/excretory, reproductive
Function: Stability, grounding, physical energy, will, security and ability to work devotedly on the physical plane.
Malfunction: Obesity, constipation, sciatica, hemorrhoids
Sense Organ: Nose/smell
Emotions: Fear, obsessive-compulsive, protective instincts

" I Have"
Color: Red or black to open,
Herbs: Valerian, red clover, lotus root, hawthorn, Lotus root
Oils: Cedar wood, vetivert, rosewood, patchouli
Vibrational Essences: Burdock/geranium, mullein, sumach, brown tourmaline
Food: Proteins, meat
Gemstone: Ruby, garnet, black tourmaline, smokey quartz, bloodstone, obsidian, rhodonite

THE SECOND CHAKRA

The second chakra, located between the lower abdomen and naval, is associated with emotions, creativity and sexuality. Its element is water.

Organs: Urinary/reproductive glands and organs.
Function: Creativity, sexuality and reproduction, healing, desire, emotion, intuition
Malfunction: Impotence, frigidity, uterine, bladder or kidney problems, stiff lower back
Sense organ: Tongue/taste
Emotions: Desire, jealousy

"I Feel"
Color: Red or orange to open
Herbs: Damiana, gokshura, marshmallow, uva ursi, saffron
Oils: Neroli, clary sage, ylang ylang
Vibrational Essences: Calendula, geranium, citrine
Food: Liquids
Gemstone: Coral, carnelian

THE THIRD CHAKRA

The third chakra, also known as the solar plexus, is associated with personal power and metabolic energy. Its element is fire.

Organs: Stomach/liver/pancreas/spleen/small intestine.
Function: Assimilation of experience, digestion, positive use of personal power, manifestation of goals, intellect, ambition, personal power and protection
Malfunction: Ulcers, diabetes, hypoglycemia
Sense organ: Eyes/sight
Emotions: Warmth, nurturing, fiery nature

"I Can"
Color: Orange or yellow to open
Herbs: Cayenne, cinnamon, calendula, chamomile, goldenseal
Oils: Lemon, tangerine, juniper, lemongrass
Vibrational Essences: Calendula, chamomile, herkimer diamond
Food: Starches
Gemstone: Citrine, amber, topaz, sulphur

THE FOURTH CHAKRA

The fourth chakra, located over the sternum, is associated with love. Its element is air.

Organs: Lungs/thymus gland
Function: Release emotionally suppressed trauma, emotional balance, soul/heart consciousness, expressing love and emotion, compassion, universal consciousness
Malfunction: Asthma, high blood pressure, heart disease, lung disease
Sense organ: Hands/touch
Emotions: Love, compassion, protectiveness

"I Love"
Color: Green or pink to open
Herbs: Rose, passionflower, lotus seed, motherwort
Oils: Rose otto, melissa
Vibrational Essences: Bee balm, foxglove
Food: Vegetables
Gemstone: Emerald, rose quartz, malachite, kunzite, pink tourmaline, green tourmaline

THE FIFTH CHAKRA

The fifth chakra, located in the throat and neck, is associated with communication and expression. Its element is sound.

Organs: Thyroid/vocal cords.
Function: Ability to verbalize, self-expression, communication, divine guidance
Malfunction: Sore throat, stiff neck, colds, thyroid problems, hearing problems
Sense organ: Ears/sound
Emotions: Honesty, dishonesty, criticism

"I Speak"
Color: Blue to open
Herbs: Bayberry, skullcap, calamus
Oils: Frankincense, benzoin, calamus
Vibrational Essences: Peach, sugilite
Food: Fruits
Gemstones: Lapis lazuli, aquamarine, turquoise, chrysocholla

THE SIXTH CHAKRA

The sixth chakra, located between the eyes, is associated with clairvoyance, intuition and imagination. Its element is light.

Organs: Medulla oblongata / pineal gland
Function: Seeing, psychic abilities and power, spiritual awareness, intuition
Malfunction: Blindness, headaches, nightmares, eyestrain, blurred vision
Sense organ: Intuition
Emotions: Imagination, idealism, love
"I See"
Color: Indigo or violet to open

Herbs: Basil, star anise, mugwort
Oils: Lavender, hyacinth, calamus
Vibrational Essences: Datura, belladonna
Food: Mind-altering substances. The higher chakras are not linked with bodily processes, but with mental states. Sometimes, a lack of food for a short time is beneficial for the sixth charka.
Gemstone: Lapis lazuli, quartz, amethyst, sapphire, sugilite

THE SEVENTH CHAKRA

The seventh chakra, located on the top of the head, is associated with knowledge and understanding. Its element is thought.

Organ: Beyond the sixth chakra one enters the "non-describable"
Function: Personal identification with infinite, Oneness with universe, peace, wisdom, spiritual center, enlightenment, cosmic consciousness, perfection
Malfunction: Depression, alienation, confusion, boredom, apathy, inability to learn or comprehend
Sense organ: Self-Realization
Emotions: Emotional imbalance

"I Know"
Color: Gold, white or purple to open
Herbs: Calamus, gotu kola, basil, lotus
Vibrational Essence: Edelweiss
Oils: Lavender, angelica, amethyst
Food: Fasting
Gemstone: Clear quartz, gold, diamond, selenite, black tournmaline

CHINESE HERBAL PATENT FORMULAS

Abundant Yin Teapills
See Da Bu Yin Wan

An Mien Pian
Traditionally used for insomnia due to heat or congestion in the liver with agitation to heart and mind. Anxiety, mental exhaustion, red or irritated eyes, restless dreaming, and poor memory.

An Shen Bu Xin Wan
Traditionally used as a natural tranquilizer for anxiety, irritability, and insomnia. Treats emotional troubles i.e. anxiety, irritability, emotional upsets, panic attacks, manic depression, bipolar disorders, uncontrolled emotions and resulting physical effects such as palpitations, insomnia, troubled sleep and dizziness.

An Shui Wan Teapills
Traditionally used for insomnia. Frequent waking with anxiety, irritability, excessive thinking or worry, fatigue. Reduces mental agitation and restlessness. Calms the mind to implement sleep and staying asleep. No side effects, i.e. hangover. Improves digestion.

Aplotaxis Amomum Pills
See Xiang Sha Liu Jun Zi Wan

Aquilaria Pills
See Chen Xiang Hua Qi Wan

Bai He Gu Jin Wan *(Lillium Teapills)*
Traditionally used for stopping cough, dry throat and coughing with blood. Used for chronic lung problems in which there has been a long-term cough, cough with blood or chronic dry, sore throat. Moistens dry lungs and replenishes vital fluids in the lungs and throat. Symptoms include chronic cough, coughing with blood, wheezing, night sweats, a red cracked tongue, hot palms and soles of the feet and dry and/or sore throat.

Bai Zi Yang Xin Wan
Traditionally used as a tranquilizer. Calms restlessness. Treats insomnia. Good for dream-troubled sleep, anxiety, forgetfulness, mental confusion. Symptoms include irritability, insomnia, difficulty sleeping and palpitations.

Bao He Wan
Traditionally used for indigestion, gas, bloating and motion sickness. Used when an individual overindulges in food or drink, which causes an upset stomach. Used when mildly contaminated food is consumed which results in diarrhea. Good for children with upset stomachs or who do not assimilate their food and remain skinny and underdeveloped. Symptoms include belching, heartburn, nausea, vomiting, little or no appetite, and possible diarrhea.

Bi Xie Sheng Shi Wan *(Subdue The Dampness Teapills)*
Traditionally used for cloudy, difficult urine, chronic ulcers on the legs, ankles or feet, vaginal discharge and enlarged prostate. Blocked fluids in lower burner.

Bi Yan Pian
Traditionally used for allergies and nasal congestion. Dries mucus and helps to open nasal passages. Kills pathogenic bacteria. Clears stuffy nose.

Bojenmi Tea
Traditionally used for reducing fat and promoting urination. Weight reducing herbal tea that maximizes nutrient absorption, and dispels fats, phlegm, and excess water. Removes atherosclerotic plaque in the blood vessels, reducing high blood pressure and lessening the chances for heart disease and stroke.

Bu Zhong Yi Qi Wan *(Central Chi Pills)*
Traditionally used for strengthening digestion, lifting prolapsed organs, and stopping chronic loose stool. Taken when a person is weak from illness or is just weak. For anemia in women with spotting between menses, or recurrent menses. Chronic diarrhea or chronic loose stools with undigested food in the stools, not due to bacteria. Prolapsed organs, such as stomach, rectum, uterus, bladder, or hemorrhoids. Other symptoms include chronic fatigue, fear of cold, pale face, pale skin. Cold hands and feet, chronic nosebleeds and little or no energy for basic functions such as speaking or exercise.

Bu Tiao Tablets
Traditionally used for regulating menses. Builds blood, harmonizes a woman's body, supports the kidneys, regulates the liver which controls the flow of blood, and warms the internal organs. Alleviates cramps, insomnia, headaches associated with menses, moodiness and irregular cycles.

Calm Spirit/Gan Mai Da Zao Wan
Excessive emotions, loss of self-control, impulsiveness, mood swings, melancholy, crying spells, inappropriate laughter, deep sighing or frequent bouts of yawning, restless sleep. In severe cases, symptoms may include manic behavior or disorientation. Tongue is red with a scanty coat or no coat. Pulse thin, rapid.

Calm In The Sea Of Life Teapills
See Tong Jing Wan

Central Chi Pills
See Bu Zhong Yi Qi Wan
Chen Xiang Hua Qi Wan *(Aquilaria Pills)*
Traditionally used for bad breath, constipation, abdominal fullness, belching, hiccups. Relieves pressure in the chest and abdomen. Symptoms include tight, constricted chest with pain and stuffiness, a feeling of fullness in the stomach. Also included are pale face, fatigue, shortness of breath and poor digestion.
Chien Chin Chih Tai Wan
Traditionally used for leucorrhea, stopping vaginal discharge, especially from deficiency of blood and Qi, which means a woman's body is not strong enough to control the fluids in her body allowing them to leak out the vagina. It is primarily a digestive problem because it controls and disperses body fluids.
China Tung Hsueh
Traditionally used for promoting blood circulation, benefits heart and kidney, enriches sexual function and counters fatigue. Tonic for aged and debilitated patients. Useful for poor memory, senility, fatigue, poor resistance to disease and strengthening the heart.
Ching Fei Yi Huo
Traditionally used for lung infection and bronchitis with yellow phlegm. Can be used as antibiotic, to fight lung infections such as bronchitis and in the aftermath of illness to clear up residual sticky phlegm.
Chuan Xin Ling
Traditionally used for sore throat, tonsillitis, ear infection, bladder infection. Popular with women who get bladder infections, especially those who get them repeatedly. Natural anti-biotic for sore throat, swollen tonsils and swollen lymph glands. For bacterial and viral infections.
Cinnamon And Poria
See Gui Zhi Fu Ling Wan
Curing Pills
Traditionally used for upset stomach. Relieves almost any type of simple stomach discomfort. Taken after meal of overeating or for bloating from weak digestion, nausea, gas or indigestion, relieves minor food poisoning
Da Bu Yin Wan
Traditionally used for nourishing the liver and kidneys. Also clears heat. Afternoon fevers, intense heat on the head, hot flashes, flushed face, night sweats, irritability, heat and pain in the knees and legs.
Du Huo Ji Sheng Wan *(Solitary Hermit Teapills)*
Traditionally used for lower back pain, sciatica and arthritis. Especially beneficial for the elderly or weak. Treats many types of body pain, including lower back, sciatica, ruptured discs, and knee problems, alleviates rheumatic arthritis, bone disorders, chronic osteoarthritis, any type of condition that affects bones. Strengthens kidneys.

Eight Flavor Rehmannia Teapills
See Zhi Bai Di Huang Wan
Eight Immortals Teapills
See Mai Wei Di Huang Wan
Emperor's Teapills
See Tian Wang Bu Xin Dan Wan
Er Chen Wan
Traditionally used for cough and clear or white phlegm in the lungs. Removes excess phlegm and dampness from the lungs, to stop a cough and relieve a congested chest. Symptoms include thick and easily coughed up damp phlegm which is either white or clear. Taken also for bloating, nausea, vomiting and dizziness, which is associated with poor digestion. Treats difficult chronic bronchitis with knotted phlegm in order to facilitate healing.
Er Long Zuo Ci Wan *(Er Ming Zuo Ci Wan) (Tso-Tsu Otic)*
Traditionally used for ringing ears (tinnitus) and deafness, caused by too little yin and too much yang.
Fargelin
See Hua Zhi Ling Wan
Four Gentlemen Teapills
See Si Jun Zi Tang Wan
Free and Easy Wanderer
See Xiao Yao Wan
Free and Easy Wanderer Plus
See Jia Wei Xiao Yao Wan
Fu Ke Zhong Zi Wan
Traditionally used to stop bruising, stop spotting between periods, calm a restless fetus and to promote fertility. Nourishes and regulates blood as well as strengthen the kidneys. Promotes fertility, by warming the womb, promoting the production of blood, plus harmonizing and regulating female hormones. Calms restless fetus.
Gan Mao Ling
Traditionally used for the common cold. Treats colds and flu. Take within first few days. Sudden, unexplained fatigue, chills and fever, sore throat, body aches, neck aches and swollen glands.
Ge Gen Wan *(Kudzu Teapills)*
Traditionally used for the common cold with associated neck pain and achy muscles. Symptoms include chills, slight fever without sweating, headache, body aches, upper back pain, stiff neck and stuffy nose with clear or white mucus. This formula causes sweating. Also used for any kind of neck pain not associated with cold or flu.

Ge Jie Da Bu Wan *(Gecko Tonic Teapills)*

Traditionally used for weakness, fatigue and reducing wheezing and asthma. For those who are weak and suffer shortness of breath, dizziness, fatigue, ear ringing, weak lower back, cold hands and feet and poor appetite.

Goldenbook Teapills

See Jin Gui Shen Qi Wan

Great Corydalis

See Yan Hu Suo Wan

Great Mender, The

See Jin Gu Die Shang Wan

Gui Pi Wan

Traditionally used for stress, over-work, pensiveness, anxiety, anemia. Over thinking and over studying. Used when studying exhausts the body and mind. Upset stomach and impaired digestion.

Gui Zhi Fu Ling Wan *(Cinnamon and Poria Teapills)*

Traditionally used for dissolving nodules, fixes abdominal masses, endometriosis, ovarian cysts and fibroids. Also used for dysmenorrhea.

Huang Lian Jie Du Wan

Traditionally used as a natural antibiotic, treats skin infections, dysentery, sore throat and ear infections. Symptoms include strong fever, irritability, dry mouth and dry throat, incoherence and insomnia accompanied by some type of skin lesion, carbuncle, boil or other skin infections with pus. Jaundice, septicemia, pneumonia.

Huang Lien Sheng Ching Pian

Traditionally used for tonsillitis, mouth sores, bronchitis, ear infections, red eyes, sore gums and swollen glands. Hot inflamed skin problems, skin rash, poison oak, hives, carbuncles and boils.

Hua She Jie Yang

Traditionally used as a replacement of Trisnake itch-removing pills. Skin itching conditions including pruritis, dermatitis, eczema, acne, and fungal infections. Also useful for leucorrhea. Skin itching, skin rash, poison oak, dermatitis, eczema, etc.

Hua Zhi Ling Wan *(Fargelin)*

Traditionally used for the healing of Hemorrhoids.

Jai Wei Xiao Yao Wan *(Free and Easy Wander Plus)*

Traditionally used for PMS, anger and irritability. Similar to Xiao Yao Wan with added herbs for emotional signs of PMS. Symptoms also include red face, night sweats, red eyes, or dry mouth. Good for women who experience anger, short temper and irritability.

Jian Pi Wan
Traditionally used for Anorexia, weak digestion, strengthens digestive system. Symptoms include loss of weight, poor appetite and bloating, indigestion, loose stools, diarrhea, sometimes with undigested food particles, and/or constipation. When food sits in stomach.

Jiao Gu Lan *(Panta Teapills)*
Traditionally used for hypertension (high blood pressure) and high cholesterol.

Jie Geng Wan *(Platycodon Teapills)*
Traditionally used for chronic cough, smoker's cough, weak lungs. Strengthening and aids in digestion and helps stop coughs. Taken also for hoarseness or sore throat.

Jin Gu Die Shang Wan *(The Great Mender Teapills)*
Traditionally used for minor sprains, strains, cuts, bruises and abrasions. Reduces pain, swelling and inflammation. Repairs acute traumatic injury such as broken bones, muscle strains, knee and ankle strains. Stops internal bleeding, reduces pain and helps to repair damage cause by many different types of injuries.

Jin Gui Shen Qi Wan *(Goldenbook Teapills)*
Traditionally used for impotence, infertility and prostate problems. Replenishes vital life force energy of the kidneys. Symptoms include lower back pain, cold legs, cold lower back, and tenderness of the lower abdomen, weakness, frequent urination especially at night, incontinence, impotence and infertility.

Huan Shao Dan Wan *(Return to Spring Teapills) (Return to Youth Teapills)*
Traditionally used for impotence, old age and fatigue. Replenishes youthful energy. Used by men or women to assist in replenishing sexual energy and vigor.

Kang Gu Zeng Sheng Pian
Traditionally used for arthritis, where both small and large joints are sore and stiff. Restore dislocated discs, eliminate pain from dull achy joints and strengthen tendons and bones to support the joints more effectively. Used for upper and middle back pain.

Kudzu Teapills
See Ge Gen Wan

Left Side Replenishing Teapills
See Zuo Gui Teapills

Li Fei Pian
Traditionally used for weak lungs, shortness of breath, chronic cough, improves breathing and eliminates shortness of breath. This formula is for those who smoke or who have smoked either tobacco or marijuana because it helps to repair the damage caused by heat and smoke. Used for chronic cough or one who is easily winded. Strengthens the function of the lungs and can be used long term by anyone who has lung deficiency.

Lilium Teapills
See Bai He Gu Jin Wan

Liu Jun Zi Wan *(Six Gentlemen Teapills)*
Traditionally used for improving digestion and draining dampness. Treats spleen deficiency, weak digestion, sluggish digestion, dull appetite, nausea, belching, bloating and loose stool. Also used for morning sickness.

Liu Wei Di Huang Wan *(Six Flavor Tea Pills)*
Traditionally used for one that has a busy, over active lifestyle, caused by excessive coffee drinking, excessive sexual activity, eating hot, spicy foods, not getting enough rest, excessive consumption of alcohol and drugs, cigarette smoking and other speedy activities. Good for burn outs. Good for yin deficiency.

Long Dan Xie Gan Wan *(The Snake and The Dragon Teapills)*
Traditionally used for migraines, herpes, irritability, hepatitis and jaundice. Clears heat from the liver created by stress and intense constricting emotions which create obstructions in the liver. It can move down to cause problems in the genital area, or up to the head to cause red eyes and headache, or can stay in the liver area and affect the gallbladder and liver. Originally used for serious diseases such as hepatitis, gallstones and gallbladder inflammation. It can be used for less severe symptoms i.e. irritability, red eyes, migraine headaches and herpes outbreaks and ear ringing. Other symptoms from the liver and gallbladder include gallstones, inflamed gallbladder, jaundice and hepatitis. Symptoms affecting genitals include herpes, external genital discharge, vaginal discharge (foul smelling), urinary tract infection, kidney infection, testicle swelling or discomfort.

Loquat And Fritillary Syrup
Traditionally used for cough, nourishes and strengthen the function of the lungs and helps to loosen sticky phlegm. Frees sticky phlegm so that it can be coughed up and no longer impede normal lung function. Good for chronic and acute cough, emphysema, asthma and difficult breathing.

Lycium-Rehmanhia Teapills
See Qi Ju Di Huang Wan

Ma Zi Ren Teapills
Traditionally used as a laxative for dry stools, constipation, and temporary relief of constipation from loss of body fluids, such as after childbirth or any type of heat condition which dries out the stool.

Mai Wei Di Huang Wan *(Eight Immortals Teapills)*
Traditionally used for dry cough, chronic cough and bronchitis, weak lungs, dry skin. Helps to improve the functioning of the lungs, producing fluids for those with chronic dry cough, chronic bronchitis, excessive thirst and dry skin problems. Good for elderly patients.

Margarite Acne Pills
Traditionally used for relieving swollen masses, promoting blood circulation, acne, furuncles, skin itching and rashes, including hives. Adolescent acne.

Ming Mu Di Huang Wan
Traditionally used for blurry vision, dry, shaking eyes, light sensitive eyes and night blindness.

Minor Bupleurum Teapills
See Xiao Chai Hu Tang Wan

Nu Ke Ba Zhen Wan *(Woman's Precious Teapills) (Women's Eight Treasure Teapills)*
Traditionally used for nourishing blood, improving digestion, and regulating the menstrual cycle. This formula nourishes all aspects of blood including red blood cells, white blood cells, platelets, plasma, fluid in the blood, etc. Improves the body's own ability to manufacture blood and assimilate the nutrients to build healthy blood. Anemia.

Peach Kernel Pills
See Tao Ren Wan

Pe Min Kan Wan
Traditionally used for allergies and nasal congestion. Dries phlegm and opens nasal passages, eliminating stuffy nose, hay fever, sneezing and allergies. Hay fever, cold formula to clear the nose of stuffiness and mucus.

Ping Chuan Pian
Traditionally used for relieves symptoms of wheezing and asthma. Clears phlegm and heat that contribute to wheezing.

Platycodon Teapills
See Jie Geng Wan

Qi Ju Di Huang Wan *(Lycium Rehmannia Teapills) (Lycii Chrysanthemum Teapills)*
Traditionally used for benefiting the eyes. Symptoms include blurry vision, dry and painful eyes, pressure behind the eyes, and poor night vision, dizziness, headaches, pain behind the eyes, outbursts of anger, heat in palms, restlessness and insomnia.

Qi Ye Lian
Traditionally used to stop pain. Analgesic and anodyne properties. Good for all kinds of pain including arthritis, headache, sciatica, trigeminal neuralgia, carpal tunnel, and other types of physical discomfort, internal and external. Takes a few days to feel effects.

Qing Qi Hua Tan Wan *(Pinellia Teapills) (Clean Air Teapills)*
Traditionally used for bronchitis, treats hot phlegm, stagnation in the lungs and bronchitis, both acute and chronic. Used to treat pneumonia and asthma with hot and yellow, sticky phlegm that is difficult to cough up and clear out of the lungs. Causes coughing and wheezing, pain in the chest with possible bloating or fullness in the chest.

Return To Spring Teapills
See Huan Shao Dan Wan

Return To Youth Teapills
See Huan Shao Dan
Right Side Replenishing Teapills
See You Gui Teapills
Run Chang Wan
See Tao Ren Wan
Sang Ju Yin Wan *(Clear Wind Heat Pills)*
Traditionally used for common cold, especially in children. Treat common colds. Especially good for children because it is mild and because children are more likely to have complications along with a cold. Early stages of cold or flu (2-3 days). Colds accompanied by cough, headache or red eyes.
Shen Qi Da Bu Wan
Traditionally used for fatigue, lack of energy and low immune system. Improves digestion and strengthens lung function so that the body can better utilize oxygen. Generates blood which nourishes all the organs and the skin, carrying nutrients and vital fluids to every cell in the body.
Shen Qi Wu Wei Zi Wan
Traditionally used for improving energy, boosting immunity and stopping excessive sweating. Lifts energy, reduces excessive sweating—night sweats, spontaneous sweating, sweating easily from exertions—while calming nervousness and strengthening the immune system.
Shou Wu Essence
Traditionally used for restoring normal hair color and building blood. Replenish sexual energy. Supports liver and kidneys. Strengthens knees and lower back, supports the softening of tendons and strengthens the function of the kidneys which support all the organs of the body.
Shou Wu Pian
Traditionally used for darkening hair color, lifts energy, reverses the graying process that occurs with aging. Builds blood, therefore improving energy levels.
Shu Gan Wan *(Soothe Liver Teapills)*
Traditionally used for reducing stress, aiding digestion, normalizing menses and reducing PMS. Designed to alleviate emotional congestion which traps the warmth of the body internally and will not allow it to flow to the hands and feet. Can be taken for emotional stress which is affecting digestion, causing alternating diarrhea and constipation, bloating, chest pain or pain in the liver and gallbladder area.
Si Jun Zi Tang Wan *(Four Gentlemen Teapills)*
Traditionally used for improving digestion and strengthening the immune system.

Six Flavor Teapills
See Liu Wei Di Huang Wan

Six Gentlemen Teapills
See Liu Jun Zi Wan

Snake Of The Dragon, The
See Long Dan Xie Gan Wan

Solitary Hermit
See Du Huo Ji Sheng Wan

Soothe Liver Teapills
See Shu Gan Wan

Suan Zao Ren Tang
Traditionally used for insomnia. Nourishes the liver, calms the heart and clears heat from the liver to sedate the mind, encouraging the eyes to close. Anxiety and insomnia. Relieves stress, allowing peaceful sleep.

Subdue The Dampness
See Bi Xie Sheng Shi Wan

Tao Ren Wan *(Peach Kernel Pills) (Run Chang Wan)*
Traditionally used as a laxative, treating problem of dry stool or constipation in the elderly or
chronically sick whose bodies do not produce enough fluid to moisten the stool. Relieves the constitutional problem of a deficiency of body fluids and blood. Symptoms include dry mouth, unquenchable thirst, dull skin, dull hair and nails, and constipation.

Tian Ma Wan
Traditionally used for arthritis, rheumatism and headache. Eliminates minor complains of aches and pains. Treats neck and shoulder pain, low back pain, joint pain and pain caused by minor arthritis.

Tian Wang Bu Xin Dan Wan *(Emperor's Teapills)*
Traditionally used for regulating and calming the heart and mind. Treats minor complaints associated with the heart—insomnia, palpitations, excessive dreaming or dream disturbed sleep, forgetfulness, difficulty concentrating, burning urination, and mouth or tongue ulcers

Tong Jing Wan *(Calm In The Sea Of Life Teapills)*
Traditionally used for regulating difficult menses. Help facilitate menstruation. Breaks up clots.

Women's Eight Treasure Teapills
See Nu Ke Ba Zhen Wan

Women's Precious Teapills
See Nu Ke Ba Zhen Wan

Wuchi Paifeng Wan
Traditionally used to build blood and regulates menses. Helps produce Qi and blood lost in menstruation. Produces normal flow.

Xiang Sha Liu Jun Zi Wan *(Aplotaxis Amomum Teapills)*
Traditionally used for improving digestion, draining dampness and spleen deficiency

Xiao Chai Hu Tang Wan *(Minor Bupleurum Teapills)*
Traditionally used for lingering common cold. Second stage of the common cold (trapped between interior and exterior). Symptoms include alternating fever and chills, an internal struggle between the body and the disease tries to penetrate more deeply. Dry throat, bitter taste in the mouth, dizziness, irritability, bloated chest, shallow breathing, low appetite, nausea and perhaps vomiting. Women who get a common cold during menses.

Xiao Yao Wan *(Free and Easy Wanderer)*
Traditionally used for PMS, stress, anemia. Enriches blood and helps regulate the liver which controls the movement of Qi and blood. PMS symptoms include distress, upset and anxiety, bloating, fatigue, headache, dizziness, blurry vision, dry mouth and throat, reduced appetite and an irregular menstrual cycle, including cramps.

Yan Hu Suo Wan *(Great Corydalis Teapills)*
Traditionally used for stopping menstrual cramps. Difficult or painful menstruation, stopping sharp, piercing abdominal pain and spasms. Can be used for similar discomfort, especially abdominal pain not associated with menses.

Yang Rong Wan
Traditionally used for easy bruising, spotting between periods and spotting when pregnant. Treats conditions of excessive menstrual bleeding. Nourishes blood, improves digestion to make more blood to promote energy. Symptoms include spotting between periods, post-partum bleeding, pale face, pale skin, small, short periods with pale, thin blood without clots, fatigue, easy bruising, a pale tongue or a period that continues for a week or longer.

Yin Chiao Tablets *(sugar coated)*
Traditionally used for the first day or two of a wind-heat attack (flu). Swollen lymph nodes, sore throat, aching body, fever with chills, headache, sore shoulders and stiff neck. Promotes sweating. Excellent when taken immediately. Useful for skin itching due to allergenic reactions (hives).

Yin Chiao Chien Tu Pien
Same as above but sugar-free.

You Gui *(Right Side Replenishing Teapills)*
Traditionally used for impotence, exhaustion, age-related problems. Symptoms include sore lower back, sore knees, cold hands and feet, general overall malaise, exhaustion and poor digestion. Good for people over 40. NOT for those who are simply tired or worn out.

Yu Dai Wan
Traditionally used to stops vaginal discharge. Damp heat in lower burner. Discharge should have a yellow color; there could be associated itching, pain and/or strong smell. Other symptoms include burning urination, lower abdominal pain, a bitter taste in the mouth and dry throat.

Yunnan Pai Yao *(Yunnan Bai Yao)*
Traditionally used to stop bleeding, heal injuries, stop pain and ease pain from trauma and injury. Anytime after minor injuries including bruising, abrasions, minor accidents and other trauma. It helps to stop internal bleeding and to ease pain. Can be applied directly to a cut or wound to stop bleeding, can be taken orally to heal internal bleeding or hemorrhaging from internal injuries. Emergency medicine.

Zhi Bai Di Huang Wan *(Eight Flavor Rehmannia Teapills) (Zhi Bai Ba Wei Wan)*
Traditionally used for night sweats, hot flashes, menopause. Symptoms include tidal fever, night sweats, hot flashes, heat in soles of feet or palms, insomnia, restless sleep, or high blood pressure.

Zi Sheng Wan
Traditionally used to improve digestion. Improves the quality of life by improving digestion. Loose stool, low appetite, gas, nausea, abdominal pain, mal-absorption of food, belching, bloating and the feeling of fullness after eating.

Zuo Gui Teapills *(Left Side Replenishing Teapills)*
Traditionally used to fortify kidney function. Treats lower back pain. Symptoms include heat conditions, night sweats, dry mouth, thirst with a desire to drink cold fluid, as well as weak legs, dizziness, ear ringing and blurry vision.

FINDING YOUR ELEMENT

	EARTH	METAL	WATER	WOOD	FIRE
Affinities	Spleen and Stomach, change of seasons, sweet tastes, the muscles and the lips/mouth, yellow, childlike voice, damp weather and damp conditions	Lungs and large intestine, fall, pungent or aromatic tastes, the skin, body hair, the nose and smell, the color white, a crying voice, dry weather and dry conditions	Kidneys and bladder, winter storage, salty, the bones, teeth and ears, hearing, the color black, a groaning voice, cold weather and cold conditions	Liver and gallbladder, spring, sour tastes, tendons, eyes, the color green, a shouting voice, wind and movement	Heart and small intestine, summer, growth, bitter tastes, the complexion, tongue, speech, the color red, a laughing voice, hot weather and hot conditions
Prone to	Tiredness, poor muscle tone and flabbiness, easy bruising, varicose veins, pale sallow complexion, digestive and bowel problems, eating disorders, yeast infections and food intolerance, poor memory and concentration, worry.	Colds, airborne allergens, selfishness, coughs, asthma, dry skin, constipation	Back problems, bladder problems, weak bones or teeth, hormonal changes, poor development	Mood swings, depression, IBS, period problems, eye problems, gallstones, alcohol and substance abuse, insomnia with nightmares, violent behavior.	Anxiety, over stimulation, poor circulation, broken Veins, bad complexion, restless sleep, dreaming, indecision, feeble memory, lack of communication skills, talking too much, hyperactivity

Key Herbs	**Ren Shen, Fu Ling, Bai Zhu, Yi Yi Ren, Shan Yao, Dang Shen, Chen Pi, Hou Xiang, Sha Ren**	**Huang Qi, Dang Shen, Mai Men Dong, Bei He, Chen Pi, Bei Mu, Huang Qin, Sheng Jiang**	**Shu Di, Gou Qi Zi, He Shou Wu, Gui Pi, Du Zhong, Huang Bai**	**Dang Gui, Dai Shao, Gou Qi Zi, Ju Hua, Chai Hu, Xiang Fu, Yu Jin.**	**Suan Zao Ren, Bai Zi Ren, Hou Ma Ren, Yuan Zhi, Ling Zhi, Dan Shen, Lian Zi, Huang Qin, Hong Hua**
Recommended Foods	**Grains, naturally sweet vegetables, orchard fruits, warm spices**	**Grains, Root Vegetables, pears, nuts, and seeds, some pungent spices**	**Seaweed, naturally salty food, warm fluids**	**Green Veggies, oily fish, red and orange root veggies, green tea, organic liver, olive oil, sesame oil.**	**Oily fish, salads with bitter leaves, dates, longan fruit**
Foods to Avoid	**Sweet foods that include processed sugars, excess of tropical fruit, large quantities of fruit juice, to much cold fluid, dairy products, wheat**	**Too much baked or barbecued food, smoked food, dairy produce**	**Cold foods and fluids, excessive salt**	**Alcohol, coffee, hot spicy and greasy foods, large amounts of pickles and vinegar**	**Stimulants, excessive spicy foods**
Cultivate	**A liking for breakfast, an early dinner, eat until only 2/3 full, aerobic muscle toning exercise**	**A regular aerobic exercise, your spiritual side, tolerance of the weakness of others**	**An exercise routine that will keep the knees and back strong, a moderate love life, the correct fluid intake**	**Relaxing activities, painting, Tai Qi, or Yoga**	**A quiet pastime that will keep your feet on the ground such as gardening, the qualities of leadership, empathy, and compassion, an early bedtime**

CLAYS AND MUDS

Used Internally

Clays have been ingested as nutritional supplements and detoxifiers throughout the world for thousands of years. Naturally absorbent and extremely gentle on the system, clays can treat many ailments. For as long as I can remember, my grandmother would mix one teaspoon of French clay (Argile) in 6 oz of distilled water every night before going to bed. In the morning she would stir it up and drink it all at once.

Caution: Not all clays can be taken internally.

Used Externally

Clays are absorbent, drawing, cleansing, thickening and tightening agents, which makes them useful in facial masques, body powders, deodorants and creams. There are many varieties of clays available. Their function depends on their place of origin and mineral composition.

How To Make A Medicinal Clay Pack

Mix your selected clay with an appropriate liquid, such as water, hydrosols, teas, extracts, etc. Make sure it is not too runny. You may also add essential oils. Apply directly to affected area, cover with a clean cloth and plastic bag. You may leave it on overnight or until the clay is dry. If this is your first time, please check for skin sensitivity. This clay pack is beneficial for sprains, strains, and parts of the body that is swollen due to injury. May also be used for water retention in the feet and legs. Do not apply this pack if the skin is broken.

Toothache Poultice

Mix bentonite clay with enough of the following herbal powders: goldenseal, echinacea, st. john's wort, spilanthes, charcoal and 2 drops of clove essential oil. Add enough distilled water to make a thick paste. Place this paste on a small piece (2x2-inch) white paper towel or gauze, roll into cylinder shape and apply directly to the affected tooth area. Change the poultice every 6-8 hours and do this for at least 3 days. Take amalaki and rosehips for Vitamin C, to bring back health to the tooth and gum. Call your dentist!

Individual Clays And Muds

Ayurvedic Mineral Clay
In ayurveda, mineral rich clays have been used for thousands of years to cleanse the body. This clay is collected during the monsoons from the marshy tropical ponds, seasonally flourishing with lotus flowers. Additionally, 33 herbs have been combined in the tradition of ayurveda and added to this clay, for cleansing the body and providing nourishment. The clay's natural drawing action helps to pull dirt out of the pores, leaving the skin cleaner than if conventional soap were used. The lingering, all-natural fragrance will leave you with a sensation of well being, while the treatment itself will leave your skin glowing, vibrant and radiant. Daily use will leave the skin supple, alive and vibrant. Try this clay and feel the skin tingle with joy.

Bentonite Clay
Bentonite clay was first discovered in Fort Benton, Wyoming, hence its name. The source of bentonite clay is basically weathered volcanic ash. Traditionally used as an internal supplement to assist in mineral deficiencies and to help bind toxins making them more soluble. Because of its naturally soft nature, this clay also makes an invigorating skin and facemask. This is the strongest pulling clay. Can be used internally!

French Blue Clay
French blue clay is a potent medicinal clay, having similar benefits as red clay, but is bluish gray in color. Used in cosmetics as a natural color additive. French blue clay is effective in drawing out oils and toxins from the skin, and is best suited for oily skin and hair. This clay whitens the skin.

French Green Clay
French green clay has enormous absorbent powers due to the constitution of its micro molecules. It literally "drinks" oils, toxic substances, and impurities from the skin. Its toning action stimulates the skin bringing fresh blood to damaged skin cells, revitalizing the complexion while tightening pores. French green clay is marvelous for treating acne, disturbed skin and for mature skin as it has an anti-aging effect. Use daily, by applying onto troubled spots and allowing to dry for 15-20 minutes. Mined from bedrock quarries in France.

French Red Clay

French red clay is high in Iron. Very stimulating and is used only for the body, NOT the face.

French Pink Clay

French pink clay heals, disinfects and soothes. It is recommended for dehydrated or delicate skin. Pink clay has softening, moisturizing, purifying, regenerative and re-mineralizing properties.

French White Clay

French white clay is similar to green clay, but milder particularly for sensitive and dry skin. White clay has softening, moisturizing, purifying, regenerative and re-mineralizing properties.

Fullers Earth

Fuller's earth is widely used as a skin-lightening agent and best known for its ability to be applied as "facial bleach". Because of its enormous drawing capabilities, fuller's earth is the number one choice for oily skin and those prone to acne. It literally draws oil from the skin and has been used industrially for this exact purpose.

White Kaolin Clay *(China Clay)*

White kaolin clay is the mildest of all clays and frequently found in powders, body packs, skin care products, and deodorants. It has an astringent effect and removes impurities from the skin while cleansing, improving lymphatic flow and increasing blood circulation to the area. For oily and normal skin.

Yellow Kaolin Clay

Yellow kaolin clay is mild and suitable for sensitive skin. It helps stimulate circulation to the skin while gently exfoliating and cleansing the skin. It does not draw oils from the skin excessively and can therefore be used on most dry skin types. It can be used in soap and body powders.

Rhassoul Clay

Rhassoul is a super fine ancient clay that comes from deep below the Atlas Mountains in Morocco. Although it is difficult to obtain from the deep clay beds, the ancient people of Rome and Egypt have used it for centuries. Rhassoul clay is rich in minerals such as silica, magnesium, iron, calcium, potassium and sodium. It helps detoxify the skin while it exfoliates gently. Rhassoul is used by the finest spas around the world.

Red Earth Clay
Enjoy this red earth clay from the American southwest. This clay is beneficial for use by all ages and skin types as it leaves the skin feeling fresh, clean and healthy. Red earth clay is soothing in the bath and relaxing when used in a footbath.

Rose Clay
Rose clay is a pale reddish powder used in facemasks and colored cosmetics. It derives its color from its iron oxide content. Rose clay is a mild clay, which will gently cleanse and exfoliate the skin. Rose clay is also used as a colorant in soap making or to make speckled soap.

Sea Clay
Sea clay has a high content of minerals and helps to draw oils from the skin while mineralizing the skin and body. Good for all types of skin. This is a dark clay ideal for facemasks and mud mask applications. Color ranges from gray to dark gray due to its high content of minerals,

Dead Sea Clay
Dead sea clay comes from the dead sea and is very high in minerals and other micronutrients.

The Basics For A Clay Facial Mask

2-3 oz cosmetic clay
1-2 oz powdered herbs
Water or hydrosol
1-2 drops essential oil.

Choose cosmetic clay and herbs that are suitable for your skin type. For example, neem powder is anti-bacterial; citrus peel powder adds astringency; rose petals powder adds moisture and fragrance, etc. Experiment with other ingredients, such as pureed strawberries, which will act like an alpha-hydroxy. Cucumbers cools the skin, yogurt cools and softens the skin, milk removes dead skin cells and softens the skin, and sea vegetable help revitalize the skin. In a small bowl mix powdered ingredients with enough warm water or hydrosol to make a paste. For dry skin you may add vegetable glycerin, honey and/or oil. Add a drop or two of essential oil if desired. Apply to the skin in a gentle circular motion, and leave it to dry for about 15 – 20 minutes. Wash off with warm water. If the skin feels tight, light oil such as camelina or hazelnut can be applied afterwards.

Individual Muds

Dead Sea Mud

Dead sea mud is a natural extract from the Dead Sea, which contains a high percentage of magnesium, potassium, bromine and other important minerals and trace elements. Dead Sea mud supports the metabolism and revitalizes the natural functions of cells. It has anti-inflammatory and anti-rheumatic effects. Worldwide, this mud is used as a supporting cure for skin and rheumatic diseases. It is also recommended as an overall regenerative and in beautification masks. Dead sea mud has long been advocated for its healing benefits for those with psoriasis. While not a true "medical therapy", many psoriasis patients claim that the use of mineral mud helps soften their skin and diminish the presence of scaling. Great for the scalp too! If you wish to use Dead Sea mud on the face, please try out on a very small facial area first and note any reactions you may have.

Moor Mud

Moor mud is one of the world's most prized ancient medicines. It has been used for centuries to balance, detoxify and tone the body. Historical reports reveal the many uses of moor mud in the treatment of human diseases. Even animals have been observed using moor mud for its curative properties. Moor mud is the unique product of time and nature that started with the retreat of the last Ice Age. A very fertile valley brimming with plant life was formed and isolated from the rest of the world. These plants became submerged under a lake formed by the melting glaciers. Over time, this area became a rich, live deposit of organic substances with all the properties of the plants intact. Analysis of moor mud shows that it contains over 1000 organic botanicals, trace minerals and elements, enzymes, natural anti-biotics, vitamins and phyto-hormones. Today moor mud is being re-discovered to heal a wide range of disorders. Moor mud is also being used by the world's finest spas for complete body care. In addition to its cosmetic use as a natural exfoliant, detoxifier and cellulite reducer, moor mud can be used in poultices to reduce swelling, reduce inflammation, draw out abscesses, and to promote healing with minimized scar formation.

MEDICINAL DESERT PLANTS

Agave
(Agaves spp)
Indigestion, chronic constipation, gas, this plant is spiny.

Brittlebush
(Encelia farinose)
Analgesic, expectorant, incense, sore joints and muscles.
Tribes: Cahuilla, Mojave, Pima, Papagao, Seri.

Buckwheat Bush
(Erioganum)
Colds, coughs, sore throat
Tribes: Cahuilla, Mojave, Pima, Papagao, Seri.

Bursage
(Ambrosia deltoidea)
Cramps, allergies
Tribes: Seri

Catclaw
(Acacia spp.)
Dysentery, diarrhea, astringent, arthritis
Tribes: Widely used by all Native Americans

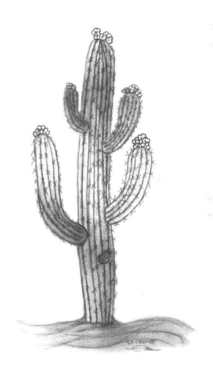

Saguaro

Creosote Bush (Chaparral)
(Larrea tridentata)
Antioxidant, antiseptic, anti-microbial, hair tonic, arthritis, blood cleanser, skin, tumors, cysts, drawing salve, cancer.
Tribes: Pima, Papago, Seri, Cahuilla.

Crucifixion Thorn
(Castela emoryi)
Uses: Inhibits intestinal protozoa, traveling long distance, styptic.
Tribes: Seri

Desert Barberry (Oregon Grape)
(Mahonia trifoliata)
Uses: Edible berries; stem and root bark as a bitter tonic, anti-microbial for skin and intestinal tract, liver tonic, yellow dye. Berberine.
Tribes: Navajo, Seri.

Desert Mistletoe
(Phoradendron californicum)
Uses: Nervine, anti-spasmodic, tonic.
Tribes: Seri, Pima, Papago, Zuni, Navajo.

Desert Sage
(Artemisia spp.)
Uses: Anti-microbial, astringent, disinfectant, sore throats, sweat baths, smudging.
Tribes: Cahuilla, Comanche, Navajo.

Desert Tabacco
(Nicotiana trigonophylla)
Uses: Analgesic poultices, pain-relieving in a bath, as a liniment, smoking.
Caution: Do not use internally.

Desert Willow
(Chilopsis linearis)
Uses: Flowers are a good general tonic, for coughing, chest and lung tiredness. Leaves and bark are antiseptic, anti-fungal, re-balancing intestinal flora.

Evening Primrose
(Oebothera biennis)
Uses: The roots were boiled and eaten like potatoes. The young leaves were cooked and served as greens. The shoots were eaten raw. A tea was made as a dietary aid or stimulant to treat laziness and "over fatness". A hot poultice made from the pounded root and applied externally to treat piles and boils. A cold poultice from the entire plant was used for bruises. The roots were chewed and rubbed onto the muscles to improve strength. The plant was also used for menstrual pain as well as bowel pain.
Tribes: Cherokee, Iroquois, Ojibwa, Pottawatomie.

Globe Mallow
(Sphaeralcea ambigua)
Uses: Demulcent, colitis, ulcers, sore throats, for mild urinary tract irritations.
Tribes: Seri, Pueblo, Navajo.

Jimsonweed (Thornapple)
(Datura stramonium)
Uses: Leaves were smoked for bronchial spasms (mixed with desert sage).
Caution: Not for internal use, narcotic.

Jojoba
(Simmondia chinensis)
Uses: Astringent, sore throats, colitis, vaginitis, ulcers, hemorrhoids, coffee replacement, nuts are high in oil, great for skin, scalp and hair.
Tribes: Seri, Pima, Papago.

Juniper (Cedar Berry)
(Juniperus monosperma)
Uses: Urinary tract infections, cystitis, saunas, incense, increases HCL, diabetes, clears bad vibes.

Larkspur
(Delphinium amabile)
Uses: Kills body lice.
Tribes: Used by the entire Western world for a hundred years.

Mesquite
(Prosopis julifera, glandulosa, pubescens)
Uses: Anti-microbial, astringent, demulcent, nutritive, eyewash, fuel, chewing gum, dye.
Tribes: Pima, Papago, Seri.

Mesquite Flour

The seeds inside the mesquite pods are very hard, therefore remove them before grinding. Although the seeds are the main contributor of protein to any mesquite flour, they have a bitter aftertaste, and can also ruin your grinder. The pods are sweet and delicious.

- Toast pods in oven for 40 minutes at 250 deg F
- Grind them in a food processor or grinder
- Sift through a fine mesh once, twice for a nicer flour

Mesquite Bread Recipe

- 1 cup + 2 tbsp warm water
- 1 cup mesquite flour
- 3 cups unbleached white flour
- 1 ½ tsp yeast
- 1 ¼ tsp salt
- Mix all ingredients and bake as you would your other breads

Mormon Tea
(Ephedra nevadensis)
Uses: Bronchial dilator, decongestant, coffee replacement, stimulant.
Tribes: Pima, Papago, Navajo, Zuni.

Ocotillo
(Fouquiera splendens)
Uses: Pelvic lymphatic system, benign cysts and tumors, bladder infections, sore throats, fatigue, heart problems, shelter, fencing. Ocotillo is helpful in cases of portal congestion resulting from poor fat breakdown and absorption in the small intestine. It is a liver stimulant and blood cleanser. Ocotillo stimulates better visceral lymph drainage and improves dietary fat absorption. This means there is less tendency for the blood to back up (portal hypertension) and less stagnation in the pelvis and upper thighs. Mexican folk tradition includes its use as an anti-tumor remedy, especially for soft, cyst-like accumulations of fatty matter generally found in the pelvic area, thighs and buttocks. It is appropriate when bowel movements and urination are boggy with dull pain. Use it when the uterus or prostate are "cold" and dull, with rheumatoid-like pains emanating from those areas.
Tribes: Pima, Papago, Cahuilla, Apache

To Make Your Own Ocotillo Bark Tincture

Take fresh, finely cut ocotillo bark and place into a clean glass jar. Cover with a good quality brandy, making sure the bark is completely covered. Let it sit for about one month or more, shaking the bottle at least once a day. Strain, discard the used bark, and store the tincture in a dark brown bottle. Use approx. 10 – 30 drops 1 - 3 times a day.

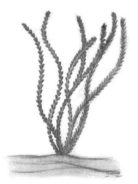

Ocotillo

Prickly Pear
(Opuntia phaeacantha)
Uses: Nutritive, demulcent, first aid, anti-inflammatory, jam, hydrophilic, diabetes, flowers are high in bioflavonoid. The pads are eaten as food – called nopales or nopalitos.

Ratany
(Krameria lanceolata, grayii, parviflora)
Uses: Astringent, topical hemostat, sore gums, abscesses, mouth sores, sore throat, diarrhea.

Sagebrush
(Artemisia tridentate)
Uses: Flu, diaphoretic, fevers, disinfectant, smudging incense.
Tribes: Paiute, Zuni, Navajo

Saguaro
(Cereus giganteus)
Uses: Nutritive, for making fences, ceilings, etc.

Yucca
(Yucca spp.)
Uses: Anti-inflammatory, urethra, bladder, prostate, shampoo, nutritive, basket crafts, digestive problems, New Mexico State plant.

An Easy Way To Extract
The Juice From The Prickly Pear Fruit

The easiest way to extract the juice from the prickly pear fruit is to harvest the fruit carefully with tongs kitchen utensil and place it directly into a container, preferably plastic. Stick this container into the freezer overnight. In the morning the fruits will be frozen. Take the container out of the freezer and let the ocotillos fruits thaw until you see the juice flowing out. Strain the juice and use it for making jellies, wine, syrups, ice cubes, etc.

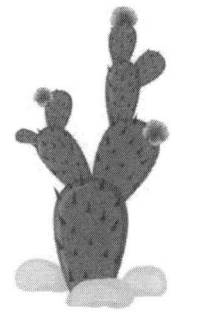

Prickly Pear

DIFFERENT FORMS OF HERBAL MEDICINES

Infusion
An infusion is the method used for preparing the delicate parts of plants, such as leaves and flowers. Use glass or enamel containers and distilled or "good water". Use one teaspoon dried herbs, or three teaspoons fresh herbs per one cup of water. Pour freshly boiled water over the herbs and let it steep for approximately 20 minutes, then strain. Add a little honey if desired and drink warm. The same rule applies for sun or /and lunar tea.

Decoction
A decoction is the method used for preparing the harder parts of plants, such as roots, bark and seeds. Use glass or enamel containers and distilled or "good water". Use one tablespoon per 1-½ cups of water, bring to a boil then turn down the heat and simmer for approximately 30 minutes. Strain, and add a little honey if desired and drink warm.

Sun or Lunar
A sun or lunar tea is used to capture the energy of the sun (yang, heating) or the moon (yin, cooling). Fill a clear gallon jar with distilled water. Add one cup of herbs of your choice, set in sun or moonshine for approximately 4-6 hours. You can also use colored jars, introducing color therapy. Add sweetener or juices before serving.

Tinctures
A tincture is an alcoholic or hydro-alcoholic herbal preparation providing a dry herb strength ratio of 1:5. A tincture is made by macerating one part of dried herb in 5 parts of brandy or vodka. Macerate for approximately 1-3 months.

Liquid Extracts
A liquid herbal extract is an alcoholic or hydro-alcoholic preparation providing a dry herb strength ratio of 1:2. Thus, extracts represent a herb strength of one part herb for every two parts brandy. Macerate for approximately 1-3 months.

Solid Extracts
A solid extract is an evaporated liquid herbal extract providing a dry herb ratio of 4:1. This represents four parts herb for every part of extract.

Vinegar-Based Tinctures

Vinegar-based tinctures are made with vinegar instead of alcohol, and are good for people who want to avoid alcohol. Also, macerating herbs in vinegar dissolves more of the minerals contained in herbs compared to the ones that are macerated in alcohol. Vinegar-based extracts are excellent for people who need easily absorbable minerals. Macerate for approximately 1-3 months.

Glycerin-Based Tinctures

A glycerin-based tincture is made with vegetable glycerin (one part) and water (one part) as the menstruum Glycerin is both a solvent and a preservative. It is good for children because it tastes sweet. Macerate for approximately 1-3 months.

Sugar Or Honey Based

Syrups are the most delicious way of all herbal preparations. To approximately one pint of concentrated infusion or decoction, add one cup of honey, maple syrup, agave syrup, sugar or vegetable glycerin. Warm the liquid and sweetener together and mix well and gently simmer for 20 minutes. You can also mix one part of tincture to three parts of syrup. Store in refrigerator.

Oil-Based, Infused Oil (For Internal Use)

To make an infused oil, use any edible vegetable oil as the menstruum. Let fresh or dried herbs infuse in your chosen oil for about two weeks, then strain. Infused oils can be used internally, for example in salad dressings.

Oil-Based, Infused Oil (For External Use)

To make an infused oil, use any vegetable oil as the menstruum. Let fresh or dried herbs infuse in your chosen oil for about two weeks, then strain. Infused oils can be used externally for dry skin, rashes, scrapes, and wounds. Infused oils absorb slowly through the epidermic layer deep into the body and internal organs. This is convenient when a person needs herbal treatments but is unable to take herbs by mouth. Apply to underarms for quick action.

Powder-Based

Grinding up dried herbs easily makes powders. Powders can be used in drinks, shakes, soups, and capsules. Capsule size "00" holds about 0.5 grams or 500 mg. of powder. Tablets are compressed powders. Lozenges are made by mixing powdered herbs with a liquid (e.g., infusion, decoction, syrups) to a dough like consistency. Roll out with a rolling pin, cut lozenges with an apple corer tool, or cookie cutter. Let them dry for a couple of days. Great for soothing sore throats.

Salves And Ointments
Salves and ointments are made with infused oils and beeswax, and they are good for nourishing the skin, for diaper rash, strains, sprains, infected wounds, burns, cuts, insect bites, sunburns, bruises, and skin irritations. Salves and ointments can also be used to carry herbs for a specific therapeutic effect, such as vapor balms for decongesting or drawing out splinters or glass.

Suppositories/Boluses
These herbal preparations are for rectal insertion/vaginal insertion. Melt cocoa butter in a sauce pan, stir in the herbs until mixture stiffens and can be worked into small cylinders approximately ¼ in diameter and one inch long, lay on plate, cover with paper towel, and refrigerate to harden.

Baths
When you take a bath it is like immersing yourself into a giant cup of tea. Add one pint of strong infusion or decoction to the bath water, or hang a cotton bag filled with herbs under the tap and let the hot water run through it. Use the bag of herbs to wash yourself. If there is no time for a complete bath make a footbath with your favorite herbs. Use in the same way for postpartum perineal sitzbath or hemorrhoids.

Liniments
Liniments are herbal extracts for external uses. Macerate herbs in denatured alcohol as the menstruum for approximately one to three months. Liniments can be massaged into affected areas. (For external use only).

Douches/Enemas
To prepare a douche infuse your selected herbs in distilled water. For enemas infuse selected herbs in distilled water or oil.

Compresses/Fomentations
Soak a cloth in a hot infusion or decoction and place over the affected are, e.g., ginger over the stomach for a stomachache. Cold compresses can be used for eyes, to reduce fevers, and to prevent swelling.

Poultices
Poultices are external applications of the whole plant. Dampen the dry or fresh herbs with hot water. Lay over the affected body part as is, or between two pieces of thin gauze. Soothing, healing, regenerates tissues, draws out toxins or foreign particles.

Vapors and Steams

Vapors and steams are useful for decongesting the lungs and sinuses and detoxifying the skin. To steam the skin, drop essential oils, herbal extracts or hydrosols into freshly boiled distilled water. For respiratory problems place a few drops of essential oils on a handkerchief and inhale. You can also drop essential oils in a light bulb ring, or vaporizer. For your convenience there are many different kinds of diffusers available now.

Lotions

A lotion is an emulsion of oil and water. Add the water phase to the oil phase (include essential oils in the oil phase) while mixing.

To Make A Basic Lotion

With Beeswax

8 oz almond or grapeseed oil
½ oz beeswax
11 oz orange blossom hydrosol
essential oils

Melt beeswax in almond oil, stirring occasionally. Let cool to body temperature. Pour hydrosol, a little at a time, into almond oil/beeswax and beat vigorously until creamy and thick. Add essential oils and beat again.

Without Beeswax

2/3 cup rose hydrosol
1/3 cup aloe vera
¾ cup jojoba or almond oil
1/3 cup cocoa butter or shea butter
1 teaspoon lecithin liquid
essential oils

Mix together rose hydrosol and aloe, in a blender. Warm cocoa or shea butter in jojoba oil. Add rose hydrosol mix, a little at the time, to the oil/butter mixture, and blend vigorously. Add lecithin and essential oils, blend until creamy and thick.

You can produce an assortment of lotions based on these basic lotion formulas by using different herbal infusions for the water part and different carrier oils for the oil part, as well as by varying the essential oils. Store homemade cosmetics in the refrigerator.

DOSING

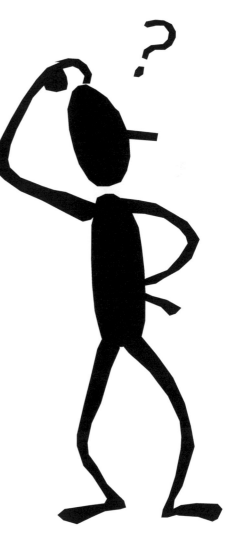

To determine the correct dosage of an herbal remedy can be confusing and not easy to figure out due to personal metabolism, dietary habits, stress levels and other differences of our individual bodies. Dosage guidelines are nevertheless important. It is better to err on the side of insufficient dosage, than to overdose. As a general rule, a large and robust person requires greater dosages than a small and frail individual. A calm and laid back person can get away with a lesser dosage than a more stressed, active and hyper person.

Children require less; the following rule is often used: Divide the child's weight in pounds by 150 to give the approximate fraction of the adult dose. Example: A fifty-pound child will require 50/150 or 1/3 of the adult dose. The same formula applies for animals.

When an herbal formula is not working it is either because the herbs being used are of inferior quality or insufficient dosage. Research the herbs that your are using to determine if there is any known toxicity from using them, then it is perfectly appropriate to increase the dosage as necessary. Ultimately, you must trust the wisdom of your own body; listen to your sense of knowing and it will guide you.

Chronic problems: Tea: 3-4 cups daily 3-4 months or longer
                   Extract: ½-1 teaspoon 3 times a day
                   Capsules 2 "00" capsules 3 times a day

Acute Problems: Tea: ¼ cup every ½ hour until symptoms subside.
                   Extract: ½-1 teaspoon every ½-1 hour until symptoms subside
                   Capsules 1-2 capsules every 3-4 hours until symptoms subside

EAR CONING

Ear coning is a healing technique that has been around for centuries. It dates as far back as biblical times when hollow reeds from swamp areas were used. It has been passed down for many generations by the Egyptian, Oriental and European cultures. Unfortunately, it is almost unknown today. The process had been basically lost for many years but has come back into practice once again and is being used by a wide cross section of people.

It is a simple but effective home remedy. It involves the use of cones made from unbleached cotton, beeswax, herbs, essential oils, herbal extracts and flower essences. The large end is lit with a match, and the small end is placed on the edge of a person's ear.

Ear coning may provide these benefits:

- Detoxification of Sinus and Lymph
- Sore Throats
- Swimmer's Ear
- Chronic Headache
- Ear Aches
- Allergies

- Hearing Improvement
- Vision Improvement
- Sharpening of mental functioning, Smell, taste and color perception
- Emotional clearing
- Spiritual opening
- Auric cleansing

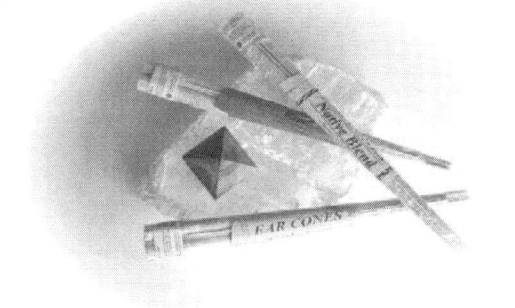

Why and How to Ear Cone

Let's look at our incredible ear. Most people think of it only as an organ of hearing. But our ears enable us to perceive sound waves, sending impulses to the brain that tell us which direction is "up," and therefore function as a balancing mechanism. They also let the brain know of movements made by the body in three-dimensional space. The ear is thus an organ of both hearing and equilibrium. The ears are structured as intricate labyrinth of canals, tubes, tiny bones, nerves, hairs and glands that are all interrelated and interconnected. They serve as one of several microsystems in our physical makeup, where a miniature map of the entire body can be found.

Treating the ears has a profound effect on different parts of our body, as does massaging of the feet in the art of reflexology. When the cone is lit, the air involved takes on a whole different composition, mixing with herbs that contain natural antibiotics, decongestants and balancing properties. The air and herbs combine to make smoke in a special way, traveling gently and non-intrusively in more-or-less the same manner that sound enters the ear canal, having an effect on the entire system. Air, in this instance, is carrying the geometric code in the shape of a spiral and, along with herbal mixtures, consists in fact, of particles of perfect spiracle form. The spiral itself symbolizes the process of coming to the same point again and again but at a different level, so that everything is seen in a new and different light. The results are a new perspective on issues, people, places and on yourself. The simplest way to explain the spiral of the ear cone is that it signifies change and balance.

Coning acts as a catalyst to clear out debris accumulated on the nerve endings. When nerve endings are blocked by earwax or fungus yeast growth, vibrational frequencies cannot be transmitted to the nerve endings. When these endings are clear, on the other hand, this allows for easy vibrational flow to the corresponding areas of the mind, body and spirit, and actually clears the way for other methods of healing.

Ear Coning Instructions
Supplies

2 hand towels
Small bowl of water
Scissors
Herb Stop Ear Oil

Matches or candles
Plastic bag or paper (to place under your bowl)
Q-Tips
Cotton balls

Procedure

1. Create a pleasant mood, and relax. Put on soothing music and dim lights. Lay the person on either side with head on small pillow OR lie flat on back (with pillow under knees).

2. Place one towel on the pillow and one to cover hair and neck to protect from possible wax drip.

3. Light the wide end of the cone and tap until smoke spirals out the small end of the cone.

4. Gently place small end on the ear canal, angle the cone away from the face 45 degrees angle. Adjust cone to seal the ear canal. No smoke should escape out of the ear canal.

5. Let the wide end burn about 2 inches down, remove from ear, cut burned section into bowl of water, and leave one fourth burning.

6. Turn the cone upside down, ream out with skewer into bowl of water. Turn up and tap until smoke resumes coming out of small end. Return to ear and seal again. Repeat. Burn half way down. Entire procedure takes three cuttings. Three inches of the cone is left to discard.

7. Cut flame off, or dowse in bowl. Place cone down on plastic bag. Break skewer in half (to make sure you do not re-use it for hygienic reasons). One skewer per cone.

8. The active force in coning is the smoking spiral in the ear canal. We need as much smoke as possible pouring in. If the wax is properly emptied out each time you cut the cone you continue the strong flow of smoke.

9. Clean out the ear with Q-Tip dipped in ear oil. Do not go deep. Gently swab only what you can see of the ear canal. This soothes the nerve endings. If one ear still feels plugged you can follow with another coning.

10. Balance the ears. Position yourself at the head of the person lying down. Place your hands lightly on both ears and wait for the energy pulse between your palms. Release (silently) the person's energy field from yours. Bring hands from ears to top of head to close auric field. Put cotton in the ears to protect from wind if going outdoors. Clean and sanitize bowl. Remove wax from scissor with fire and wipe with paper towel.

11. Most people will need at least three initial conings, seven to ten days apart. More may be necessary; your body will tell you if you listen carefully.

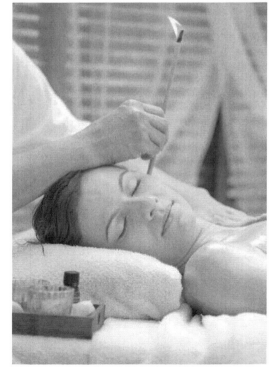

ESSENTIAL OILS AND ATTARS

Essential oils are the fragrant essences of plants in their purest, most concentrated form, which are either steam distilled, solvent extracted, cold pressed or CO2 extracted. Essential oils are the plant's soul extracted from flowers, leaves, spices, fruits, woods and roots, each with its own benefits to the body and mind. They are the foundation of aromatherapy. Their health-enhancing, beautifying and mood elevating properties can easily be incorporated into one's lifestyle.

Aromatherapy is the study of how odors affect us. The mechanism in processing odors is quite complex and highly evolved. At the bridge of our noses is the olfactory epithelium. About the size of a penny it contains 20 million hairs that protrude through a thin layer of mucus membranes. These hairs are actually nerve cells that translate odors into nerve messages. The messages travel to a part of the brain responsible for emotions, moods, feelings, and memories. Odors can also stimulate the release of neuro-chemicals and hormones. University research in Milan, Italy, has found that vanilla can treat anxiety and depression. In Russia, eucalyptus oil has cured a certain flu strain, and American and Japanese researchers are studying the effects of inhaling fragrances to relax claustrophobics, improve productivity in the work place, and even ward off subway violence.

Essential Oils Can Be Enjoyed In Many Ways:

Diffuser (electric)	Facial masks (essential oils with clay)
Humidifier (disinfectant, colds, bronchitis)	Ceramic ring (when traveling)
Inhaler (sinus congestion or infection)	Facial steam (skin)
Sauna	Compresses (opens pores before facials)
Bath	Massages
Footbath	Facial Spray
Cooking and Baking (caution)	Laundry, house-cleaning products

Individual Essential Oils

Agar wood *(see Oud)*

Allspice
(Pimenta dioica)
This warming essential oil has an overall calming influence, improves digestion, enhances mental clarity, promotes restful sleep, reduces pain, helps in the reduction of cellulite deposits, and inhaling the vapors allows for better breathing. Use a tiny amount in massage oil for chest infections, and for severe muscle spasm to restore mobility quickly, or where extreme cold is experienced.

Aloes Wood *(see Oud)*

Amber
(Pinus succinifera)
A fossilized tree resin, amber has warming, calmative, analgesic, antispasmodic and expectorant properties.

Amyris
(Amyris balsamifera)
Amyris is cooling and calming, releases anxiety and promotes a peaceful state of mind. Amyris has been used as an economical substitute for the more pricy sandalwood in the perfume industry. Used as a fixative for fragrances.

Angelica
(Angelica archangelica)
Angelica is added to some skin care products for its soothing effect on irritated skin conditions, psoriasis, as well as to brighten up dull and congested skin. Internally, angelica is helpful for arthritis, gout, rheumatism, and water retention, respiratory and digestive ailments. Removes accumulated toxins in the body, which improves the health of the immune and lymphatic system. It also eases muscle spasms, nervous tension and calms anxiety. Fine liquors are made from angelica.

Anise

(Pimpinella anisum)

Anise seeds have a warm, pleasant and sweet flavor. Added to massage oils, anise essential oil can be used to increases breast milk production, with a calming and antispasmodic effect on both mother and baby. This warming, stimulating oil eases muscle spasms, coughing, and digestive disturbances. It is especially effective to relieve menstrual cramps and to induce menstruation if it is due to hormonal imbalance. It is known for its strong calming and relaxing effect on the nervous system. Additionally, it has a reputation to be an aphrodisiac. A veterinarian who specializes in horse's teeth problems came to the see me one day and was looking for anise essential oil. She uses the scent of this essential oil to calm a horse before a dental examination. According to her experiences the scent of anise essential oil alleviates aggression and fear response. A horse that is being introduced to a new group, the scent of anise essential oil can ease the transition. (Synergy Equine LLC, Prescott, Arizona).

Armoise *(see Mugwort)*

Basil, Sweet

(Ocimum basilicum)

There are about 150 different varieties of basil. Usually, the essential oil is made from ocimum basilicum. Basil has been used since antiquity for respiratory infections, including bronchitis and whooping cough, fevers, digestive problems, jaundice, as well as for headaches, migraines and head colds. It is also an excellent cephalic, second only to rosemary in its clarifying effect on the brain, so it is great for mental chatter. The scent of sweet basil is uplifting and refreshing, and mainly used for poor memory, confusion, indecision, depression, fear, paranoia, mental stress and fatigue. I like to add a few drops of basil essential oil in my car diffuser when traveling long distances, to keep my mind calm, but alert. Sweet basil improves digestion, increases lactation, neutralizes toxins from insect bites, and reduces cellulite. It also sharpens the senses, improves meditations, and helps with dream recall.
Caution: Avoid if you have sensitive skin.

Basil, Holy (Tulsi)

(Ocimum sanctum)

In India, people consider tulsi the most sacred of all plants. They plant it around their homes, temples, and graves. Tulsi balances right and left brain; therefore it is being used for deep meditations and spiritual awakening. It has a calming effect when the mind is overactive. It is interesting to notice how popular this plant became around 2012.

Bay (Laurel)
(Laurus nobilis)
Sweet bay's warming quality improves circulation, increases mental clarity and alertness, sharpens the senses, reduces stress, and relieves aching limbs and muscles. Added to massage lotions it promotes lymphatic drainage. In ancient Greece, bay was used to encourage prophetic visions.

Bay Rum
(Pimento racemosa)
West Indian bay is a tropical evergreen tree native to the West Indies. During Victorian times, men used bay rum as an aftershave. Over the years, bay rum has been used as a hair loss remedy, and to treat scalp conditions, dandruff, greasy and lifeless hair. Bay rum's aroma is light, spicy, and sweet, the aroma of "Old Spice", a popular fragrance added to aftershave lotions. Bay rum may act as an appetite stimulant and to settle stomach pains, relieve general aches and pains, as well as rheumatic pains.

Benzoin
(Styrax benzoin)
Benzoin is extremely thick and gooey with a sweet vanilla-like fragrance. It can actually be substituted for the more expensive vanilla essential oil, but for its fragrance only, not the medicinal qualities. Benzoin is warming and acts as a decongestant for the lungs. It is also a relaxing oil for nervous tension and stress. Inhaling the scent of benzoin soothes a sore throats and the loss of voice. It can be used for eczema, dry or cracked skin. Because of benzoin's ability to stimulate and at the same time soothe, it seems to get things moving in the body, whether it is clearing mucus, stimulating circulation, expelling gas or increasing the flow of urine. Benzoin sends out a comforting feeling to ease grief and loneliness. For people who are sad and lonely, depressed or anxious, combine with rose essential oil, especially during a crisis.

Bergamot
(Citrus bergamia)
This relaxing, refreshing and uplifting citrus oil comes from the peel of a small, pear-shaped Italian fruit, and was named after the town of Bergamo in Italy. It reduces inflammation, enhances immunity, and cools fevers. Bergamot inhibits certain viruses, especially herpes simplex virus, which causes cold sores. Mix with eucalyptus and dab onto the sore, either neat or diluted in a little alcohol at the first sign of eruption. It reduces the discomfort and pain of chicken pox and shingles. Bergamot has been used to relieve anxiety, nervous tension and depression. It is the bringer of freshness and joy. Earl Grey tea is black tea with added bergamot essential oil, which makes a delicious and uplifting cup of tea, or a cup of liquid joy!

Birch, Sweet
(Betula lenta)
The essential oil from the bark of this beautiful tree is a circulatory stimulant, with warming and pain relieving, anti-inflammatory and febrifuge properties. Due to its methyl salicylate constituent, best known in its synthesized form as aspirin, it is highly effective in relieving the pain of sore muscles, joints, tendons, sprains, arthritis and rheumatism. Birch essential oil drains toxins in case of arthritis and rheumatism, which are the cause of pain. For tendons that have become inflamed because of overuse (repetitive tasks) especially of the ankles and wrists, birch oil is the choice remedy. Dramatic results have been seen in treating cellulite, when all other essential oils have not been successful. The diuretic action reduces edema by removing toxins. It can also be used as a skin softener. Added to a hair tonic or shampoo sweet birch can prevent or eliminate dandruff.

Birch Tar
(Betula alba)
Birch tar is extracted by slow distillation from the bark, and is a very old, well-known, old-fashioned product that is still used in healing lotions and ointments for dermatitis, dull or congested skin, eczema, psoriasis, arthritis, cellulite, edema, and poor circulation. Birch tar is also being used by leather manufacturers.

Black Pepper
(Piper nigrum)
Black pepper is warming and stimulating and has been used to increase energy. As a single essential oil or in formulas black pepper is helpful for pain, poor circulation, poor muscle tone, chills, catarrh, earaches, loss of appetite, nausea, colds and flus. To make an effective earache remedy, place three 3 drops black pepper and three drops of lavender on a cotton ball and place gently into the ear.

Bois de Rose *(see Rosewood)*

Cade
(Juniperus oxycedrus)
Cade is an evergreen shrub native to the Mediterranean region and North Africa. The essential oil is obtained from the wood chips and branches of the shrub. Cade is also known as prickly juniper or prickly cedar. Throughout time cade oil has been used for snakebites, leprosy, to soothe toothaches, kill lice and their eggs, and heal skin problems, such as dermatitis, psoriasis, chronic eczema, parasites, dandruff and hair loss. Veterinary practitioners use the oil for parasitic skin problems.

Cajeput (White Tea Tree)
(Melaleuca cajeputi)
Cajeput produces a sensation of warmth and quickens the pulse. Highly esteemed in the East, it is used for colds, headaches, throat infections, toothache, sore and aching muscles, fever and rheumatism. It is a powerful germicide. Cajeput is used in inhalations for colds and respiratory infections. It repels insects, gets rid of head lice, and acts as a natural flea repellent for pets.

Calamus
(Acorus calamus)
Calamus essential oil rejuvenates the brain and nervous system (especially after a stroke), improves cerebral circulation, sharpens memory, and enhances awareness. In Sanskrit it is named "vacha," which means speaking the power of the word, intelligence and self-expression. Calamus can be used for nervous complaints, vertigo, headaches, gastritis, intestinal colics, anorexia, and gastric ulcers. In India it is sold as a candied rhizome for dyspepsia, bronchitis and coughs. In China, calamus is used to treat deafness, dizziness, and epileptic seizures. When my husband was two years old living in a remote area on the Navajo Indian Reservation, he contracted meningitis. Without access to proper health care, he was unable to receive immediate treatment which resulted in scarring in a portion of his brain. This scarring has resulted in him having epileptic seizures. During these episodes, I rub a couple drops calamus oil under his nose and on top of his head, which lessens the duration of his seizures, and "brings him back".

Camphor, White
(Cinnamomum camphora)
Camphor is useful to loosen congestion in the respiratory system, for colds, coughs, and the flu. Camphor reduces inflammation and can be massaged into sore muscles and joints to warm and relieve pain. A few drops in a closet or drawers can repel moths. Camphor is sometimes referred to as "Borneol" because this tree is native to Borneo and Sumatra. The wood of the various camphor trees is used in temple building and in the making of religious icons (Buddhas).

Caraway
(Carum carvi)
Caraway is an old and safe traditional remedy to relieve dyspepsia, flatulence, intestinal colic, menstrual cramps, poor appetite, laryngitis and bronchitis. It also promotes the production and quality of breast milk. During World War II mothers would eat caraway soup (caraway seeds mixed in water) every day to increase the amount and quality of breast milk. As a result they would have enough milk to feed their own babies, as well as orphaned babies.

Cardamom

(Elettaria cardamomum)

Cardamom is a digestive aid, easing nausea, heartburn and flatulence. It is also helpful for diarrhea, as it eases the gripping pains. Cardamom is very popular in Arab countries. They add cardamom seeds when preparing coffee, which negates coffee's harmful effects. While in Saudi Arabia, our sponsor gave us cardamom pods to carry with us in our pockets, just like all Saudis do. After a meal, they chew on these little seeds to help digestion, eliminate bad breath, and to awaken the brain, when one feels sleepy. Cardamom has carminative, antispasmodic, disinfectant, expectorant, refreshing and uplifting properties, with a wonderful fragrance. It also has a reputation to improve physical, as well as sexual strength.

Carrot

(Daucus carota)

Carrot essential oil is made from the wild carrot seeds, otherwise known as Queen Anne's lace and is used primarily in skincare, to revitalize and tone mature skin, lessen wrinkles, and for rashes, dermatitis, eczema, and psoriasis. Carrot essential oil stimulates proper liver function and is being used for indigestion, digestive and urinary disorders, retention of urine, arthritis, rheumatism, accumulation of toxins, gout, edema, and to promote menstruation.

Cassia

(Cinnamomum cassia)

Cassia is a carminative, an agent that helps to break up intestinal gas and can be used for digestive complaints such as flatulence, colic, diarrhea and nausea. Cassia is also effective in treating the common cold, rheumatism, kidney and reproductive system complaints. In a diffuser, it dispels depression, apathy and exhaustion. Cassia is the bark of an evergreen tree that belongs to the laurel family, a relative of cinnamomum zeylanicum, the "true" cinnamon. Cassia's flavor is slightly bitter, while cinnamon is warm and sweet.

Catnip

(Nepeta cataria)

Researchers at Iowa State University have found that catnip essential oil is about ten times more effective at repelling mosquitoes than DEET, the compound used in most commercial insect repellents. Catnip essential oil can also repel cockroaches! To keep your summer bug-free, all you need to do is add 25 drops of catnip essential oil to 4 oz of water. Spray it in your home, especially the crucial areas, where insects live or where they like to enter your home. You can also add catnip essential oil to your lotions, body mists, shampoo, conditioner, or bathwater. This oil is totally non-toxic, and completely safe, for children too.

Cedarwood
(Juniperus virginiana)
Cedarwood is an evergreen tree native to North America. Cedarwood is calming and grounding, relieving anxiety and nervous tension. It is known for its antiseptic mucolytic/anti-catarrhal properties (pulmonary and genito-urinary). In skincare, it can be used for acne, dandruff, eczema, oily hair and skin. It is an excellent insect and vermin repellant (mosquitoes, moths, wood worms, as well as rats. Cedarwood was once used commercially with citronella, as an insecticide. Native Americans use cedar extensively, both for medicine and for spiritual purification.

Cedarwood, Atlas
(Cedrus atlantica)
The Atlas cedar is closely related to the biblical cedar of Lebanon. The oil from the Atlas cedar is a powerful antiseptic and is used particularly for bronchial infections. It breaks down mucus, which makes it useful in treating chronic bronchitis. It is very effective for cystitis and vaginal infections and discharges. The Atlas Cedarwood oil has astringent and antiseptic properties and is used in skincare to treat acne, dandruff, dermatitis, eczema, fungal infections, greasy skin, and hair loss. It is used in men's toiletries, especially aftershave where both the astringent and antiseptic properties are useful, though its popularity as a masculine perfume may be connected with its reputation as an aphrodisiac. It undoubtedly has a tonic and stimulant action on the whole body, while at the same time reducing stress and tension.

Celery Seed
(Apium graveolens)
The essential oil of celery seeds is used mainly as a spice in cooking to prevent indigestion and liver congestion. Blended with other essential oils it is excellent for cellulite and lymphatic congestion, to support the body in clearing out toxins, as well as to relax and relieve muscle soreness.

Chamomile, German
(Matricaria recutita)
This is an excellent skin care remedy, with similar qualities as roman chamomile, except that it's anti-inflammatory properties are greater due to the higher percentage of azulene. Azulene is one of its constituents, not found in the whole plant, but is produced during distillation, when reactions take place between various plant constituents and the steam used in distilling. It gives it a beautiful blue color. Azulene prevents discharge of histamine from the tissues by activating the pituitary-adrenal system, causing the release of cortisone. Azulene stimulates liver regeneration. For all states of tension and the symptoms that arise from it, such as a nervous digestive system, tension headaches, sleeplessness. G. chamomile calms without depressing.

Chamomile, Maroc *(see Chamomile Wild)*

Chamomile, Roman
(Anthemis nobilis)
Roman chamomile is very relaxing, and increases awareness. It is used for anxiety, nervous tension, anger, depression, hypersensitivity, impatience, irritability, panic and hysteria. It contains less Azulene than German chamomile. It brings inner peace, serenity, understanding and spiritual cooperation.

Chamomile, Wild
(Ormenis multicaulis)
Distinctly different from German or Roman chamomile, wild chamomile cannot be considered as a replacement for them. Wild chamomile contains antispasmodic, anti-inflammatory, cholagogue, emmenagogue, hepatic, sedative and tonic properties. Emotionally and mentally, wild chamomile creates a shield for the sensitive person. Valerie Ann Worwood says "Wild chamomile is for the sweet and tender-spirited person who has been overlooked by society in favor of those with a more forceful nature."

Champaca
(Michelia champaca)
Champaca essential oil is warming, and calming, reduces stress and promotes a peaceful state. This evergreen tree is native to Asia, and in India it is planted around temples to supply flowers for religious ceremonies. It is known to ease inhibitions and stress, and transports one to a blissful, relaxed state. This essential oil has also been used in romantic massage oils. Champaca is also known as frangipani.

Cinnamon Leaf
(Cinnamomum zeylanicum)
Cinnamon leaf essential oil has antiseptic, analgesic, and warming properties, stimulating circulation, as well as relieving menstrual cramps. It is good for weakness and debility. In Chinese medicine cinnamon is included in many remedies, as a tonic for depression, a calmative, and a strengthener for the heart. Emotionally, cinnamon warms the heart, encouraging clearer expression of our innermost feelings. The smell of cinnamon from candles containing the essential oil gives a room a warm and welcoming atmosphere.

Cistus *(see Labdanum)*

Citronella
(Cymbopogon nardus)
Citronella is a popular insect repellant. Some people say that it works and some say it doesn't work. At any rate, if you use citronella when camping in the woods you may repel mosquitoes but may attract bears; they love the scent of citronella. Citronella is slightly disinfectant, uplifting, and cooling. It also relieves mental fatigue.

Clary Sage
(Salvia sclarea)
Clary sage contains sedative, hormonal balancing, soothing, and relaxing properties. It is known to contain a hormone similar to the one produced by females. It is useful in helping women with sexual problems, menstrual cramps, PMS, postpartum depression and menopausal hot flashes. It is an adrenal stimulant. It is used for anxiety, panic attacks and paranoia. Clary sage rejuvenates skin cells, calms the complexion and reduces dandruff. It is known for its inspirational and euphoric effect on the psyche. Clary sage encourages calmness and tranquility.

Clove Bud
(Syzygium aromaticum)
Clove oil is warming, stimulating, antiseptic, analgesic, anti-parasitic, and anti-fungal. It is a well-known oil to treat toothaches, numbing the pain. Since it has a numbing effect, clove oil can be applied to painful areas, or diluted in vegetable oil or cream. In a diffuser it stimulates and revives a tired mind and body. In parts of Central America, it is believed that clove dispels the demons of diseases. Some people say that it repels moths.

Coffee
(Coffea arabica)
This oil is delicious, stimulating and rich. Place a few drops on a light bulb for a quick pick-me-up. Great added to lip balm. Before a fashion show, runway models rub their body with coffee body polish to eliminate unsightly cellulite. Fill an 8 ounce jar halfway up with salt. Add grape seed oil to cover salt by about ½ inch, and then add 20 drops of coffee essential oil. Stir the whole thing, and close the jar with an airtight lid. Treat yourself anytime to a spa-like treatment. Stand in the shower or bathtub, take about one tablespoon of body polish and rub vigorously all over your body (not the face) until your skin is slightly red. Rinse with cool water and dry yourself. You will feel invigorated. Your skin will be smooth, hydrated and glowing. (Body polish is also named salt glow because it makes your skin glow). This treatment cleanses your skin as well as the lymphatic system. Don't use coffee essential oil body polish before going to bed; it will keep you up. Coffee is absorbed through the skin and has a stimulating effect, similar to drinking several cups of coffee.

Copaiba
(Copaifera officinalis)
The balsam harvested from this rainforest tree, is harvested by natives using bamboo tubes which are driven into a hole in the trunk. The liquid is clear and flows out easily. Copaiba has a calming and uplifting effect, and can enhance your meditations. It opens breathing passages and allows for deeper breathing, especially when there is a pulmonary infection. Additionally, it has a healing effect on the skin. Copaiba can also be used as a fixative for fragrances.

Coriander
(Coriandrum sativum)
Coriander is a sweet, warm and spicy essential oil known for its carminative, sedative, analgesic, antispasmodic, tonic and regenerative properties. Because of its stimulating digestive properties, coriander relieves nausea, indigestion and an upset stomach. Coriander is analgesic, and good to use for migraine headaches, neuralgia and rheumatic pain. It can also be applied to clear blackheads and for oily skin. Coriander encourages good memory, confidence, and optimism.

Cypress
(Cupressus sempervirens)
Cypress contains anti-rheumatic, cleansing, mucolytic/anti-catarrhal properties. It is healing and balancing to the reproductive system, used for PMS, menopause and menstrual disturbances, as well as to stimulate circulation. It is used for varicose veins, hemorrhoids, and cellulite. Its styptic action is useful for small wounds and bleeding gums. Cypress promotes lymphatic drainage. It also reduces oiliness of skin. Cypress trees are often grown around graveyards, because of their association with the passing of a soul, and to bring comfort to those left behind. Jesus' cross and Noah's ark are thought to have been made from the cypress tree.

Davana
(Artemisia pallens)
Davana essential oil is made from a native Indian annual herb. With its mucolytic properties it has been used for coughing attacks with thick, ropelike mucus ("toux grasses et spasmodiques").
Caution: Do not use on babies, children or pregnant women. Considered a nerve toxin and abortive.

Dill
(Anethum graveolens)
Dill is a soothing digestive aid for indigestion, gas, and colic, especially in children. It can also be used to bring on menstruation. Dill promotes the flow of milk in nursing mothers.

Elemi
(Canarium luzonicum)
Elemi is a tropical tree native to the Philippines and closely related to those that give us frankincense and myrrh. The Egyptians used elemi for embalming. It has a long history of being used in skin care products and for respiratory complaints. In more modern times it was often used to replace the expensive and scarce frankincense. Elemi relieves congestion, dry coughs, and irritated throats. Elemi is effective for chest infections when there is a lot of phlegm. It is rejuvenative for mature and wrinkled skin, as well as healing for infected cuts, wounds, and scars. During an emotional crisis, elemi offers comfort and strength, reconnecting all parts of our being, our mind, body and spirit. When around dense energy, elemi keeps the auric field clear, offering protection, grounding and centeredness.

Eucalyptus, Lemon
(Eucalyptus citridora)
This lemon scented eucalyptus is useful for colds, flu, and fevers. Lemon-scented eucalyptus is also being used for athlete's foot and other fungal infections, as well as for candida, cuts, dandruff, herpes, scabs, and to repel insects. Diffuse in a sickroom in the evening to calm, relax, and encourage sleep while fighting infection.

Eucalyptus, Blue Gum
(Eucalyptus globulus)
Eucalyptus is cooling and stimulating. It is a pectoral tonic, expectorant and anti-infectious. Inhaling eucalyptus opens the sinuses and breathing passages. Place one to two drops on your pillow before bedtime to help you breathe freely. Eucalyptus is refreshing, energizing, and improves mental clarity and alertness. It can be applied to blisters, cuts, herpes, insect bites, lice, or skin infections. Added to massage oil it can alleviate muscular aches and pains, due to sprains and poor circulation.

Eucalyptus, Radiata
(Eucalyptus radiata)
This species of eucalyptus is strongly antiviral and expectorant (more than E. globulus) and is indicated for the respiratory system. It's also useful for vaginitis, acne, and sinus infections.

Everlasting *(see Helichrysum)*

Fennel
(Foeniculum vulgare)
Fennel stimulates digestion, promotes adrenal function, increases the flow of milk in nursing mothers, and allows for lymphatic drainage. It has diuretic and detoxifying properties, making it useful for water retention and cellulite. It is considered a carminative to relieve gas, nausea and indigestion.

Fir
(Abies albla)
Fir has antidepressant, expectorant, analgesic, antiseptic, tonic and stimulating properties. When used in massage oil it stimulates circulation and relieves muscle aches and pains. Fir encourages protection, grounding, compassion, clarity, strength and inner unity.

Frangipani *(see Champaca)*

Frankincense (Olibanum)
(Boswellia carteri)
Frankincense contains cleansing, strengthening and rejuvenating properties. It is revitalizing for mature, dry or scarred skin. Frankincense can ease depression, confusion, indecision, impatience, irritability, dwelling on past unpleasant events, and when there is an inability to free the mind. Frankincense has a grounding effect when you are lost in your mind. It slows and deepens the breath making it helpful for mediations, tension and coughing spasms. At one time this richly perfumed resin was as valuable as gold, for the spirit of frankincense evokes the divine.

Galangal
(Alpinia officinarum)
Galangal is a reed-like plant, whose rhizomes are used as a spice in the essential oil industry. Related to ginger and cardamom, galangal has been used for dyspepsia, flatulence, colic, nausea and vomiting. It contains antiseptic, carminative, diaphoretic, stimulant and stomachic properties. Galangal is sometimes used to treat the pancreas.
Caution: Do not confuse with galanga or false ginger.

Galbanum
(Ferula galbaniflua)
Galbanum is similar to frankincense, obtained from an herb in the same family as the carrot. It is generally used for treating wounds, inflammations, skin disorders, but it is also for respiratory, digestive and nervous complaints. Galbanum heals scar tissues, tones the skin, and helps soften fine lines and wrinkles.

Garlic
(Allium sativum)
Due to its unpleasant and pervasive smell, garlic oil is not often used externally. However, garlic powder in capsules may be taken internally for respiratory and gastro-intestinal infections, urinary tract infections, heart and circulatory problems and to fight infectious diseases in general.

Geranium
(Pelargonium graveolens)
Geranium is stimulating, uplifting and energizing. It has a special affinity to the female body, and is used for PMS, anxiety, tension, and depression. Geranium is also useful for respiratory problems, healthy immune function, and to improve circulation. Geranium brings comfort during great transitional times, such as during puberty or menopause.

Ginger
(Zingiber officinale)
Ginger is warming, carminative and stimulating and therefore useful for all sorts of digestive complaints. It is indicated for indigestion, nausea and gas, as well as for use in massage oils to ease muscle and joint pain, poor circulation, and cramps. Ginger has a reputation for enhancing pelvic circulation and relieving pelvic congestion. In some instances ginger has been used to eliminate parasites.

Grapefruit, White
(Citrus paradisi)
Grapefruit essential oil is depurative for oily skin, promotes lymphatic drainage and removes toxins. Added to massage oils it is known to reduce cellulite and water retention. Food grade grapefruit essential oil can be added to water for a delicious and refreshing morning wake-up drink, afternoon pick-me-up, or during a long car trip to relieve anxiety and fatigue. Grapefruit promotes joy, a positive attitude and is uplifting.

Grapefruit, Pink
(Citrus paradisi)
Very similar to white grapefruit, pink grapefruit essential oil is known for its antidepressant, antiseptic, diuretic, disinfectant and stimulating properties. It uplifts and revives the spirit and is supportive in times of stress and depression. Grapefruit may also have an effect on obesity and fluid retention. With its detoxifying properties it is ideal for treating cellulite. It also has a stimulating effect on the digestive system. Added to a skincare routine grapefruit can clear the complexion, and is valuable in treating acne and congested, oily skin. Some people have experienced relief in cases of migraine headaches, premenstrual tension and jet lag. In a spray blend it is refreshing and ideal for disinfecting rooms.

Guaiacwood
(Bulnesia sarmienti)
Guaiacwood is used for poor circulation, muscle and joint complaints, arthritis, gout, and rheumatoid arthritis. Added to massage oil it acts as a stimulant and lymphatic decongestant, specifically to decongest the pelvic area.

Helichrysum (Everlasting) (Immortelle)
(Helichrysum angustifolium)
This is the best oil for treating scars and aiding skin healing. Helichrysum is also effective for bacterial infections, inflammation, cough, muscular aches, and rheumatism. It is used for depression. A pilot told me once that he was losing his hearing and was going to be let go from his job with the airline company. An aroma therapist advised him to put one drop of helichrysum in each ear daily. Within three months his hearing came back.

Ho Wood
(Cinnamomum camphora)
Ho Wood essential oil is used as an excellent substitute for the endangered rosewood. The chemical composition is very similar, making this the first choice for perfumes, as well as for its medicinal action. Ho Wood is traditionally used as an anti-depressant, anti-microbial, anti-septic, aphrodisiac, tissue regenerative, soothing agent and has even been used for epilepsy.

Hops
(Humulus lupulus)
Hops essential oil has hypnotic, sedative, nervine, and estrogen-like properties. Hops has been used for tachycardia, nervous gastritis, and insomnia. This oil has also been used to reduce sexual over activity.
Caution: Do not use if there is a tendency toward depression or during menopause.

Hyacinth
(Hyacinthus orientalis)
Hyacinth is specifically for the nervous system, indicated for stress, mental fatigue, and for developing the creative side of the brain. On an emotional level, it promotes forgiveness, self-esteem, perseverance, trust, faith and courage. It has a quality unlike any other, as is can make someone feel dizzy and lightheaded, inducing visions and prophecies. In Switzerland, when a visitor brings hyacinth flowers to a patient in the hospital, the nurse will routinely take them away for the night, because the patient may overdose on the fragrance, which causes headaches, dizziness and nausea.

Hyssop
(Hyssopus officinalis)
This is a helpful essential oil for severe colds, sinusitis, congestion, and sore throats. It is especially helpful in bronchitis and pneumonia. Put one drop in a glass of warm water or vinegar and gargle in case of tonsillitis. It is strongly antiviral and anti-bacterial, as well as useful for fever blisters and other skin irritations. To regulate blood pressure, ease anxiety, and to revitalize the nervous system, hyssop can be diffused into the air, or added to massage oils for an exhilarating massage. For digestion problems, hyssop can be added to a carrier oil and massaged in the stomach area. Add one drop to a little honey and let this melt in your mouth to ease indigestion and colic. Hyssop can also be used for bruises, earaches and toothaches.

Immortelle *(see Helichrysum)*

Jasmine Absolute
(Jasminum officinale)
Jasmine essential oil is a precious oil. The flowers are carefully picked during the night being careful not to bruise them, and then processed right away into an essential oil. People have successfully looked to jasmine to help them overcome depression, anxiety, stress and lack of libido. Jasmine increases self confidence and creativity. The higher end cosmetic companies blend this exquisite oil into creams and lotions to treat dry, greasy, irritated and sensitive skin. Because of its euphoric and aphrodisiac properties, jasmine is extensively used in the perfume industry.

Juniper
(Juniperus communis)
Juniper encourages circulation and the elimination of fluid waste. Juniper is helpful for acne, oily skin and cellulite, as well as for muscle discomfort, menstrual cramps and rheumatism. It is used for poor memory, mental stress and fatigue, jet lag, apathy and lack of energy.

Juniper, Taos
(Juniperus scopuiorum)
Taos juniper from the southwestern United States is used in Native American ceremonies. It has a purifying effect, facilitating the transmission of thoughts and prayers to the divine. It brings enlightenment and humility.

Kewda
(Pandanus odoratissimus)
This essential oil is made from the flower of a well-known Hawaiian tree, recognized for its beautiful scent. Hence, it is used in the perfume industries, as well as in the making of delicious beverages.

Labdanum (Rock Rose)
(Cistus ladaniferus)
Labdanum is a small evergreen bush. The oil is used in skincare for mature and wrinkled skin. It is also used for colds, cough, bronchitis and rhinitis.

Lavender
(Lavendula angustifolia, Lavendula officinalis)
Lavender is known for its balancing, relaxing, pain-relieving and anti-inflammatory properties. It is used for nervous tension, depression, headaches, hiccups, insomnia, impatience and irritability. Use neat on insect bites, as it neutralizes poisons. Lavender can also be used for various types of skin conditions such as acne, to soothe burns, for hair and skin care, and in men's cosmetic products. It can be used in the birthing room with a diffuser during childbirth. For gallbladder attacks, an essential oil blend of one part lavender and one part rosemary in a little olive oil, massaged over the gallbladder area, can be most helpful to relieve the pain.

Lavandin
(Lavendula hybrida)
Lavandin is a hybrid plant that can be used in a similar way as true lavender, but it is more penetrating and rubefacient with a sharper scent – good for respiratory, circulatory or muscular conditions. Lavandin has a higher yield of oil than true lavender during the steam distillation process.

Lemon
(Citrus limon)
Lemon essential oil can improve digestion, in particular when bloated with a heavy feeling after a greasy meal (lemon can cut through fat). Lemon is well-known for its ability to increase circulation, eliminate cellulite, move lymphatic congestion, balance oily skin, and to clear acne. Lemon is refreshing, cooling, depurative, as well as anti-viral and anti-bacterial. It contains anti-oxidant and preservative properties. Lemon has a "clean" feeling; the scent is uplifting and refreshing with a positive effect on the psyche, promoting mental clarity.

Lemon Balm *(see Melissa)*

Lemongrass
(Cymbopogon citrates)
Lemongrass is used in Thai cooking for its fragrant flavor. It increases circulation and is detoxifying, effective for cellulite, muscle and joint pain. As an effective insect repellent it is often combined with citronella and catnip. Lemongrass has a revitalizing action when one experiences fatigue, exhaustion, depression, and jet lag. Lemongrass is added to cosmetics to treat acne and skin infections, as well as to hair products to stimulate hair growth.

Lemon Tea Tree
(Melaleuca citridora)
Lemon tea tree is used in the same way as tea tree oil, but is not as strong. It has a fresh lemony scent.

Lemon Verbena
(Aloysia triphylla)
This beautiful fragrant plant is known for its antiseptic, antispasmodic, aphrodisiac, digestive, emollient, insecticide and stomachic properties. It is famous for banishing depression due to its tonic, soothing effect on the parasympathetic nervous system. Lemon verbena regulates the digestive system, especially for easing stomach spasms and cramps, and for nausea, indigestion and flatulence. With its lemony scented fragrance it can stimulate a healthy appetite. Lemon verbena has a cooling action on the liver, which can ease inflammation and infection, as in cirrhosis, and could be beneficial in cases of alcoholism. It is helpful for bronchitis, or asthmatic coughs, as well as nasal and sinus congestion. It calms heart palpitations and may relieve nervous insomnia. Its reputation as an aphrodisiac probably stems from its ability to calm underlying tension. Lemon verbena has been used in the cosmetic industry to reduce puffy eyes.

Lime
(Citrus aurantifolia)
Lime is used mainly for colds, flu, fever, infection, digestion and cellulite. It is uplifting, stimulating and refreshing. Blend with other citrus oils to freshen up a sickroom, to remove cooking odors, or to create a festive mood.

Linden Blossom
(Tilia vulgaris)
Linden tea is a popular beverage in Europe to unwind and relax after a busy day. The essential oil has been used for the digestive system, to relieve cramps, indigestion and liver pains. Linden can also be used for nervous tension, headaches, insomnia, migraine, and stress related conditions. Due to its calming properties linden can prevent hypertension and the development of arteriosclerosis, especially when these are associated with stress and nervousness, tension and anxiety. Many classical poets wrote about the emotionally healing properties of the linden tree. It is said, sitting under the linden tree brings healing to the emotional heart, when life seems rough, harsh and uncaring, when people seem to be unfeeling and cold. It is good for nursing a broken heart, calming a restless baby, and soothing the elderly.

Litsea Cubeba (May Chang)
(Litsea cubeba)
Commonly also known as may chang, litsea cubeba is similar to lemongrass. It is known for its antidepressant, anti-inflammatory, antiseptic, astringent, insecticide, calming and sedative properties. It may be also helpful in cases of bronchitis and asthma. This essential oil is greatly uplifting and stimulating. Litsea cubeba can also be used as an insect repellent on its own or mixed in with other essential oils.

Lovage
(Levisticum officinale)
Lovage has a celery scented fragrance and has long been used to flavor fine liquors and digestive bitters. Lovage stimulates a healthy appetite for those who have lost interest in food, promotes strong digestion, relieves a congested liver, relieves water retention, and improves circulation. The French consider lovage to have powerful antitoxic actions against poisons. Lovage has also been used for psoriasis, parasites, and as a vermifuge, especially against tapeworm. Lovage blended with grapefruit in a little carrier oil or lotion is helpful in reducing cellulite. It is also known for its euphoric and mood uplifting properties, as well as to improve mental clarity and alertness.

Mandarin
(Citrus reticulata)
Mandarin has a calming effect, relieves tension and anxiety, as well as insomnia. The next time you go on a road trip add a few drops of mandarin essential oil to your car diffuser or on a cotton ball placed in the car ashtray, to alleviate travel fatigue and calm down restless children. Also, your car will smell nice! Mandarin encourages uplifting feelings, inspiration and tranquility. It may have a rejuvenating effect on dull and congested skin. Mandarin originated in China, and the fruit was traditionally offered as gifts to the Mandarins. The names mandarin and tangerine are both used to describe the same oil, with a tendency to use the name mandarin in Europe, and tangerine in America.

Mandarin, Red
(Citrus reticulata)
Red mandarin has similar properties as mandarin.

Mandarin, Yellow
(Citrus reticulata)
Yellow mandarin has similar properties as mandarin.

Manuka
(Leptospermum scoparium)
Manuka has strong anti-microbial properties, 20-30 times stronger than tea tree oil. It is sometimes referred to as New Zealand tea tree, as it is distantly botanically related to tea tree. Manuka is effective against bacterial and fungal infections and can be used for acne, eczema, ringworm, skin rash, itching, dandruff, athlete's foot, nail infections, foot odor, as well as for muscle and joint aches. It is particularly suggested against gram-positive organisms.

Marjoram
(Origanum majorana)
Marjoram has a soothing and calming influence on body and mind. This is mainly the reason why it has an influence on blood pressure, regulating it. As a mild analgesic and antispasmodic oil, it has been used for menstrual cramps. Marjoram boosts the immune system and fights viruses. Marjoram can be emotionally supportive to the person who suddenly finds themselves alone, such as after the death of a close family member.

May Chang *(see Litsea cubeba)*

Melissa (Lemon Balm)
(Melissa officinalis)
Melissa or lemon balm essential oil has strong anti-viral properties making it useful for colds, coughs, and cold sores, and is active against the herpes virus. Place one drop on affected area several times a day. It is calming, yet uplifting, and has been used successfully for insomnia, hysteria, nervous crisis, irritability and great anger. Women have looked to melissa to regulate the menstrual cycle. Breathe in this lemony scent to calm a nervous stomach and digestion, and to lower blood pressure. It is also an effective insect repellant.

Mimosa
(Acacia dealbata)
Mimosa is used in cosmetics for sensitive or oily skin, and for other skin problems caused by stress. Inhale the fragrance for nervous tension, sensitivity and anxiety.

Mugwort (Armoise)
(Artemisia vulgaris)
Mugwort can be used to remove warts as well as internal parasites (for external use only; do not ingest). When added to massage oils it can soothe aching joints and muscles, or aid in painful and delayed menstruation. It enhances prophetic dreams and visions, and at the same time protects against negative influences. It keeps you alert to your surroundings especially when added to rosemary essential oil.

Myrrh
(Commiphora myrrha)
This is an ancient oil and has been used for thousands of years. It is the best essential oil for healing the skin, especially when inflamed, weepy, or cracked. It is used as well for mature skin to reduce wrinkles. Myrrh contains antiseptic and anti-fungal properties, to relieve sore throats and coughs, athlete's foot or toenail fungus. Myrrh's other known constituents are anti-viral and hormone-like. It moderates the thyroid, is an-aphrodisiac, and anti-inflammatory. To fight gum problems add to mouthwash or tooth powder/paste. Myrrh is a calming oil used in religious ceremonies, as it assists meditation and strengthens spirituality. The ancient Egyptians burned it at midday in praise of the sun god Ra; it was also used in their Kyphi incense, and in embalming.

Myrtle
(Myrtus communis)
Since myrtle is less stimulating than eucalyptus, it is sometimes a better choice to use for children and the elderly to relieve colds, coughs, and flu. It is a decongestant for catarrh, opens nasal passages, and promotes restful sleep. Myrtle is also used in skin-care products to balance oily and blemished skin. It has a sedative effect on the psyche, balancing and soothing the emotions.

Narcissus
(Narcissus poeticus)
The name derives from the Greek word "narkao" – to be numb – due to its narcotic properties. It is an anti-spasmodic, aphrodisiac, emetic, narcotic, and sedative. Narcissus's exquisite fragrance is used almost exclusively in high-class perfumes of the narcotic/floral type.

Neroli
(Citrus aurantium)
Neroli has a wonderful scent and considered one of the precious oils. It is relaxing, soothing and rejuvenating, used for anxiety, depression, nervous tension, fear, panic, shock and hysteria. Women have reported neroli being supportive during labor and childbirth. Added to skin-care products, neroli nourishes all skin types, especially dry, mature and sensitive skin. Because of its exquisite fragrance, neroli is being used in the perfume industry. Neroli is the bringer of joy!

Niaouli
(Melaleuca viridiflora)
Niaouli is a great substitute for tea tree essential oil. It is softer and sweeter scented with the same strong anti-viral, anti-bacterial, and anti-fungal properties. Used for colds, flu, cold sores, bronchitis, coughs, and as an analgesic for sore muscles and joints. Relieves congestion, clears the mind, and eases allergic conditions. Niaouli assists in the healing of burns, cuts, and insect bites.

Nutmeg
(Myristica fragrans)
Nutmeg essential oil alleviates arthritis, gout and muscular aches and pains. It also relieves digestive problems, such as flatulence, indigestion, and nausea. It is also used for bacterial infections, nervous fatigue, frigidity and impotence.

Oakmoss
(Evernia prunastri)

Oakmoss is an important ingredient in high-end perfumes for its earthy, mossy scent. It is an excellent fragrance in romantic blends. The medicinal properties of oakmoss have a positive effect on people experiencing asthma, bronchitis, cough, and nasal congestion. Oakmoss has a balancing and calming effect on the mind.

Olibanum *(see Frankincense)*

Opopanax
(Opopanax chironium)

Opopanax is very similar to myrrh, possessing anti-inflammatory and anti-parasitical properties. This essential oil is indicated for dysentery, skin ulcers, and parasitical infections in the gut.

Orange, Bitter
(Citrus sinensis)

Bitter orange essential oil is cooling, calming, stress-reduces, and promotes restful sleep. It is a mood elevator and improves mental clarity and alertness; calms angry and irritable children. It can be used in cooking, if the essential oil is food grade.

Orange, Sweet
(Citrus sinensis)

Sweet orange is an antidepressant and encourages a positive outlook. It relieves emotional tension and stress and is good to use during the winter months to lift your spirits. It moves energy (Chi) in the body. It promotes proper immune function, and assists digestion.

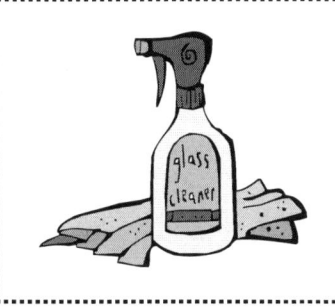

Window Glass Cleaner

This environmentally friendly cleaning product is an excellent degreaser;
Cleanses and sanitizes non-wood items. Keeps bugs away too!
Mix all ingredients together. Shake before use.

50 ml white vinegar   10 ml denatured alcohol
65 ml distilled water   10 drops orange & 5 drops lemon essential oil

---

Oregano
(Oreganum vulgare)
This is the "true" oregano and considered a tonic for the entire system. It is a traditional remedy for digestive upset, respiratory problems, colds and flu. Oregano can be added to massage blends for achy joints. For inflammation of the mouth and throat place one drop on the tongue. If this is too strong, mix one drop with some honey, place on the tongue, and let it "melt" slowly. My friend Chris had an ear infection with a perforated ear drum. Antibiotics did not stop the infection and doctors did not know what to do. Frustrated, she took the matter into her own hands and placed a few drops of oregano oil on a cotton ball and placed it in the ear. The pain went away and within two weeks the infection was completely gone. Oregano can be used to prevent "catching" a cold, flu or fungal infection, especially when going into large crowds, schools, or hospitals, by placing one drop of oil on the tongue.

Ormenis Flower *(see Chamomile Wild)*

Oud (Aloes Wood) (Agar wood)
(Aquillaria malaccensis)
Oud is the Ahaloth mentioned in the Bible as "Aloexylum". It is an evergreen tree native to northern India, Laos, and Vietnam. When the tree dies and has fallen to the ground a fungus begins to grow upon causing a dark resin to form within its heartwood. This resin, oud, is a stimulant, tonic, aphrodisiac, diuretic, carminative and antimicrobial. It is being used for digestive and bronchial complaints, shortness of breath, asthma, abdominal pain, diarrhea, nausea, liver congestion, chills, for illness during and after childbirth, and for weakness in the elderly. Oud is highly psychoactive. It is used for spiritual journey, enlightenment, clarity and grounding. Buddhists use it for transmutation of ignorance. Tibetan monks use it to bring energy to the center and calm the mind and spirit. Oud enhances mental clarity and opens the third eye as well as all the upper chakras. It drives away negative energy and exhaustion, and calms the nervous system. It is useful in nervous disorders such as obsessive behavior and other neuroses. Oud is a great companion during times of solitude.

Palma Rosa
(Cymbopogan martinii)
Palma rosa is calming, refreshing and clarifying. It contains anti-viral, anti-bacterial and anti-fungal properties, useful for colds, flu, sinusitis and coughs. It also eases morning fatigue and mild depression. Palma rosa is nourishing, balancing and regenerative for all skin types, and promotes skin healing, helpful for scars, rashes, and wrinkles. This oil also regenerates and regulates oil production of the skin and is great for dry skin.

Parsley
(Petroselinum sativum)

Parsley essential oil is useful in massage oils for sore muscles and joints, cellulite and detoxification. Parsley has an influence on the urinary system and prostate gland. It can be applied on insect bites. Some people like to use it for indigestion. Parsley calms nerves and relieves mental fatigue.

Patchouli
(Pogostemon cablin)

Every old hippie knows the scent of patchouli. It promotes friendly, sociable feelings. This essential oil regenerates tissues, closes large pores, soothes itchy skin, aids scars and reduces wrinkles and inflammation. It can be used as a deodorant. Patchouli repels moths and other pests.

Pennyroyal
(Mentha pulegium)

Pennyroyal essential oil is a mucolytic, tonic and stimulant. With its emmenagogue properties, pennyroyal can bring on the menses, especially when there is congestion in the pelvis. It is an excellent insect repellent.
Caution: Considered an oral toxin and uterine abortive.

Peppermint
(Mentha piperita)

Peppermint is cooling, refreshing and stimulating. One drop placed on the tongue can relieve digestion problems, nausea and motion sickness. Peppermint is also helpful for colds, flu, bronchitis and coughs, easing congestion and fighting infection. For headaches place one drop on the temples and back of the neck. If you experience poor memory, depression, melancholy, confusion or indecision you may want to infuse your environment with peppermint. A diffuser or spray bottle makes this easy, or you can add a few drops to simmering water. For a cooling effect during hot summers, add a few drops of peppermint to your lotion, or to your bath, shampoo, and conditioner. A foot massage with a peppermint lotion can revitalize tired, painful and swollen feet. Interestingly, peppermint can be effective in warding off mice. Place a few drops of peppermint on a cotton ball and place it into a plastic bag, then make a few holes in the plastic bag. Now, place this bag into the places where you suspect the mice may be coming in.

Peru Balsam
(Myroxylon pereirae)
Peru balsam is a slow-growing tree native to Central America. Peru balsam is also known as black balsam or Indian balsam. When the tree is wounded, a dark brown resin begins to flow. The fruit also yields a balsam. Peru balsam has warming, stimulating, anti-microbial, and antiseptic properties, useful for various skin conditions, and to promote healthy growth of the epithelium when mixed with castor oil. Use neat as a disinfectant for eczema, pruritis, to relieve itchiness from scabies, and for sores and ringworm. Relieves dry and chapped skin, and can also be useful to toughen nipples in preparation for nursing. Add a little alcohol if the oil gets too thick.

Petitgrain
(Citrus aurantium)
Petitgrain comes from the leaves and twigs of various citrus plants. It soothes inflamed and irritated skin tissues, and reduces skin blemishes. It is refreshing and uplifting and calms the nerves, relieves anxiety, tension and mental stress. Use it in a diffuser before meditation to improve mental alertness and clarity. The scent of petitgrain gives strength during emotional times, when you are feeling vulnerable and fragile, giving you self-confidence, strength and joy.

Pine Needle
(Pinus sylvestris)
Pine needle essential oil has mild analgesic properties and is good for muscular aches and pains, rheumatism, arthritis and neuralgia. It is useful for respiratory complaints, fatigue, nervous exhaustion and stress-related conditions. Pine needle oil can be used for cuts, sores, excessive perspiration, scabies and lice. It deodorizes, kills germs, and is refreshing.

Pine, Pinion
(Pinus edulis)
Pure essential oil from the southwest used in Native American ceremonies for strength.

Pine, Ponderosa
(Pinus ponderosa)
The ponderosa pine tree is the state tree of Montana, USA. This gentle giant can grow over 200 feet and can live over 500 years. The essential oil has been used to treat a wide range of skin issues, cuts, wounds, and burns. It can be used topically for lung ailments and respiratory infections, as well as massaged into joints, muscles and tendons to increase flexibility. It has also been used in the treatment of worms in the digestive system. The essential oil of the ponderosa tree can be placed into a room

diffuser to boost the immune system, alleviate respiratory problems, and to regenerate the lungs and kidneys. It is also high in vitamin C. Some massage therapists find this oil to benefit the spine, relaxing the surrounding muscles to open the flow of energy. As with all tall trees, ponderosa pine assists in meditation, opening oneself to receive ancestral help and information, as well as a sense of peace and protection. Diffuse this oil with spruce and orange to kill airborne germs.

Ravensara
(Ravensara aromatica)
Ravensara aromatica is a tree that grows on the island of Madagascar and by its features can be compared to the bay leaf. It is an exceptional immune system stimulant, excellent to use at the beginning of a cold or when feeling run down. It is a neurotonic acting deeply, even in low dosages. Ravensara reduces stress, relieves aches and pains, improves mental clarity, and is uplifting. It is also of great use for sinusitis, loosening tight muscles, relieving menstrual discomfort, for aches and pains, shingles, mononucleosis, genital herpes, cold sores and wounds.

Rock Rose *(see Labdanum)*

Rose Absolute
(Rosa centifolia)
Rose essential oil is a superb skin care oil, especially for mature and sensitive skin to rejuvenate skin cells. It is relaxing, antidepressant and relieves stress and anxiety. It is also an aphrodisiac, regulates menstrual cycle, and increases sperm count. Rose encourages inner vitality, confidence, passion, fulfillment and a sense of freedom. Nurturing and comforting, it is the best choice for grief or to heal a broken heart.

Rose Otto
(Rosa damascena)
The ultimate oil for all skin types to balance and rejuvenate. Rose is considered a cellular regenerative, good for damaged and wrinkled skin. Emotionally, rose is relaxing, uplifting and soothing. It is used for anger, shock, grief, jealousy, anxiety, nervous tension, depression, melancholy, sadness and emotional transitions.

Rose Geranium
(Pelargonium graveolens)
Rose geranium is used for acne, bruises, broken capillaries, congested skin, cellulite and poor circulation. It balances the function of the oil glands, and therefore can be used for both dry skin and oily skin. It is good for the female body due to its

hormone-regulating properties. This oil is also an adrenal cortex stimulant, and may be inhaled by those with adrenal function problems, such as people with asthma, or menopause. It has a balancing effect on the emotions, reducing mood swings when treating PMS and menopausal problems.

Rosemary
(Rosmarinus officinalis)

Rosemary is invigorating and refreshing. It is good for respiratory problems, as it loosens congestion and boosts the immune system. Add it to witch hazel to create a tonic for oily hair, oily scalp, and dandruff. Rosemary oil has great skin healing properties, especially for chronic problems. It is ideal for dry or mature skin to gently regenerate and stimulate glandular function, or for acne prone skin to fight infection. It can be used to relieve headaches and an upset stomach. This oil is excellent to use for poor memory, mental strain, and when there is an inability to concentrate, fatigue and for low mental and physical energy. It can be used during a gallbladder attack to relieve pain. Massage an essential oil blend of one part rosemary and one part lavender in a little olive oil over the gallbladder area. It can also be used for inflammation of the gallbladder.

Queen Of Hungary Water

The Queen of Hungary was known for her most beautiful skin. Rumor has it that she used a rosemary herbal blend to treat her skin. There are many tales about her exact recipe. Here is one recipe I like and have used on and off over the years:

Mix 4 drops rosemary essential oil, 6 drops lemon essential oil, 2 drops orange essential oil, 1 tbsp orange flower water, 1 tbsp rose water, and 4 tsp vodka. Stir the essential oils into the vodka, and then blend in the orange blossom and rosewater. Shake well every day, as the potion matures for about two months or longer.

Rosewood (Bois de Rose)
(Aniba roseaodora)

Rosewood oil rejuvenates skin cells, and is useful for scars and wrinkles. It is gentle enough to use on children and elderly to stimulate the immune system and for colds, flu and coughs. Rosewood helps relieve jet lag, and has uplifting, strengthening qualities. It supports and promotes courage during stressful times. Rosewood is an aphrodisiac, and can restore libido.

Sage, Dalmation
(Salvia officinalis)
Sage is cleansing and purifying. It balances women's hormones and reduces breast milk. Nursing mothers can wean off their babies easily by massaging sage essential oil mixed in a carrier oil. Babies do not like the taste of sage. Sage activates the nervous system and the adrenal cortex, making it useful both for asthma and to regulate hot flashes. It is mucolytic and anti-catarrhal. Sage is a great deodorant. Make your own natural and effective deodorant by adding 15 drops of sage essential oil to 1 ½ oz distilled water and ½ oz denatured alcohol, filled into a spray bottle. It reduces perspiration and oiliness of skin. Sage also encourages new hair growth. It is excellent to use in foot baths for tired, aching and sweaty feet.

Sage, Desert
(Artemisia tridentata)
This is a pure essential oil from the desert sage of southwestern United States. In Native American cultures the smoke from desert sage is an essential part in ceremonies to dispel negativity.

Sage, White
(Salvia apiana)
White sage has been used in Native American ceremonies to dispel negativity and confusion. White sage raises the vibration in any location. The essential oil of white sage is an excellent substitute when smudging (smoke) is not tolerated or allowed (smoke sensitive people, at work, in hospitals, prisons).

Sandalwood
(Santalum album)
Sandalwood cools inflammation and is excellent for sore throats, laryngitis, and dry coughs. All skin types benefit from sandalwood, as it softens the skin. It is exceptional for dry and mature skin. This oil has a gentle lasting stimulation, is a mood elevator, brings out emotions, euphoric, clears the mind, helps one dream, and increases the ability to meditate. Sandalwood is a good choice for centering and to relieve anxiety, nervous tension and melancholy.

Sassafras
(Sassafras albidum)
Sassafras is useful for various skin problems, skin inflammation and infections. It can be used for general weakness, and to treat mental problems of all sorts.

Savory, Winter
(Saturaia montana)
Winter savory is a wild species. It is a culinary herb since antiquity used much in the same way as summer savory. Recent research has shown superior anti-microbial properties, compared to thyme, rosemary and lavender. Winter savory is known in Germany and Switzerland as "Bohnenkraut" (green bean herb) and is usually added to fresh and dried green bean dishes as a flavoring agent. Caution: Do not use winter savory essential oil on the skin at all.

Savory, Summer
(Saturaia hortense)
Summer savory is a cultivated species used in cooking. Aids digestion, makes the stomach feel good, relieves digestive spasms, and expels parasites. Used for tough phlegm in the lungs. Summer savory is hotter than winter savory. Caution: Do not use summer savory essential oil on the skin at all.

Spearmint
(Mentha spicata)
Spearmint is a good alternative to peppermint, but it is less stimulating. It is cooling and anti-inflammatory properties, and is a good choice for migraines and itchy skin conditions. It is a mental stimulant, as well as a carminative for digestive upsets, gas and bloating.

Spikenard
(Nardostachys jatamansi)
In ancient times spikenard was known as "Nard". It is a superb skin care oil, as it can rejuvenate mature skin, calm allergic reactions, and promote healthy skin. It is also helpful for dandruff. With its antiseptic and anti-fungal properties spikenard is recommended for athlete's foot and toenail fungus. Additionally, spikenard has grounding and relaxing qualities to relieve anxiety, insomnia, and stress.

Spruce Hemlock
(Tsuga canadensis)
Spruce essential oil breaks up congestion in the respiratory system, and is effective for respiratory weakness. For muscular aches and pains, as well as poor circulation, spruce essential oil can be added to a carrier oil or lotion for an invigorating massage. Inhaling this essential oil can relieve anxiety and stress-related conditions. Spruce's fragrance enhances animated meditations, such as yoga and tai chi.

Star Anise
(Illicium verum)
Star anise is an evergreen tree native to Asia and can grow over 35 feet in height. The leaves are shiny green, and the small flowers develop into star-shaped fruits. The brown seeds also are star-shaped. The fruits are edible, but the leaves are poisonous. Star anise essential oil can be used to improve digestion, calm the nervous system, promote restful sleep, open the sinuses when congested, relieve menstrual discomfort, and increase lactation in nursing mothers.

St. John's Wort
(Hypericum perforatum)
St. John's Wort essential oil is used for nerve damage, especially in the extremities, fingers, toes, tailbone, etc., and for neck and back injuries. It can be blended in a carrier oil for a full-body massage to calm and strengthen the nerves.
Caution: Causes photo-sensitivity.

Styrax (Storax)
(Liquidamber orientalis)
Styrax is the sweet resin taken from a tree also known as sweet gum, red gum and alligator tree. It has antiseptic, anti-tussive, expectorant and nervine properties. It can be used somewhat like benzoin. Styrax oil is used to make "amber resin" by mixing with labdanum gum resin. Styrax removes lymphatic toxins, breaks down cellulite, has a calming, soothing, harmonizing and uplifting effect to combat stress and anxiety.

Tagetes
(Tagetes minuta)
Also known as French marigold, it is useful for skin inflammations, cuts, and bruises. It has strong anti-fungal properties.

Tangerine
(Citrus reticulata)
Internally, tangerine oil can be used as a digestive stimulant and for all sorts of digestive problems. Externally, tangerine oil is used in various carrier oils as a massage oil to break down cellulite and pockets of fat, as it helps to stimulate lymphatic drainage, especially when mixed with fennel. Reduces stretch marks. It is a muscle relaxant with calming and sedative properties. Blend together with marjoram and ylang ylang when you feel anxious and worried.

> # Adding Essential Oils to Paint
>
> Tangerine essential oil can be added to paint, either to paint your house or on your canvas, for a wonderful and uplifting "feel". Add 15 – 20 drops of tangerine essential oil to one gallon of paint. Mix well. Other essential oils work well for this purpose, such as lime, lemon, orange, grapefruit and mandarin.

Tarragon
(Artemisia dracunculus)
Tarragon is also known as estragon. Inhaled, it relieves intestinal spasms, hiccups, and aids in the passing of gas. It improves mental clarity and alertness, as it stimulates circulation. Added to massage oil tarragon relieves aches and pains, and menstrual pain.
Caution: Considered to be abortive! Not to be used internally.

Tea Tree
(Melaleuca alternifolia)
Tea tree essential oil is an effective antiseptic, anti-viral and anti-fungal essential oil. It is a powerful killer of all sorts of bacteria. It is non-toxic to the body, and produces no negative side effects. It can be used externally on deep wounds, fungal infections, head and pubic lice, pimples, sinus congestion, and much, much more. Tea tree is an immune tonic, as it strengthens the immune system. For ringworm, apply single drops on affected areas. In a short time you will notice the ring breaking up and disappearing. One mother told me that tea tree oil relieves growing pain. To one tablespoon of lotion add 5 to 10 drops tea tree oil and massage affected areas. Tea tree oil protects the skin from radiation burns during cancer treatments.

Thuja (Cedar Leaf)
(Thuja occidentalis)
Thuja is a powerful essential oil for rheumatism, gout, warts, fungal and bacterial infections.

Thyme, Red
(Thymus zygis)
Red thyme oil is the crude distillate. It is anti-viral and used topically for warts. It also contains anti-bacterial and anti-parasitic properties and can be used to fight colds, flu, coughs, sore throats, and fungal infections. It is effective for a wide

variety of infectious diseases. It is also helpful for indigestion, sore muscles, and poor circulation. Red thyme is a highly skin penetrating oil good for cellulite and sports injuries. Thyme's greatly stimulating scent helps dispel fatigue, giving renewed strength.

Caution: Both red thyme and white thyme are skin irritants; do not use neat!

Thyme, White
(Thymus vulgaris)

White thyme oil is produced by further re-distillating red thyme. Both thymes are used externally as an antiseptic and antibiotic anywhere on the body or face. It has been used to kill parasites, for hair loss, and as a mouthwash. It is stimulating and strengthening. Inhaled, white thyme is used for tension headaches; emotionally, it helps balance the emotions.

Throat Lozenges

Most throat lozenges contain sugar, which is not what you need when you have a cold. This recipe is actually not a lozenge, but a honey mix, which slowly melts in your mouth. It is easy to do and effective for a sore throat, tonsillitis, or a cough. Make sure you use food-grade essential oils for this recipe. Into one tablespoon of honey mix in thoroughly three drops eucalyptus essential oil, two drops hyssop essential oil, and one drop white thyme essential oil. Let this honey mix melt slowly in your mouth.

Tuberose
(Polyanthes tuberosa)

Tuberose is used mostly in high-end perfumes. Inhaled, the oil is euphoric and an aphrodisiac; it centers the emotions, and is slightly narcotic.

Tulsi (see Basil, Holy)

Turmeric
(Curcuma longa)

This oil is useful to aid sluggish digestion, for liver congestion and for anorexia. Its analgesic and anti-inflammatory properties are helpful for sore muscles and joints, rheumatism, arthritis, and to heal skin wounds.

Tolu Balsam
(Myrosperum toluiferum or Toluifer balsamum)
Toll balsam is much used in the same way as peru balsam. Both tolu and peru balsam are produced from the injuries made to the trunks of trees. The balsam seeps out, hardens and then processed into an essential oil. It is used for dry, chapped and cracked skin, eczema, rashes, and sores. It soothes and heals laryngitis, bronchitis, croup, and removes catarrh.

Valerian
(Valeriana officinalis)
Valerian essential oil is useful for nervous headaches, restlessness, tension, indigestion and muscle spasms. It relieves insomnia, soothes panic, and eases stress. It has a calming effect during an emotional crisis. Mix with lavender essential oil for total relaxation and a good night sleep.
Caution: Do not drive after using this oil.

Vanilla Oleoresin
(Vanilla planifolia)
Vanilla essential oil is sensual, warm, and an aphrodisiac. It has the ability to evoke warm memories, calm the emotions, and ease tension and grief. It is useful for children to ease homesickness and brighten their mood. In massage oils it has been used for impotent or frigid people. Mixed with a carrier oil it is lubricating for vaginal dryness.

Vetivert
(Vetiveria zizanoides)
Vetivert is a scented grass native to Asia. The essential oil is distilled from the roots. Vetivert relieves muscular pain and stiffness, improves digestion, revitalizes and strengthens the body. It is also known to stimulate the immune system and increase the ability to withstand stress without becoming ill. The oil is used for oily skin and acne, especially when the liver is involved. But most of all, vetivert is deeply relaxing during stressful times, as it calms anxiety, relieves depression, and promotes restful sleep. No wonder people in India call this oil "the oil of tranquility". It is wonderful for grounding spacey, nervous or emotionally exhausted individuals, due to its stabilizing, earthy quality. Add 5 – 10 drops of vetivert essential oil to a bath for the most de-stressing experience. A massage with vetivert added can be beneficial for those who focus excessively on intellectual activities to the exclusion of the physical, and for anybody who at times feels a bit insecure. It would be a good oil to use after a shock or during a traumatic period in life, such as bereavement, divorce, or separation.

Violet
(Violet odorata)
Violet leaf and flower is known for its analgesic, anti-rheumatic, decongestant, diuretic and soporific properties. It has healing and soothing properties valuable in treating skin problems, especially acne, oily skin, large pores, as well as for capillary fragility, and for baby's diaper rash and cradle cap. Very expensive!

Wintergreen
(Gaultheria procumbens)
Wintergreen is a small North American plant. Native Americans chewed the leaves to improve breathing. Wintergreen essential oil contains a high amount of methyl salicylate, which is similar to salicylic acid in aspirin. It is therefore a mild analgesic and anti-inflammatory mainly for joint and muscular problems such as lumbago, sciatica and neuralgia, and to relieve the discomfort of arthritis. It has also been used for respiratory problems such as chronic mucous discharge and for coughs. It is one of the ingredients in "Olbas". In the United States it is extensively used as a flavoring agent for toothpaste, chewing gum, root beer, Coca-Cola, and other soft drinks.
Caution: Do not take internally! Many people are allergic to methyl salicylate, formed during the distillation process.

Yarrow
(Achillea millefolium)
Yarrow essential oil is used in creams and salves to calm severe skin rashes, for wounds that will not heal, skin irritations and allergic skin reactions. It is an excellent anti-inflammatory with soothing and healing properties. Yarrow's beautiful blue color is due to it's azulene component. It regulates menstrual cycle and eases menopausal imbalances.

Ylang Ylang
(Cananga odorata)
Ylang ylang is an evergreen tree native to Asia. The name means "flower of flower". There are pink, mauve and yellow – flowered varieties and the best oil comes from the yellow flower. The first part of the oil which is extracted during the steam distillation process is of the highest quality, and sold as ylang-ylang, while that which comes from the latter part of the process – known as the "tail" of the distillate – is of a poorer grade and is usually sold under the name of cananga. In either case, the therapeutic properties are the same, but the perfume of cananga is less refined. Ylang ylang has the ability to slow down over-rapid breathing and over-rapid heartbeat. These symptoms may appear when somebody is in shock, frightened or anxious, and sometimes when extremely angry. The immediate use of ylang-ylang can be very helpful. It also reduces high blood-pressure, often associated with tachycardia. Just as jasmine and rose, ylang ylang is antidepressant, aphrodisiac, euphoric,

sedative, relaxing and calming. The calming and relaxing effect of ylang-ylang may be responsible for its designation as an aphrodisiac, as it can be used to break the vicious cycle of anxiety about sexual inadequacy. In skin care, the oil has a balancing effect, and therefore suitable for all skin types. It can be added to shampoos or conditioners for a luxurious treatment. Ylang-ylang also balances the nervous system and can be used for stress, insomnia, depression, low self-esteem, anger, rage, panic and pre-test anxiety.

Attar Oils

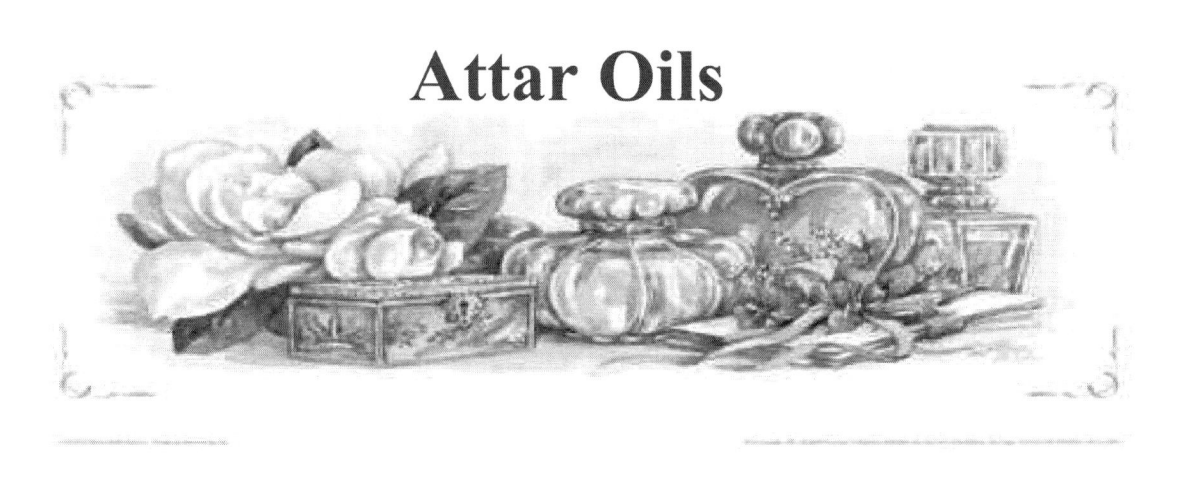

Attar is a Persian word meaning "fragrance, scent or essence". Attar perfume oils are a specific type of fragrance product derived from natural plant substances, both single ones, and those blended together carefully to produce remarkably rich scents. These perfumes are of East Indian and Persian traditions that have been worn by women and men of the East for centuries creating a truly spiritual sensuality. The word perfume comes from the French "par fume", meaning "through smoke". It was common to burn the oils in order to gain access to the essential etheric qualities released by burning. Although, some attars are simply individual oils, which on their own are suitable for fragrance use, such as amber, sandalwood, patchouli, they are usually composed of careful blends of various oils, resins and concretes placed in a natural base or carrier oil.

The beauty of wearing attar oils is that they create an aura of tranquility, confidence and mystery. Because they do not contain any alcohol, the scent "clings" within one or two feet of your body, in the "zone of intimacy".

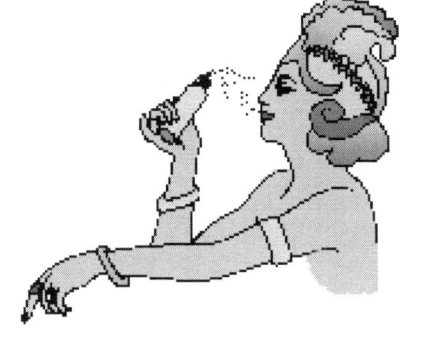

Amber attar
Amber attar is a sweet and warming fragrance. It improves ojas (glow and health), and acts as an aphrodisiac.

Hina attar
Hina attar is a warming and luscious fragrance. It strengthens mind and body and nourishes the heart. Hina also relieves anger, frustration and discontent. Hina attar encourages hair growth, leaving it lustrous.

Nag Champa attar
Nag champa is a sweet and light fragrance. It removes heavy moods, promotes ojas, and strengthens the aura. It is used in meditation and yoga.

Rose attar
Rose attar is a cooling and rich fragrance. It increases love, compassion and devotion. Rose attar opens the mind and heart for the purpose of spiritual enlightment.

Especially for Him
Bay Rum After Shave
1 tsp whole allspice
1 tsp whole cloves
1 tsp cinnamon
1 tsp cardamom pods
1 handful bay leaves
½ cup rum
orange flower water
10 drops sandalwood

Place first five ingredients in a clean glass jar and cover with rum. Soak for 2 weeks, shaking daily. Strain and dilute liquid with equal part orange flower water. Add sandalwood and shake well.

Especially for Her
Cleopatra's Perfume

1/8 oz neroli essential oil
1/8 oz rose otto essential oil
1/8 oz jasmine essential oil
1/16 oz sandalwood essential oil

Find a beautiful perfume bottle, and fill it with the above essential oils. Let the perfume "age" for approximately 9 weeks or more. The scent gets more and more exquisite as the various parts meld. This perfume is not diluted, therefore only 1 – 2 drops are needed at one time.

Especially for your Pet
Flea Collar
2 tbsp peppermint essential oil
½ cup rosemary essential oil
2 tbsp cedarwood essential oil
¼ cup citronella essential oil
2 tbsp eucalyptus essential oil

Blend the oils together and store in a glass jar. To make the flea collar, measure a heavy cotton wick that will tie comfortably around your pet's neck. Soak the wick in the above-prepared oil, then let it dry for several hours. Tie collar around your pet's neck, removing it at night to offer a break from the strong smell.

Minimum-Maximum Drops Of Essential Oils	Into Measurement Of Base Oil
0-1 drop	1/5 teaspoon
2-5 drops	1 teaspoon
4-10 drops	2 teaspoons
6-15 drops	1 tablespoon
8-20 drops	4 teaspoons
10-25 drops	5 teaspoons
12-30 drops	2 tablespoons

1 teaspoon = 5 mL
2 teaspoons = 10 mL
1 tablespoon = 15 mL

20 drops = 1/5 tbsp.
40 drops = 2/5 tsp.
60 drops = 3/5 tsp.
Etc.

EXFOLIATING NUT MEALS

These pure, natural seed/nut meals make great exfoliants in body and face scrubs. They are rich in their respective oils and therefore lend nutritive value to skin formulations. Mix with vegetable oils, essential oils, oatmeal, salt or sugar for a moisturizing body polisher. Use an anti-oxidant, like vitamin E oil, to keep the nut meal stable. These meals also make a nice additive in soaps. The shelf life on these meals is approximately 6 months. Store meal in glass and refrigerate if possible.

Almond Nut Meal
Almond Nut Meal is a good source of vitamin D. It is suitable for all skin types, but is especially good for dry or irritated skin.

Rough Skin On Elbows, Knees And Feet?

Take 1 cup of almond nut meal and mix with warm whole milk or cream to a paste. You may also add honey and/or essential oils. Apply to elbows, knees or feet. As soon it is dry, just simply rub off.

Apricot Kernel Nut Meal
This exfoliating nut meal is taken from the kernel of the apricot seed. It is an excellent softener for delicate skin.

Borage Seed Meal
This nut meal contains an abundance of gamma linoleic acid (GLA), an essential fatty acid that the body uses to manufacture prostaglandins - hormone like substances that balance and regulate cellular activity. This meal is ideal for the face and body, gently removing dead skin cells, which may reduce the aging process of the skin.

Colloidal Oat Meal

Good for individuals who cannot use soap. This is cosmetic grade oatmeal. The coarse grain makes it useful in soaps, scrubs, facials and cleansing grains.

Corn Cob Granules

This is an abrasive exfoliating agent ideal for gardeners and mechanics.

Evening Primrose Seed Meal

Evening primrose is a rich source of GLA and is useful for the relief of many skin conditions, PMS and tender breasts. Evening primrose meal gently removes dead skin cells from the surface of the skin.

Flaxseed Meal

Flaxseed meal is rich in essential fatty acids, lecithin and contains all of the essential amino acids and almost every known trace minerals. It can be used to make face and body scrubs. It is moisturizing to the skin.

Hemp Seed Meal

Hemp nut meal is a rich source of GLA and is useful for the relief of many skin conditions.

Moisturizing Facial Scrub

- 1/8 cup borage seed meal
- 1/8 cup evening primrose meal
- 12 drops rosehip seed oil
- 1 teaspoon jojoba oil
- 2 drops rose essential oil
- heavy cream as needed

Mix all ingredients together, using enough cream to make a thick paste. Massage the paste into the skin in a circular motions. Rinse with warm water.

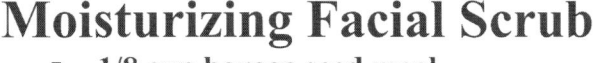

Hand and Foot Scrub

- ½ cup colloidal oatmeal
- 2 tablespoon milk powder
- 1 tablespoon rose petal powder
- Heavy cream

Mix dry ingredients and add enough cream to form a wet paste. Apply and let it sit for 10 minutes. Rub the paste into the skin until it forms into dough and falls off. This is an extremely nice moisturizing treatment.

Other Exfoliating Ingredients

Jojoba Wax Beads
Jojoba wax beads are excellent for dry, sensitive and mature skin. Add jojoba wax beads to cleansers and exfoliating creams for a gentle, non-drying exfoliating treatment. You may just simply add jojoba wax beads to jojoba oil.

Jojoba Cleansing and Exfoliating Cream

7 oz jojoba oil
½ oz grated beeswax
10 oz distilled water or hydrosol
1 teaspoon borax
25 - 50 drops essential oils
1-2 oz jojoba wax beads

Completely melt beeswax with oil. Dissolve borax in hydrosol. Add the hydrosol/borax phase slowly to the oil/beeswax phase by beating vigorously. Add jojoba wax beads and essential oils.

Exfoliating Fruit Seeds

Fruit seeds have been isolated from the fruits, milled and sterilized so that they can be used on the skin without the chance of contamination. They make excellent and gentle exfoliants.

Black Raspberry Fruit Seeds
(Rubus occidentalis)

Blueberry Fruit Seeds
(Vaccinium myrtillus)

Cranberry Fruit Seeds
(Vaccinium macrocarpon)

Grape Seeds
(Vitis vinifera)

Raspberry Fruit Seeds
(Rubus idaeus)

Strawberry Fruit Seeds
(Fragaria vesca)

Strawberry Face Scrub

This recipe may be used as a facial scrub or mask. You can add fresh strawberries, pureed, which will act like an alpha-hydroxy.

Mix together:

- 1 teaspoon honey powder
- 1 teaspoon rose petal powder
- 1 teaspoon strawberry seeds

Add enough water or hydrosol to make a thick paste.

Apply to the face and gently massage in a circular motion. You may then wash it off with warm water, or you may leave it on, as a mask for 15-20 minutes, or until dry.

THE GIFTS FROM THE HONEY BEE

Busy as a Bee
For one pound of honey one single bee has to travel approx. 120,000 km, equals 3 times around the earth.
For a person it would take 6 years, working 8 hours a day.

Bee Pollen is a complete food and is often referred to as nature's "perfect" food containing all ingredients necessary for life. With 22 amino acids, it contains more protein than beef. Athletes using bee pollen report an increase in strength and energy. Used for building the immune system in cases of allergies. Start with one grain and over several months build up to 1 tablespoon a day.

Honey is an instant energy food with all the essential minerals necessary for life, 7 b-complex vitamins, amino acids, and other vital ingredients. Most processed honey has been heated and filtered which destroys its nutritional value.

Royal Jelly is nature's rejuvenator. Royal jelly is fed by the bees to an ordinary worker larva to make it become a queen that lives for 5 years instead of 3 months. She produces twice her own weight in eggs each day. Royal jelly is an excellent source of nutrients and is gentle to the system. Although royal jelly has been traditionally known to prolong youthfulness and improve the skin beauty, evidence indicates that this substance increases energy, alleviates anxiety, sleeplessness, moodiness, memory loss, and bolsters the immune system.

Propolis is the most sterile place in the beehive. Propolis is responsible for neutralizing any bacteria, fungi or virus that enters the hive and is one of the most powerful germ fighters in nature. European studies have found propolis to be a powerful food for the immune system.

Beeswax is a natural secretion of honeybees. Natural beeswax has a beautiful sweet smell of honey and a rich golden color. It adds many wonderful properties, including anti-biotic properties, to various body care products.

How To Make Fragrant Herbal Honeys

Fragrant honeys are useful in both the kitchen and medicine chest. They can be used as drinks, spread on toast and fruits, or used in any recipe that calls for honey. Try using bay leaf, cinnamon, clove, ginger, grapefruit, jasmine, orange, lavender, lemon, mint, rose, rosemary, sage, tangerine, ylang ylang, or combine them to charm your taste buds.

1.)
Loosely pack a fancy jar full with herbs and pour honey over it to fill the jar. Let the mixture steep for several weeks.

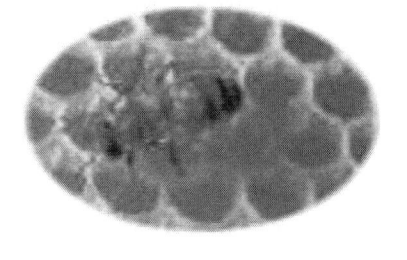

2.)
To a pound of honey add 3 drops of essential oils, stir, and let marinate for about 24 hours.

3.)
Instead of sucking on cough candies next time you have a scratchy throat, try the following recipe:
Mix the following essential oils very well into 1 tablespoon of honey:
3 drops of eucalyptus, 2 drops of tea tree, and 1 drop of thyme essential oil
Take a small amount and let the honey mixture slowly melt in your mouth.

HENNA AND MENDHI

Henna is a potent natural dye, derived from the dried, crushed leaves of the *Lawsonia inermis* shrub. It is henna, which produces the lovely reddish hair color favored by many Middle-Eastern and North African women. It is also used to paint designs upon the body, traditionally the palms and soles, for the purposes of beauty and spiritual benefit. The art of henna painting, also known as mendhi, has become fashionable worldwide and for good reason. Besides its beauty, henna is safe, temporary and painless. The dye, which is permanent on fabric or wood, lingers anywhere from 2-12 weeks on the skin. Henna is believed to improve the texture of hair and skin. On a spiritual level, henna is believed to bestow happiness, good fortune.

Mendhi Paste

This is a basic recipe for creating mendhi paste. Take this one and experiment: you can add espresso coffee, blue or black malva, rose petals petals, safflower, or hibiscus flowers.

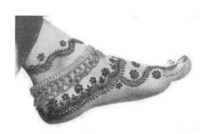

One teaspoon henna powder
Two teaspoons strong black tea or coffee
5 drops of essential oils of clove and eucalyptus

In a glass bowl mix all ingredients stirring in one direction to dissolve lumps. The texture should be akin to toothpaste: add extra powder or liquid, a little at a time, to achieve this consistency. Once the paste is smooth, cover the bowl with a towel and let it sit overnight in a warm place before using.

Henna For The Hair

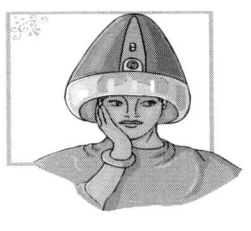

This is a basic recipe for creating natural hair dye. Take this one and experiment.

2 oz of henna (choose a color of your choice)
2 cups boiling water and 2 tbsps vinegar (red wine vinegar for red hair, balsamic for black, apple cider for light, etc.)
For added color use malva flowers, alkanet powder, beet powder or red wine (if red hair is desired)
½ -1 lemon juiced

Mix henna with vinegar water, add color ingredient of your choice, and lemon juice, to make a paste. Mix and apply to hair. Cover your hair tightly with a garbage bag. Let it "cook" from 2 hours to 6 hours.

Your hair can also reap the benefits of henna without the color.

Neutral (colorless) henna powder may also be used to condition the nails.

THE HERB LIST

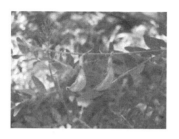 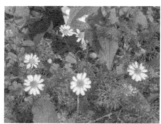 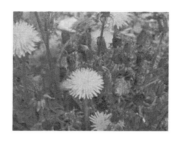 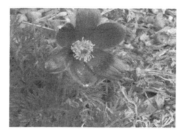 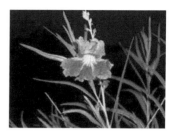

For thousands of years herbs have been used safely by people and animals. Herbs are foods with medicinal and nutritional qualities. Because they combine with our bodies the same way as foods do, herbs are able to address both, the symptoms and causes of a health problem. Botanicals are also less expensive and do not have the side effects pharmaceuticals have.

Roots, Leaves and Stalks, Flowers

Roots
Roots have an impact on the physical body, the physical structure, the atom itself in the cellular structure. Roots are for physical ailments. When you affect the physical body you influence the mind and the emotions. Roots have their greatest potency in the winter.

Leaves and Stalks
Leaves and stalks have an impact on the mind, the thoughts, affecting the physical structure through the mind. Leaves and stalks have their greatest potency in the spring.

Flowers
Flowers have an impact on the emotions, affecting the physical structure through the emotions. Flowers have their greatest potency in late spring into summer, unless they bloom in the fall.

Acacia/Gum Arabic *(Acacia spp)* – Acacia is an effective demulcent to soothe irritated mucous membranes, including throat, stomach, bowels, uterus and vaginal area. Gum Arabic's main effect is to form a protective, soothing coating over inflammations. The resin from the acacia tree is edible and nutritive. Externally, add to poultices to retain warmth and moisture.

Acerola *(Malpighia glabra)* – Acerola's western use is mostly associated with its high content of vitamin C, known to be a free radical scavenger due to its antioxidant properties. Acerola is being used in cosmetics to fight cellular aging, not just for its high vitamin content, but also for its mineral salts, which have shown to aid in the re-mineralization of tired and stressed skin, while the mucilage and proteins have skin hydrating properties and promote capillary conditioning.

Achiote *(see Annatto)*

Agar Agar *(Gelidium amansii)* – This seaweed is widely used as a treatment for constipation. It does not increase peristalsis, but works as a bulking agent. Dry agar has the ability to absorb and retain moisture. Used to make jelly, add 1 oz dried agar to 1 pint of boiling water.
Caution: Do not use internally in dried form, as it is irritating. Always mix with liquid first.

Agrimony *(Agrimonia eupatorium)* – Agrimony is high in nutrients, necessary for normal healthy body functions, especially for the colon, intestines, kidneys, liver and stomach. It is used as an astringent and homeostatic to inhibit bleeding. Restores tone to muscles, stomach and intestines; counteracts flaccidity. This herb is useful for urinary tract infections, as well as for an overactive liver after chemotherapy or drug excess. Singers have used agrimony to cut the mucus in their throats before singing. It is soothing to inflammation of the bile ducts. It is a mild liver tonic.

Aletris *(Aletris farinose)* – Aletris is a female organ tonic. For low back pain associated with pelvic prolapse or congestion.

Alfalfa *(Medicago sativa)* – Highly nutritive, it contains all known vitamins and minerals necessary for life, and therefore beneficial for all ailments, due to nutrient deficiencies. It is the basis for liquid chlorophyll, with a balance of chemical and mineral properties almost identical to human hemoglobin. Support for arthritis, rheumatism and osteoporosis; a phyto-estrogen precursor during menopausal hormone changes.

Alkanet *(Alkanna tinctoria)* – Alkanet is cultivated mostly for its dye, which is easily extracted through maceration in oil. It is employed in pharmacies to give salves a red color. It is also being used in staining wood, soaps, etc.

Aloe *(Aloe vera)* – Taken internally, aloe vera juice/gel increases digestion and absorption, as well as being excellent for promoting the growth of friendly bacteria in the colon. Balances blood pH and boosts the immune system. Dehydrated aloe vera is available in capsules form, when a strong cathartic (a strong laxative herb which causes rapid evacuation) is needed. Additionally, taken in small doses, dehydrated aloe vera increases menstrual flow. In both instances it is advisable to blend aloe vera with carminative herbs (herbs that relieve intestinal gas pain and promote peristalsis) to reduce griping. Applied externally, aloe vera promotes the removal of dead skin and stimulates the normal growth of living cells. It softens, moisturizes and balances the pH of the skin. For burns, i.e. radiation burn, thermal burns, sunburn, etc., it reduces the chance of infection and scaring, stops the pain and speeds up the healing process.
Caution: Aloe vera is a powerful herb; please consult your herbalist before taking it.

Growing Aloe Vera

All aloe plants exhibit more or less the same properties, however, the aloe vera is the easiest to use medicinally, because of its size and softness of the leaf. "Aloe" is from Arabic alloeh or Hebrew halal wich means a shining and bitter substance. "Vera" is from the Latin root verus which means true. Aloe barbadensis is the species long favorite by herbalist for it's medicinally properties. Aloe is a sun-loving plant native to warm, dry regions of the world. It likes full sun, but in the southwest desert it needs some protection from the hot afternoon sun, sandy and well drained soil, and moderate watering. It is quite hardy and can survive outdoors in zone 8 if well protected. I grow my aloe in a large pot. It lives outside during the frost-free months, afternoon shade, and occasional watering. During the winter months I take it inside and water it about once a month.

How To Prepare The Gel

Cut a firm leaf from your aloe plant. Slice it open on a plate. The gel will start oozing out. Use a spoon to scoop out the inner gel. If you want a smooth gel you can puree it in a blender. Apply the gel directly to a burn, wound, or skin irritation. It will feel cooling and soothing, as it instantaneously repairs and heals damaged tissues. Aloe gel does not keep well; therefore it is best to use it right away.

Amalaki/Amla *(Emblica officinalis)* – This is the Indian gooseberry, a fruit high in Vitamin C. One berry contains about 3000 mg of vitamin C, is 99.9% absorbable, and stays in the body for 36 hours. Vitamin C supplements are known to increase pH acidity in the body; therefore, amalaki is a better choice, as it has an alkalizing effect on the body. Amalaki enhances the vitality of every cell in the body, boosts immune response to fight colds, flu, and infections, and strengthens the blood in cases of debility. It is also an excellent tonic for the eyes.

Andrographis *(Andrographis paniculata)* – This bitter herb is a powerful antiviral. Good for colds, influenza, sore throats, hepatitis and other viral infections. It is also being used for allergies. Deemed effective in reducing headache pain, fever, irritation, congestion and general fatigue, while strengthening the body's immune system.

Angelica *(Angelica archangelica)* – This is a warming and bitter herb to support digestion, especially when there is deficient hydrochloric acid, gas, nausea and colic. Angelica regulates menses because of its hormonal balancing properties. It is effective for colds, bronchial catarrh, rheumatic pain, menstrual cramps and for cold extremities.

Candied Angelica

Collect angelica stems and place them into boiling water until they are tender enough to remove the outer skin. Return the peeled stems to the pan and again bring to a boil. Cool the stems and add an equal weight of sugar to the stems, cover and leave for two days. Then place the stems and the syrup in a pan and bring to a boil. Preheat the oven to 200 F (100C). Place the stems on a tray. Sprinkle with confectioners' sugar, let dry completely, and store in an airtight glass container.

Anise *(Pimpinella anisum)* – Anise seeds contain natural enzymes, released when they come in contact with saliva, to assist digestion and absorption. Anise warms the abdomen and breaks up blockages due to mucus accumulation, therefore stopping fermentation and gas in the digestive tract. In ancient Rome, anise seeds were used to flavor wedding cakes, which worked to prevent indigestion and flatulence from overeating. Chewing on anise seeds prevents and alleviates halitosis, and the leaves can be used to flavor spicy dishes. Anise stimulates milk production in nursing mothers. It can also control estrogen levels by stimulating female glands. It is also helpful for emphysema and coughs.

Anise, Star *(Ilicium verum)* – Star anise is an evergreen tree native to Asia and can grow over 35 feet in height. The leaves are shiny green, and the small flowers develop into star-shaped fruits. The brown seeds also are star-shaped. The fruits are edible, but the leaves are poisonous. Star anise can be used to improve digestion, calm the nervous system, relieve nausea, to promote restful sleep, and to open the sinuses when congested. It can relieve menstrual discomfort, and increase lactation in nursing mothers. In Chinese herbal medicine it is recommended for lumbago, constipation, bladder problems, and to ease symptoms of acute rheumatism.

Annatto *(Bixa orellana)* – Long used by indigenous people of Mexico and South America, known as achiote, to make body paint, a pigment for mural painting, and ink. As a food colorant, the ground annatto seeds are mixed with other spices, garlic, pepper, oregano, and sometimes a little vinegar, made into a paste and added to soups, stews, and other dishes. It can be used as a substitute for the high prized saffron. Annatto seeds are used in cosmetics for its beautiful yellow to orange color and for its emollient properties. It also has UV protection capabilities. Medicinally, it has been used as an expectorant, and because of its high carotenoid properties, as an anti-oxidant, and to protect the liver. It has also been used for high cholesterol and hypertension. Increases urination. Some people are very sensitive to annatto, even in small amounts. Next time at the movies, notice if you need to urinate more often after eating a little buttered popcorn. Annatto is added to butter to make it look yellow.
Caution: Do not eat if you have diabetes.

Apricot Seeds *(Prunus armeniaca)* – Apricot seeds are especially good for bronchitis, asthma, emphysema, and for dry cough, because of its oily nature. It is more demulcent than wild cherry bark. When there is constipation due to dryness in the colon, apricot seeds can be used as a stool softener, and a mild laxative. Laetrile is derived from apricot seeds and has been with used with success in Mexico and Germany for the treatment of cancer.

Aritha/Soapwort *(Saponaria offinalis)* – An ayurvedic herb, which has been used in India as a mild all natural cleanser for skin, hair and delicate fabrics, and to treat mild psoriasis, eczema, chronic itching, and very sensitive skin. It does not dry the skin or hair. The pulp of the soapwort fruit contains naturally occurring saponins. Good for the hair, skin, fabrics and the environment. To use as an exfoliant for face and body, wet hands, add a little powder, rub hands together to make thin paste. For hair and body wash, mix 1 tablespoon in 1 cup of boiling water, let sit for 10 minutes, cool, strain . In a bath, or for delicate fabric, dissolve 1 tablespoon in warm to hot water, stirring vigorously, add to bath water or fabric water. You will not get any foam or lather.

Arnica *(Arnica montana)* – Reduces bruising and swelling due to injuries. It also works well for muscle pain including fibromyalgia, back pain and whiplash.
Caution: For internal uses take in a homeopathic form. The herb/flower is for external use only! Do not use on broken skin!

Arrowroot *(Maranta arudinacea)* – Arrowroot is valuable as an easily digestible, nourishing herb food for convalescents, especially when there is bowel complaints.

Artichoke *(Cynara scolymus)* – Artichokes stimulate secretion of digestive juices to assist digestion, absorption and elimination. This herbal food is especially helpful for a sluggish liver, poor fat metabolism and hypoglycemia.

Asafoetida/Hing *(Ferula asafoetida)* – Asafoetida is an Asiatic spice that is also known as devil's dung, or stinking gum. The name is derived from the Persian word aza, meaning "resin" and the Latin word fetida, meaning "stinking". Just a little added to vegetarian dishes can bring out their natural flavors. It is a strong detoxifier, used for killing parasites and treating indigestion and gas. It is effective in breaking up impacted fecal matter while improving intestinal flora.

Aspen *(Populus tremuloides)* – The bark of aspen is anti-inflammatory and a fever reducer. Has aspirin-like properties, but does not irritate the stomach.

Astragalus *(Astragalus membranicus)* – Astragalus is an antiviral, specific in immune-resistance building formulas; increases overall energy and builds resistance in cases of weakness and illness. Helps reduce the occurrences of colds and shortens their duration. It is an immune system food, raises T-Cell count, increases antibodies, and nourishes the adrenal glands. It has also been used as a vasodilator. Astragalus eases chemotherapy and radiation side effects, and inhibits the spreading of tumors.

Atractylodes *(Atractylodes macrocephalae)* – Atractylodes is an effective remedy for gas, diarrhea and bloating, as it strengthens and nourishes the spleen and stomach. It is useful in treating any condition where fluid retention is a problem.

Bacopa *(Bacopa monniera)* – Traditionally used in southern India as a rejuvenative for the nerves and brain, to increase mental clarity, improve memory and promote intelligence.

Balm of Gilead/Poplar Bud *(Populus tremuloides)* – This is a potent anti-oxidant and anti-bacterial herb for upper respiratory infections and wet cough. Topically, it can be used in a carrier oil to massage into sore and tired muscles, stiff neck and arthritic areas.

Baptisia *(Baptisia tinctoria)* – Baptisia is a blood cleanser for septic conditions and degenerative diseases, as it stimulates metabolism of waste products.

Barberry *(Berberis spp)* – The uses for barberry go back to ancient Egypt, where they mixed it with fennel to prevent the plague. It contains an alkaloid called berberine which dilates blood vessels, thereby lowering blood pressure. Berberine is a strong antiseptic that is also found in goldenseal. It is a bitter tonic herb beneficial to the liver and gallbladder with mild laxative properties. Soothes sore throats, strengthens the body, stimulates appetite, promotes bile secretion, normalizes liver secretion. Can be very effective for acne, psoriasis, eczema and herpes, where constipation and mal-absorption are the cause.

Basil *(Ocimum basilicum)* – Basil has been used for the mind and nervous system. It lifts the spirit, dispelling depression, and brings clarity of thought. Basil reduces mental fog, especially when associated with drug use, and is supportive during menopausal years. This culinary herb can also be used to reduce chronic stress. It is an anti-viral, carminative and galactagogue.

Basil, Holy *(Ocimum sanctum)* – Holy basil is also known as tulsi, and comes to us from India, where it has been used for a wide variety of ailments, such as colds and flu. In addition, recent research done in the USA on this herb shows that it contains adaptogenic properties. It has the ability to modulate levels of the stress hormone cortisol to relieve tension and to improve mental focus. Holy basil balances blood sugar levels, as well as curb cravings for sugar!

Batcherlor's Button *(Centaurea cyanus)* – The American Indians used it for snakebites, insect bites and stings. It can be used to treat sensitive skin, as eyewash, and to relieve inflammation and irritation.

Bay Laurel *(Laurus nobilis)* – In ancient Greece, bay leaves were used for inflammation, to improve memory, and for insect stings. They also used it to encourage prophetic visions. In ancient Rome and Greece, bay was the symbol of glory and reward. The recipients of the crowning with the bay laurel wreath were kings, priests, prophets, victorious athletes and soldiers. Bay leaves repel insects, especially spiders. At one time, the alarm at our store would go off more than once for no reason. Our alarm service company came to check things out and noticed a spider nesting around one of the sensors, setting off our alarm. The technician recommended placing a couple of bay leaves around all sensors. It worked!!!

Bayberry *(Myrica spp)* – Bayberry improves the voice, opens the mind, and clears sinuses. It works well as a gargle for sore throats, tonsillitis, as it clears mucous accumulation in the respiratory and alimentary tract. Clears vata in the head, strengthens prana, and heals mucus membranes. For initial stages of diseases, it mobilizes the defensive energy of the body. Bayberry can also be used as a tonic, to stimulate blood circulation, to invigorate and strengthen the body, and to help raise vitality. Bayberry inhibits bacteria and therefore can be used to fight infections. To help heal ulcers, cuts, bruises, and insect bites, apply a poultice made from the root bark. Bayberry has also been used for female problems, such as excessive menstruation.

Bearberry *(see Uva ursi)*

Beet *(Beta vulgaris)* – This is a highly nutritious vegetable/herb particularly effective for the kidneys and the liver. It has been used as a blood cleanser and anti-inflammatory. It is supportive to the liver and spleen to cleanse toxic wastes and encourage healthy blood cell formation.
Caution: Do not use more than 3 days at a time, because the oxalic acid builds up in the body and can cause gout.

Beth Root *(Trillium pendulum)* – Also known as birthroot, this plant is an excellent uterine tonic. It may be used when there is excessive blood flow from the uterus. Its astringency can be utilized where there is hemorrhage anywhere in the body. Beth root contains a natural precursor to the female sex hormones, and the body may use it needs if needed, or otherwise leave unused. What a wonderful example of the normalizing powers of some herbs. It may also be used as a douche.

Bergamot *(Monarda fistulosa)* – This is a wonderful aromatic herb and good for digestive problems, stress headaches and colds. Topically, it has a cooling effect on first-degree burns.

Bilberry Berry *(Vaccinium myrtillus)* – The berry can be used for eyesight improvement, night blindness and in formulas for anemia, as well as for vascular support, such as varicose veins or easy bruising. Regenerates the retina, and slows down the development of glaucoma and cataracts. Excellent during pregnancy to strengthen veins and capillaries.

Bilberry Leaf *(Vaccinium myrtillus)* – The leaf can be used in the same way as uva ursi for urinary problems. Bilberry leaves have also been used as a sugar regulator for diabetes. Its astringent properties are useful for sinus congestion and runny nose, and for diarrhea.

Birch Bark *(Betula alba, Betula lenta)* – Anti-rheumatic, diuretic and for dissolving kidney stones. It has a mild sedative effect and can be taken for insomnia. Externally, it is known to ease muscle pain.

Birch Leaf *(Betula pendula)* – Birch leaves act as an effective remedy for cystitis and other infections of the urinary system as well as removing excess water from the body. It has also been used for gout, rheumatism and mild arthritic pain.

Birth Root *(see Beth root)*

Bistort *(Polygonum bistorta)* – One of the strongest astringent medicines and highly styptic, useful for internal or external bleeding problems, e.g. nosebleeds. It is also effective in stopping diarrhea. For sore throats or spongy gums, use as a gargle.

Bitter Melon *(Momordica charantia)* – Bitter melon has received a lot of attention in the west for its ability to take on life-threatening problems such as Aids. In clinical studies bitter melon fights viruses, lowers blood sugar and kills tumor cells. Widely used in the treatment of diabetes. Take it before meals to prevent a rise in blood sugar. Momordica in Latin means "to bite", in reference to the seeds, the edge of which appears as if bitten. In TCM, it cools the body systems, treats fevers, a tonic and purgative.

Bitterroot *(Lewisia rediviva)* – It once was a primary food source of the western Native Americans. This is the story of this plants origin: An old woman who had no food to feed her children was afraid they would starve to death. She wept each morning on the riverbanks. The sun sent a guardian spirit in the form of a red-feathered bird, which consoled her by saying that from each of her tears that fell on the earth there would rise a beautiful flower to feed her people. A legend says that the plant's silvery appearance comes from the old woman's hair and the redness of the flower is from the crimson feathers of the sunbird's wings. The plant, although a staple food, will always be bitter in flavor because of the old woman's sorrow.

Blackberry Leaf *(Rubus fructicosus)* – This astringent and styptic herb is useful for diarrhea (mix with catnip for better results). Blackberry leaf is ideal for treating mild conditions in children and infants, as it is highly nutritious. It has also been used for obstruction in the urinary system and for urinary stones. These highly nutritious leaves tonify the reproductive energy (chi). Strengthens the uterus, and has been used during the whole of pregnancy, labor and delivery. As a gargle, or just chew the leaves for bleeding gums, and to stop capillary bleeding.

Blackberry Root *(Rubus fructicosus)* – Blackberry root is more astringent and homeostatic than the leaf.

Black Cohosh *(Cimicifuga racemosa)* – Black cohosh supports and increases estrogen production, and therefore has been used for female problems, such as hot flashes during menopause, to ease menstrual cramps, and to contract the uterus when menstruation is sluggish. Black cohosh calms the nervous system, considered a nervine, because it has a tonifying effect on the central nervous system. Dr. Jack Ritchason, N.D. claims it to be effective for spinal meningitis, as well as for medulla oblongata damage, caused by hallucinogenic drugs. This root relieves nervous irritation, and is an excellent and safe sedative. It breaks up mucus and phlegm deposits, soothes local pain and headaches, although in large amounts it may cause headaches.

Black cohosh equalizes blood pressure, acts directly on the heart, (slightly lowers heart rate, while increasing the force of the pulse) lungs, stomach, kidneys, and the reproductive system. It is a smooth muscle relaxant, has anti-inflammatory properties and is being used in arthritis-, rheumatism-, and sciatica formulas.

Black Currant Juice *(Ribes nigrum)* – Black current juice, prepared from the fresh berries, is valuable for preventing colds and flus, and useful in fevers and diarrhea. *(Also see Red Currant)*

Black Currant Leaf and Root *(Ribes nigrum)* – The leaf and root carries out the specific function, and that is of eliminating uric acid from the system. Its main action is on the body's fluids and the urinary tract. It is an astringent and anti-inflammatory for injuries, gum and throat problems, and for postpartum tissue trauma.

Black Haw *(Viburnum prunifolium)* – Black haw is a uterine antispasmodic, for painful menses, clotting, and low back pain; for scanty flow, as it increases bleeding. Women have long used black haw for threatened miscarriage, mixed with false unicorn and red raspberry leaf.

Black Walnut Hulls *(Juglans nigra)* – Black walnut hulls are anti-fungal, and effective in the treatment of intestinal worms, candida, ringworm, scabies, thrush, herpes, canker sores and boils. It delivers oxygen to the blood, and thereby killing parasites. Good for "bad blood" diseases, i.e. diphtheria and syphilis. It is known to help people affected by valley fever. Black walnut hulls are high in organic iodine. Walnut can raise prolapsed conditions, stop excessive sweating, stop bleeding and relieve diarrhea and other discharges of the intestines, reproductive organs and skin. Walnut is helpful for those with bone disorders, mineral deficiencies and anemia, especially with exhaustion and muscular or skeletal weakness. By altering the internal fluid environment of the connective tissues, walnut is also able to build and nourish the blood and fluids. It has been used on patients with electrical shock.
Caution: Avoid using walnut leaf and hull with tinnitus present. Do not take internally for more than about 21 days at the time.

Black Walnut Leaf *(Juglans nigra)* – The leaf of the black walnut is best used for digestive disorders, arising from stagnant Chi or damp cold. It is also more stimulating and spasmolytic than the hulls. Walnut leaf has been explored as a growth stimulant, perhaps as a protein anabolism stimulant, in those with metabolic disorders such as retarded children's development.
Caution: Avoid using walnut leaf and hull with tinnitus present. Do not take internally for more than about 21 days at the time.

Blessed Thistle *(Cnicus benedictus)* – Because of its bitter properties, blessed thistle stimulates digestive activity. It is being used to treat gastritis and peptic ulcers. Blessed thistle is effective in treating liver stagnation, poor fat metabolism and rebellious chi (hiatal hernia, regurgitation of stomach acid, hiccoughs). It has long been used for jaundice and hepatitis, and headaches caused by liver congestion. This thorny plant is a digestive tonic (Benedictine liquor) and a diaphoretic to support skin detoxification. Blessed thistle increases oxygen uptake into the body.

Bloodroot *(Sanguinaria canadensis)* – Bloodroot is a powerful herb for any kind of skin problems, such as skin cancer, fungus, eczema, ringworm, nail fungus, venereal warts and sores and many other skin disorders. To treat such skin disorders, apply castor oil on the affected areas first, wait for about one hour, and then carefully apply bloodroot extract with a Q-tip or cotton ball. The purpose of applying castor oil first is to soften the skin to allow deeper skin penetration of the bloodroot extract.

Blueberry *(Vaccinium myrtillus)* – Taken internally, the fruit is good for tired eyes, as it regenerates retinal purple. The leaf has long been used for diabetes. The leaf also acts as a mild diuretic and urinary antiseptic.

Blue Cohosh *(Caulophyllum thalictroides)* – Blue cohosh in not related to black cohosh. It is used in PMS formulas, and to increase blood circulation in the pelvic area, and to tone the uterine tissues. It is mostly used at the onset of labor to induce labor, insure easier dilation and birth.

Blue Flag *(Iris missouriensis)* - Called a liver lymphatic, it gets natural oils to the skin. Mixed with other herbs it is good for blood toxicity. It is a strong diaphoretic and powerful liver stimulant, increases metabolism and assists in the assimilation of foods.

Blue Vervein *(Verbena hastata)* - For spasmodic nervous disorders, for menopausal anxiety, PMS, irritability associated with fevers and flu. This mellowing herb cools out acid indigestion where heartburn is present. Blue vervein has a calming, relaxing effect on the system which aids in breaking down obstructions, and with a stimulating effect helps to expel waste from the system. Good and safe for children.

Blue Violet *(see Violet)*

Boldo *(Peumus boldus)* - Stimulates bile production in the liver. It is an excellent laxative, well known in Europe.

Boneset *(Eupatorium perfoliatum)* – Boneset has tremendous healing and rejuvenating properties, used for intermittent chills that tend to appear on a regular basis, once a day, once a week, or once a month; in the Chinese system intermittent fever is described as halfway in, halfway out. It is a bitter, helpful in rebuilding the digestive system after it has been destroyed by intermittent fever. It heals broken bones and teeth. It is good for people who complain about pain deep in the bones. Matthew Wood says that chronic intermittent fever can constrict the arteries around the gallbladder causing hepatic congestion and nausea, where boneset releases the tension. It stimulates secretion of bile by the liver, as well as the gallbladder. As a fever reducer and pain modifier, it can be of service in flu symptoms where there's deep-seated, achy, muscular and joint pain. As an expectorant, and can facilitate the movement of mucus out of the lungs, when there is a weakened cough with lots of secretions but a lack of power to cough it out.

Before Massge Tea

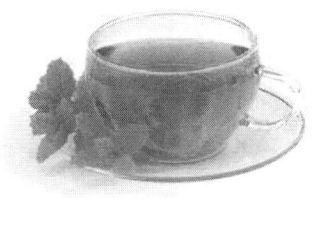

To heighten the effects of your next massage drink one cup of warm boneset tea one hour before your appointment. This tea relaxes sore and tight muscles, even strained muscles. You may add lemon balm or lemon verbena to heighten the effect.

Borage *(Borago officinalis)* – Borage soothes the mucous membranes of the mouth, throat and the digestive system. It also reduces inflammation in the respiratory system. Borage stimulates the adrenal glands, which helps restore vitality when recovering from illness. Borage expels excess mucous through the kidneys. Use it as an eyewash to soothe irritated eyes.

Brazil Nuts *(Bertholletia excelsa)* – The Brazil nut tree grows slowly, but becomes enormous, frequently attaining a height of about 150 feet. It bears three-sided nuts, containing white meat or flesh that contain 70 % fat or oil, commonly used in South American countries for cooking, lamps and to manufacture soap. In addition to protein and fat, Brazil nuts are a good source of selenium, an important antioxidant. Without it, several enzymes our body uses to destroy free radicals don't function properly. The incidence and mortality rates of numerous cancers are higher in those with low levels of selenium. And adequate selenium levels also reduce the risk of heart disease, increase immunity, and dramatically boost male fertility. One single Brazil nut exceeds the U.S. recommended daily allowance of selenium. Eat the nuts raw or grate them into your food.

Brigham Tea *(see Mormon Tea)*

Buchu *(Barosma serratifolia)* – Buchu grows in South Africa, where is has been used by indigenous people as a soothing remedy. Buchu is excellent to use for chronic kidney and bladder inflammation due to highly acidic urine, as well as pain while urinating. It absorbs excessive uric acid, increases frequent urination, as well as increased fecal solids. It acts as a tonic, astringent and disinfectant to the mucus membranes. Good for water retention and to reduce bladder irritations. One of the best herbs for treating enlarged prostate gland. (A great choice for alkalizing the system).

Buckthorn *(Rhamnus frangula)* – Buckthorn is a close relative of cascara sagrada. It stimulates the flow of bile from the liver to the gallbladder, therefore helping the bowels evacuate effectively. Buckthorn does not gripe and is actually calming to the digestive system. It is not habit forming. Do not use the fresh plant, as it acts as an irritant poison on the gastro-intestinal canal.

Bugleweed *(Lycopus virginicus)* – Bugleweed is a specific herb for an over-active thyroid gland, particularly if it is accompanied with tightness of breathing, palpitation, irregular heartbeat, elevated blood pressure, nervousness, and overly rapid GI transit times. This plant has specific qualities that regulate the body by relaxing some systems while tightening others. It strengthens the heart and circulatory system and has been used for extreme water retention. Bugleweed has also been used successfully for bleeding in the lungs and bowels, for excessive menstruation, as well as for some pain.

Bupleurum *(Bupleurum falcatum)* – This valued herb in the Chinese system is used for hepatitis and to treat all liver disorders. Bupleurum is a major chi regulating and carminative herb, helpful to raise yang vitality, to lift prolapsed organs, for moodiness and sagging spirits. It has the capacity to dredge out the old emotions of sadness and anger that may be stored in the organs and tissues of the body.

Burdock Root *(Arctium lappa)* – The whole plant (leaves, seeds, roots) can be used as a blood purifier and cleanser to eliminate long-term impurities from the blood very quickly. Excellent for skin problems, relieves congestion of lymphatic system, reduces swelling around the joints by promoting kidney function. In Europe it has been used for prolapsed and displaced uterus. It is an important herb in the metabolism of carbohydrates, because it consists of a high amount of inulin. It is one of the ingredients in Essiac, a cancer remedy.

Burdock Seed *(Arctium lappa)* – The seeds of burdock are good for dry, crusty, itchy and flaky skin conditions. Use with milk thistle and flaxseed or olive oil. Contains 45 % inulin, which is important in the metabolism of carbohydrates.

Butcher's Broom *(Ruscus aculeatus)* – This is the best remedy for restless leg syndrome (RLS), heavy leg syndrome, as well as for cramps in the legs and hands, as it improves circulation. It is for heart weakness and for low blood pressure. It improves peripheral circulation, while also increasing circulation to the brain, legs and arms. Butcher's broom strengthens each stroke of the heart, as well as the walls of the blood vessels. It also reduces cholesterol. Beneficial when there is water retention due to heart weakness. Reduces pain caused by hemorrhoids. It dissolves blood clots, and can be used for aneurysm.

Butterbur *(Petasites vulgaris)* – Butterbur root is a heart stimulant, acting both as a cardiac tonic and as a diuretic. It is an anti-spasmodic for intestinal cramps, asthma, or painful menstruations. Not only does is ease muscles spasms, but also relieves pain. Butterbur can also be used for fevers, colds and urinary complaints. Recently, butterbur has become popular among migraine and allergy sufferers.

Butternut *(Juglans cinerea)* – Butternut is a relative of black walnut. It is a mild and safe laxative without causing dependency. Mix with dandelion root for constipation and delayed transit time.

Cacao *(Theobroma cacao)* – Pure cacao is increasingly recognized as a rich source of powerful antioxidants such as catechins (the antioxidants in green tea) and proanthocyandins. Theobromine, the alkaloid contained in the beans, resembles caffeine in its action, but its effect on the central nervous system is less powerful. Its effect is primarily on muscles, the kidneys and the heart. It is useful when there is an accumulation of fluid in the body resulting from cardiac weakness.

Calamus/Sweet Flag *(Acorus calamus)* – Calamus root rejuvenates the brain and nervous system. It is used for cerebral circulation, to sharpen memory, and to enhance awareness. In Sanskrit it is named "vacha," which means speaking the power of the word, intelligence, and self-expression. Calamus can be used for nervous complaints, vertigo, headaches, gastritis, intestinal colics, anorexia, and gastric ulcers. In India it is sold as a candied rhizome for dyspepsia, bronchitis and coughs. In China, calamus is used to treat deafness, dizziness, and epileptic seizures.

Calea *(Calea ternifolia)* – Calea increases oxygenation in the brain, enhances endorphin release in the brain, and stimulates the adrenals, increasing physical energy. This is a wonderful herb to use before bedtime to enhance vivid and lucid dreams.

Calendula *(Calendula officinalis)* – The flower of the sun (petals close when there is no sun). Calendula promotes tissue repair. For inflammatory gastric problem, including ulcers, diverticulitis, gallbladder inflammation, and as an antiseptic in skin healing formulas for burns, bruises, sprains, and inflammatory eruption such as measles and chicken pox. It is also a strong anti-fungal, internal and external, for thrush, candida albicans, yeast infections, and athlete's foot.

California Poppy *(Eschscholtzia californica)* – California poppy is useful as a sedative and antispasmodic indicated for insomnia, nervous headache, muscle pain and sleeplessness due to pain and agitation. It can also be used in formulas for gallbladder and intestinal pain. It is not related to the regular poppy seeds used in baking *Papaver rhoeas*, therefore safe to use for people going for drug tests.

Cannella/Wild Cinnamon *(Canela alba)* – Canela is the inner bark of a tropical evergreen tree. It is famous for its clove and cinnamon taste. It is also used alone or in combination to assist with digestive health.

Camu Camu *(Myrciaria dubia)* – This fruit contains the highest naturally occurring content of Vitamin C found on Earth, which may be up to 4,000 times the amount of Vitamin C found in an orange. It also contains a wide variety of bioflavonoids. In comparison to oranges, camu-camu provides 30 times more vitamin C, 10 times more iron, 3 times more niacin, twice as much riboflavin, and 50% more phosphorus.

Caraway *(Carum carvi)* – Caraway seeds are a digestive aid, especially in the digestion of protein. It is an appetite enhancer. Stimulates production of breast milk in nursing mothers and eases colic in infants. Russian and German people make a delicious liquor called Kümmel. Caraway is being used in cathartic and laxative formulas to prevent cramping or griping.

Caraway Soup – Köménymag Leves

Place 2 tbsp all-purpose flour in a small saucepan and cook it, stirring, over medium heat until the flour is lightly brown. Set aside. In a separate large saucepan combine 9 cups vegetable broth and 2 tbsp caraway seeds and bring to a boil. Simmer for thirty minutes, then strain. Discard the seeds. Blend the browned flour with 2 tbsp of vegetable oil. When smooth, stir in ½ cup of cold water. Add this to the caraway broth, stirring rapidly, and bring to a boil.

Cardamom *(Elletaria cardamomum)* – Stimulates digestion, relieves gas, energizes the spleen, as an anti-mucoid it is added to lung tonics. Chew it to freshen your breath. Green: better for kidneys. White: better for lungs. Added to coffee it negates the toxic side effects.

Carob *(Jacaranda procera)* – Carob is a delicious good chocolate substitute. The pods are rich in sugars and protein. Carob also contains demulcent and emollient properties. It can be used in the treatment of coughs and diarrhea.

Cascara Sagrada *(Rhamus purshiana)* – This is a reliable non-addictive laxative and works within eight hours. Cascara sagrada is an excellent remedy for chronic constipation. It is considered not habit forming, as it cleanses and tones the colon, by increasing secretion flow of the stomach, liver and pancreas. Cascara sagrada is also helpful in gallstones and liver ailments.

Cassia *(Cinnamomum cassia)* – Cassia is not cinnamon, although it has a similar flavor and is less expensive. Cassia is the bark of an evergreen tree that belongs to the laurel family, a relative of cinnamomum zeylanicum, the "true" cinnamon. Cassia is not sold under its own name, but mixed with true cinnamon to be marketed as ground cinnamon or rolled and sold as "cinnamon sticks". Cassia's flavor is slightly bitter, while cinnamon is warm and sweet. True cinnamon sticks look like quills (a single tube); cassia sticks are rolled from both sides toward the center so that they end up looking like scrolls.

Catnip *(Nepeta cataria)* – Catnip causes euphoria in cats, but calms humans. It is a mild sedative, relieves stomach upsets and cramps. It is a nice-tasting children's tonic. Stimulates appetite and digestion and is also known as "Nature's Alka-Seltzer". To help you quit smoking and to decrease the desire for cigarettes, place a few drops on the back of the tongue. Externally, catnip has been effective as a mosquito repellant. A friend in my writer's association had an amazing healing effect with catnip tea. He was diagnosed with ulcers in his ascending colon, and his doctor recommended immediate surgery. He started drinking one to two cups of catnip tea everyday and in about 3 months his ulcers were totally healed.

Cat's Claw/Una de Gato *(Uncaria tomentosa)* – One of the most recognized plants of the rainforest because of its numerous health benefits. For more than 2000 years tribes of Peru have used cat's claw as a powerful medicine. It is a highly effective immune system stimulant; used to treat arthritis, bursitis, intestinal disorders, allergies and to ease the side effects of chemotherapy. Cat's claw has been referred to as the "opener of the way" because of its ability to cleanse the entire intestinal tract and its effectiveness in treating stomach and bowel disorders such as Crohn's disease, leaky bowel syndrome, ulcers, gastritis, diverticulitis, and other inflammatory conditions of the bowel, stomach, and intestines. In Peruvian medicine today, cat's claw is even being used in veterinary medicine to benefit dogs and cats with hip dysplasia, arthritis, cancers, Parvo virus, dermatitis and other skin disorders, tumors, FIV, and feline leukemia.

Cattail Pollen *(Typhus spp)* – Stops internal and external bleeding. Benefits blood circulation, relieving conditions of blood stagnation such as abdominal pains and menstrual pains. It is also effective for heart pains (angina pectoris). Mixed with honey, the pollen can be applied externally to painful swellings and sores to promote healing. Cattail pollen is being used by Native Americans for ceremonial purposes.

Catuaba *(Juniperus brasiliensis)* – This rainforest botanical has been used as an aphrodisiac for both male and female, and a specific tonic to the male organs. In Brazil, catuaba has been used without ill effects for many nervous conditions including insomnia, hypochondria, and pain related to the central nervous system. In Europe catuaba is considered an aphrodisiac and a brain and nerve stimulant. The tea is used for sexual weakness, impotence, nervous debility, and exhaustion. In the United States it used in much the same way: as a tonic for the genitals as well as a central nervous system stimulant, for sexual impotence, general exhaustion and fatigue, insomnia related to hypertension, agitations, and poor memory.

Cayenne *(Capsicum frutescens)* – Cayenne increases digestive fire and circulation. Rich in flavonoid, these hot fruits have anti-inflammatory and antioxidant activity. Improves circulation, strengthens heart, arteries, capillaries and nerves. Increases the power of all herbs!

Time for Cayenne

Cayenne is considered to be the most useful and valuable herb in the plant kingdom. The name is derived from the river Cayenne in French Guiana, and is also commonly called Guinea pepper. Cayenne's heat is determined by the amount of capsaicin it contains and is measured in HU + Heat Units on a scale from 0 – 200"000 HU. It is both an intense food and a medicine. Rich in flavonoids, these hot fruits have anti-inflammatory and antioxidant properties. Improves circulation, strengthens heart, arteries, capillaries and nerves. In the digestive system, cayenne is known to rebuild tissues in the stomach and the peristaltic action in the intestines. It aids assimilation and elimination as well as helping the body create hydrochloric acid (the amount of hydrochloric acid diminishes after the age of 20), which is so necessary for good digestion and assimilation, especially of proteins. All this becomes very important since the digestive system plays the most important role in mental, emotional and physical well-being, as it is through the digestive system that the brain, glands, muscles and every other part of the body are fed.

Cedar Berries *(Juniperus monosperma)* – These little blue berries restore the function of the pancreas. Dr. Christopher found that cedar berries could replace insulin injections.

Celandine *(Chelidonium majus)* – Celandine I useful for insufficient bile with clay colored stool and liver congestion. It does prevent gallstone formation. Use externally to remove or reduce warts.

Celery Seed *(Apium graveolens)* – Celery is a powerful diuretic and urinary antiseptic, removing uric acid, excellent for gout and gouty arthritis, as well as for bone spurs. Assists digestion, balances acidity in the body, reduces weight, controls dizziness and headaches, relieves incontinence, helping any type of disease of chemical imbalance in the body. Celery is a natural source of organic sodium which is needed for the lining of the stomach, joints, and the bloodstream. It lowers blood pressure, and helps regulate the nervous system by producing a calming effect.

Centaury *(Centaurium erythraea)* – Centaury promotes appetite and strengthens digestion. It strengthens the bladder of elderly people or those with urinary control problems. It acts on the liver and kidneys, purifies the blood, and is an excellent tonic. Centaury has also been used to treat bed-wetting.

Chamomile *(Matricaria recutita)* – Chamomile calms the gastrointestinal and nervous system, especially in children and the elderly. The Greek meaning is "apple on the ground". Chamomile can also be used externally for any kind of skin problems, even open wounds, as an eyewash, great for pink eyes, a toothache, and for dandruff. Chamomile is excellent for children's upset stomach, colic, to calm and induce sleep, and reportedly useful for nightmares. Chamomile can also be used on animals. Caution: People who are allergic to ragweed may also be allergic to chamomile.

Chanca Piedra/Quebra Pedra *(Phyllanthus niruri)* – Quebra pedra literally means, "stone breaker". In the Amazon jungle indigenous people have used this herb for ages to help eliminate excess calculi formation, gallstones and kidney stones. This herb is also known to support the liver.

Chaparral *(Larrea tridentata)* – This plant is also known as creosote bush. It is a strong antioxidant, painkiller and antiseptic. Chaparral cleanses deep into the muscles and tissues, rebuilds healthy tissues and tones the system. Chaparral tones the liver and increases dietary fat metabolism. It has the ability to dissolve tumors, fight cancer by constraining undesired rapid cellular growth. Chaparral prevents free radical damage and is therefore rejuvenating and anti-aging. It has a reputation to pull heavy metals out of the body. Chaparral can be used to treat rheumatism, radiation poisoning, parasites and other unfriendly bacterias/microbes. It is an excellent lymphatic cleanser.

Chaparro Amargosa *(Castela emoryi)* – Useful in amoebic dysentery and giardiasis, it acts as an active inhibitor of all intestinal protozoa. It can be used as a preventative while traveling. Use as a preventative for candida and bacterial enteritis.

Charcoal - The best charcoal is made from the finest wood, such as boxwood, the shells of coconut, willow, pine, and other woods. It is NOT BBQ charcoal. Charcoal is very useful as an antiseptic due to its absorbent and oxidizing qualities, excellent for acid dyspepsia, gas, fermentation, heartburn and food poisoning. Charcoal can absorb and condense many times its own volume, up to 250 - 350 times its own volume. Charcoal can also be used externally as a poultice for ulcers, sores, gangrene, insect bites, etc. Mixed in distilled water it can remove dust and pollen from the eyes, as well as to relieve inflammation.

<u>Internal use:</u> Take one teaspoon to one tablespoon as often as needed and depending on the condition. Put the charcoal powder in a cup, add water, enough to make a paste, dilute, and drink at once.

<u>External use:</u> Mix charcoal with water, tea or olive oil to a consistency of paste. Place directly on affected areas and leave it on for several hours.

Eye Wash Treatment

To clear pollen and dust out of the eyes, make an eye wash. Place one teaspoon powdered charcoal and place into a mini filter (small coffee filter). Pour one cup distilled water through it. With an eye wash cup, rinse out the eyes. Make sure all of your utensils are clean and sterile.

Chaste Tree Berry/Monk's Pepper *(Vitex agnus-castus)* – This spicy little pepper normalizes and balances hormones and is beneficial in treating painful and irregular menstruation, infertility, PMS, menopausal problems, and other hormonal imbalances. It has also been helpful in the treatment of endometriosis and is also useful in normalizing the system after discontinuing birth control pills. It is most effective when taken for several months or one year. Because it stimulates the production of prolactin, chaste tree is often given to nursing mothers to help ensure a healthy supply of milk.

Chia Seeds *(Salvia hispanica)* - These little seeds have an abundance of nutrients, a vast array of vitamins and minerals, and a usually good ratio of omega-3 to omega-6 oil. Chia seeds are a good source of easily digestible protein. A single seed placed in the eye before going to sleep is said to collect excess mucus.

Chickweed *(Stellaria media)* – Chickweed assists in dietary fat metabolism, removes fatty substances out of the body, as well as plaque out of the blood vessels. It strengthens the tissue lining of the stomach and the intestines due to its demulcent properties, healing gastritis, duodenal ulcers, stomach ulcers, inflamed bowels, lungs, as well as urinary inflammation. It is useful for rheumatism where the pain is shifting around. Topically, it has been used for skin inflammation, diaper rash, breast inflammation during lactation, sore eyes, swollen testes, hemorrhoids, cancer, and many other skin and mucous membrane problems.

Chicory *(Cichorium intybus)* – Chicory is a wonderful blood cleanser, as well as helping eliminate excessive internal mucus. It is a useful laxative, whenever the liver is congested, or there is a lack of bile production. It is excellent for poor fat metabolism, as well as in hepatitis protocols. Chicory relieves gout by removing uric acid. It brings relief to joint stiffness due to arthritis. Chicory has many constituents found in dandelion.

Chinese Lantern *(Physalis spp)* – The fruits or berries are used as a diuretic, for bladder problems and gout. They are also lightly laxative and can be used to appease rheumatic pain. Contains a high amount of vitamin C. Clears fevers and resolves phlegm. The roots and leaves can be used as a bitter tonic.

Chives *(Allium schoenoprasum)* – Chives are used to stimulate appetite and promote digestion especially when poor appetite is due to a cold. Like onions, garlic, and leeks, chives contain health-promoting compounds that are believed to help prevent cancer and treat high blood pressure.

Chrysanthemum *(Chrysanthemum morifolium)* – This plant is used in Chinese medicine for eye problems, headaches and dizziness. It cools dry and swollen eyes. It is also useful in treating colds, flu, fevers, headaches and pneumonia. Emotionally, it calms anger and irritability.

Cilantro *(Coriandrum sativum)* – Cilantro leaves increase heavy metal excretion, especially mercury. The seed of cilantro is coriander and is used in cooking to prevent and relieve gas and nausea.

Cinchona/Peruvian Bark *(Cinchona calisaya)* – The bark is a source of quinine. Cinchona bark strengthens the stomach and acts to stabilize the whole nervous system. It is helpful for fevers, rheumatic pain, and to treat intoxication from alcohol. Caution: Do not use during pregnancy!

Cinnamon *(Cinnamomum cassia)* – Cinnamon stimulates digestion, and assist sugar metabolism. It is a thermogenic, calms the stomach, reduces milk flow, stops excessive menstruation, and counteracts congestion. It was once used in embalming mixtures. It can control actions caused by microorganisms, especially the one which causes botulism and staphylococcus aureus. It devastates the fungus that produces aflatoxin, a potent poison and carcinogen. It suppresses E. coli and candida albicans. Cinnamon has also been used to help stop vomiting. Cassia is the bark of an evergreen tree that belongs to the laurel family, a relative of cinnamomum zeylanicum, the "true" cinnamon. Cassia is not sold under its own name, but mixed with cinnamon to be marketed as ground cinnamon or rolled and sold as "cinnamon sticks". Cassia's flavor is slightly bitter, while cinnamon is warm and sweet. True cinnamon sticks look like quills (a single tube); cassia sticks are rolled from both sides toward the center so that they end up looking like scrolls.

Citrus *(Citrus reticulata)* – The peel of citrus moves the energy in the body, when there is stagnation. It helps in the elimination of mucus in the lungs and digestive tract.

Cleavers *(Galium aparine)* – Cleavers is helpful for urinary tract inflammation, it is a non-irritating diuretic. It can also be used for enlarged lymph nodes in children and adults.

Clematis *(Clematis spp.)* – This plant can be used for migraines and cluster headaches.

Clove *(Eugenia caryophyllus)* – This warming and energizing spice dispels chills. It warms and strengthens the lower back, increases circulation, and clears the lungs to allow deeper breathing. Sugar cravings can sometimes show up when there is low adrenal energy. Clove can soothe these craving and raise energy levels. Clove can also increase the yang of the kidneys and correct weakness in this area, for example when there is excessive clear-colored urine. If sexual energy is weak, clove can be emotionally and physically warming and stimulating. Add ¼ teaspoon to one cup of warm water and drink at once. Clove has also been used for nausea, gas and bacterial diarrhea, as well as to cleanse the lymphatic system. Dentists have long used clove as a local anesthetic and anti-bacterial for certain dental problems. For a toothache apply one drop of clove essential oil with a Q-tip, then make an appointment with your dentist.

Codonopsis *(Codonopsis pilosula /tangshen)* - This plant can be used to substitute ginseng. Used for fatigue, anemia, poor appetite, immune deficiency, organ prolapse and diabetes. Codonopsis strengthens endocrine function.

Collonsonia *(see Stone Root)*

Coltsfoot *(Tussilago farfara)* – Coltsfoot sedates the cough reflex, resolves wheezing, hoarseness, bronchitis, shortness of breath. Use with horehound and marshmallow to make the best cough remedy. Coltsfoot can be used to treat asthma to stop wheezing, as a demulcent for a persistent cough, especially for smoker's cough. Dioscorides recommended smoking coltsfoot for lung problems. Even today, Native Americans prepare smoking mixture for ceremonial purposes. One of the mixtures is made with tobacco, anise, licorice, lavender, and coltsfoot.

Comfrey Leaf and Root *(Symphytum officinalis)* – Comfrey is also called the knitter, as it heals and knits tissues and bones. Pouring fluid extract of comfrey into a wound often closes the wound, thus avoiding stitches. It promotes healthy skin, and strong bones. Good externally and internally to promote the healing of sores, bones, muscles and other tissues; the root is high in mucilaginous properties. Comfrey contains allantoin, a cell proliferant, meaning that it stimulates new cell growth to support rapid healing. A lady came to see me one day and told me how she had cured her psoriasis with comfrey. Stress usually aggravates her condition and when it flares up, more often than not an indication to slow down, she bathes her hands in comfrey leaf tea. She takes a handful of comfrey leaf and adds it to 2 quarts of hot water, and lets it steep for about 30 minutes. She bathes her hands in it and watches her psoriasis disappear.

Coptis *(Coptis chinensis)* – Coptis is a rich source of anti-bacterial and anti-fungal alkaloid berberine. Known as Huang Lian in TCM, it is used for bacterial dysentery, strep throat, cystitis, sinusitis and gingivitis.

Coffee *(Coffea arabica)* - Coffee is America's most widely used herbal infusion. Coffee may help asthma attacks, boost physical stamina, may help loose weight and overcome jetlag. It is a brain stimulant, which produces sleeplessness. Coffee should be used as carefully as any other healing herb. Its active constituent, caffeine, is addictive. It can raise blood pressure, dehydrate, perpetuate wrinkles and shallow complexion, and aggravate the digestive system. On the other hand, instant coffee can be used to eliminate the odor of skunk, after being sprayed.

Cordyceps *(Cordyceps sinensis)* – This is a superb blood tonic for reducing fatigue. Stimulates endocrine function, calms nervousness, and enhances physical performance. It is useful for heart arrhythmia and for loss of libido.

Coriander *(Coriandrum sativum)* - Coriander is a sweet, warm and spicy seed known for its carminative, sedative, analgesic, antispasmodic, tonic and regenerative properties. Because of its stimulating digestive properties, coriander relieves nausea, indigestion and an upset stomach. The leaf of coriander is cilantro and is used in cooking to cool spicy foods.

Cornflower *(see Batchelor's Button)*

Cornsilk *(Zea mays)* – The silk of corn is mildly diuretic and safe to use in children and during pregnancy. It is also for a chronic inflamed bladder and for prostate problems. Cornsilk assists all phosphatic and uric acid build up and is especially helpful in treating inflammation of the urethra, bladder and kidneys, which are the cause of most malfunctions of the system due to uric acid retention. It is very helpful for children troubled with bedwetting due to uncontrollable swollen bladders.

Cornus *(Cornus officinale)* – These berries are excellent to use for the treatment of a weak body. Cornus is helpful when there is excessive loss of fluids in the body, i.e. incontinence, excessive sweating, night sweats. Benefits weak backs and knees.

Corydalis *(Corydalis ambigua)* – Corydalis is used for blood stasis with pain, and as an analgesic for painful menstruation, gallbladder spasms, angina, and insomnia due to pain.

Couchgrass *(Elytrigia repens)* – This is a soothing diuretic in urinary problems. It has both anti-bacterial and anti-inflammatory properties. It can also be used for gout, prostatitis and urinary calculi.

Cowfoot – *(See Pata de vaca)*

Cow Parsnip *(Heracleum sphondylium)* – May be helpful for acid indigestion, gas and persistent nausea. As an antispasmodic for the GI tract, it may help with spastic colitis and cramping.

Cowslip *(Primula veris)* – This beautiful plant with its yellow flower is a sedative for insomnia and restlessness. It also contains anti-spasmodic properties. It is uplifting and supportive for seasonally affected disorder (SAD). Cowslip can be used on the skin to soothe sunburns.

Crampbark *(Viburnum opulus)* – Crampbark is antispasmodic and specifically for dysmenorrhea and other rhythmic uterine pains. It is helpful for backaches and back spasms. It can also be used for smooth muscle cramps or spasms, including intestinal. It is sometimes used for threatening miscarriage.

Cranberry *(Vaccinium macrocarpon)* – Cranberries are best used to prevent urinary tract infections. The juice has shown to reduce the amount of ionized calcium in the urine by more than 50% in people with recurrent kidney stones. Also used for candida albicans. It has also been used to open bronchial tubes; works better than coffee.

Culvers Root *(Veronicastrum virginicum)* – A slow acting laxative used for liver congestion with non-obstructive jaundice, poor fat metabolism, liver headaches with constipation and clay colored stools.

Cumin *(Cuminum cyminum)* – Cumin seeds strengthens digestion, especially protein digestion.

Cyani - *(see Batchelor's Button)*

Cyperus *(Cyperus rotundus)* – This rhizome is especially effective for menstrual pain. It regulates liver chi, making it useful for symptoms of stagnation such as cramping, gas, nausea and vomiting.

Damiana *(Turnera aphrodisiaca)* – As its botanical name suggests, it is the herb of choice for helping with sexual impotence and infertility for both males and females. It is a sexual rejuvenator and a tonic for nervous depression and poor appetite; for recurring genitourinary complaints with emotional causes. It is helpful for overcoming exhaustion and for weakness in the limbs.

Dandelion Leaf *(Taraxacum officinale)* – Highly nutritious, dandelion leaf can be taken on a long-term basis as a mineral/vitamin rich food, for edema (cardiac, circulatory, PMS, pulmonary) hypertension, liver problems, including cirrhosis of the liver and uric acid. Dandelion leaf contains 7,000 units of vitamin A per ounce. Drink it as a tea or juice it to balance electrolytes. Taraxacum means disorder and remedy in Greek.

Dandelion Root *(Taraxacum officinale)* – The root of dandelion is an excellent bitter tonic to stimulate the activity of the digestive system by Increasing hydrochloric acid, bile, pancreatic and small intestine enzymes. It is indicated for chronic constipation due to poor digestion. Dandelion root stimulates the growth of healthy bowel flora. Excellent liver cleanser; lowers cholesterol and blood pressure. Clears obstructions, balances enzymes. A great liver tonic.

Dandelion Leaf & Root

Dandelions are versatile, flavorful and really, really good for you. A very tenacious plant and one of the most complete foods. The leaf of dandelion is highly nutritious, containing more beta-carotene than carrots, more potassium than bananas, more lecithin than soybeans, as much iron as spinach, and it has a wealth of other vitamins and minerals. Besides that, dandelion has long been recognized to be effective in the treatment of a wide range of medical problems, including liver ailments and digestive disorders. It is also an effective diuretic, increasing the elimination of urine without depleting potassium. It is appropriate for long-term use for edema when there is cardiac insufficiency, decreased blood circulation, hypertension due to water retention, PMS, excess water in the lungs, etc. Dandelion leaf has also been used to reduce weight and is especially good for people who retain water (kapha). Dandelion root and leaf are known to re-balance electrolytes in the body. Dandelion root can be lightly toasted in the oven then used the same way as coffee beans, for a coffee substitute. Dandelion is truly a remarkable plant!

> # Dandelion Salad
>
> **This delicious dandelion salad has been one of my favorite recipes since early childhood. You can pick your own dandelion leaves before they bloom (make sure not to harvest the greens from a pesticide-treated lawn) or you can go to the store.**
>
> 6 oz dandelion leaves
> 2 eggs, hard-boiled
> 1/3 cup olive oil
> Juice of ½ of a lemon
>
> 2 garlic cloves
> 1 teasponn mustard
> 2 anchovies
>
> **Crush anchovies, garlic and mustard into a paste. Slowly stir in olive oil until well combined. Stir in lemon juice. Chop eggs into small pieces and add to sauce. Add dandelion leaves. Serve with whole grain bread. You can also simply add a tablespoon of dried dandelion leaves to your regular salads, salad dressings, dips, sandwiches or soups for extra nutrients.**

Deer's Tongue *(Liatris odoratissima)* – The leaves are used to flavor tobacco. Deer's Tongue's perfume is largely due to its property, coumarin. Uplifting, cleansing, mood elevator.

Devil's Claw *(Harpagophytum procumbens)* – This plant is found near the Kalahari Desert of South Africa. The name, Devil's Claw, is given because of the thorny, barbed claw arrangement of the seed pod. It is a well-known anti-inflammatory, due to its possible acting on prostaglandin pathways. Devil's Claw is useful for gout, arthritis, rheumatism, and other joint inflammation. This plant can be helpful for liver and gallbladder problems, as well as for its natural cleansing effect, removing toxic impurities out of the body. Devil's Claw strengthens the body and slows down the aging process by preventing the hardening of the veins and arteries, helping them remain elastic.

Devil's Club *(Oplopanax horridum)* – Devil's Club is very effective for hyperthyroidism. It is a blood purifier, builds endurance, and has also been used for lowering blood sugar.

Dogbane *(Apocynum cannabinum)* – This cardiac stimulant should be used with caution. In small doses it acts as a vasoconstrictor, slowing and strengthening the heartbeat and increasing blood pressure. Externally, it stimulates circulation and repairs nerve damage when applied to referred pain areas, such as sciatica, uterine pain and spinal cord injuries. As a hair rinse, it stimulates hair follicle growth.

Dong Quai *(Angelica sinensis)* – Dong Quai is the ginseng for women; it strengthens and builds the female body, especially after childbirth, as a post-partum tonic. It balances female hormones, is a menstrual regulator, and prevents anemia. Increases breast size. Dr. Jack Ritchason, N.D., in his book "The Little Herb Encyclopedia" mentions an herbal combination of dong quai, chaparral and red clover to rebuild the lymphatic system, especially after cancer. Reduces high blood pressure; strengthens the heart; it is a blood tonic; increases circulation to relieve tinnitus, blurred vision and palpitation. It also enhances the use of Vitamin E.
Caution: May increase menstrual bleeding. May feed fibro-cysts.

Dulse *(Rhodymenia palmate)* – This is a common edible seaweed that is rich in minerals and other essential micronutrients. In small amounts dulse is used to stimulate an under active thyroid gland.

Eclipta *(Eclipta alba)* – This herb helps stop bleeding and strengthens liver and kidney chi. Used for nosebleeds, tinnitus, premature graying of hair and balding, blurred vision.

Echinacea *(Echinacea angustifolia)* – This beautiful plant has strong immune stimulating properties; useful in colds, flu, sore throat, infections, skin eruptions, allergies, viral disease and immune deficiencies. It blocks receptor site of the virus on the surface of the cell membrane preventing infection. Echinacea is a wonderful blood and lymphatic cleanser. It has the ability to cleanse morbid matter from the stomach.

Elder Berry *(Sambucus nigra)* – Elderberry syrup and wine is the most popular cold remedy in Europe, and it is delicious. For anemia, it is an excellent blood tonic. Elder berries and flowers have similar properties. Additionally, the berries are useful for rheumatism. For people with a sensitive and weak stomach it is too strong to use by itself. Always mix with other herbs. It increases digestive activity and secretion, materials are moved along at a better rate. Digestion is improved; congestion and stagnation are removed, decongestion of the liver is enhanced, which moves the stool. During WW II, people in Germany would gather elder along roadsides to cure diphtheria.

Elder Flower *(Sambucus nigra)* – A hot tea has diaphoretic, (sweat-inducing) properties, useful for colds, flu, fever. A cool tea affects the urinary tract with its diuretic properties. It generally detoxifies matter that has been in the body for a long time and has hardened. Soothes inflammation, heals burns and cuts. Cleanses the skin, clears complexion of freckles and eases sunburn. Has a positive effect on many kinds of skin problems, such as irritated skin, roseacea, eczema and boils.

Elecampane *(Inula helenium)* – Elecampane is an excellent expectorant. It is a traditional remedy for respiratory tract infections, relieving irritation due to excessive coughing. It brings up and dissolves phlegm. Has the highest naturally occurring source of inulin, a precursor to insulin to support the pancreas. Elecampagne lowers excessive blood sugar levels, and can prevent tooth decay and gum disease.

Eleuthero/Siberian Ginseng *(Eleutherococcis senticosis)* – This is a well-researched herb for balancing endocrine activity, promoting strength and energy, enhancing work or athletic performance. It acts on the adrenal glands to normalize stress hormone levels thereby smoothing out the peaks and valleys of energy that characterize chronic stress. Normalizes blood pressure, if high blood pressure is due to stress, strengthens immune activity, reduces fatigue, stress, depression and arteriosclerosis. Soothes the emotional ups and downs during menopause and also reduces hot flashes. It curbs irritability, helps during emotional suffering, aids in many nervous disorders, improves cerebral circulation and alertness. I call it the "Happy Pill".

Ephedra *(see MaHuang and Mormon Tea)*

Epimedium/Horny Goat Weed *(Epimedium grandiflorum)* – This herb is also known as yin yang huo, elfenblume, gokshura, puncture vine, goat head, and horny goat weed. It is a powerful remedy in Traditional Chinese Medicine and has been used for thousands of years to promote male potency, libido, increasing sperm count, and as an aphrodisiac. Modern Chinese herbal medicine uses epimedium (usually in combination with other herbs) not just to treat impotence, but also for asthma, bronchitis, cervical dysphasia, congestive heart failure, leucorrhoea, leukopenia, and viral infections of the heart. Epimedium is also used to treat menopause in women often combined with morinda. It slows down aging and promotes longevity. In Eastern Europe this herb is being used to strengthen muscles. It seems to encourage the production and reception of androgens, including testosterone, which plays an important part in increasing libido.

Eucalyptus *(Eucalyptus globulus)* – With its antiseptic and expectorant properties, eucalyptus leaves can be made into an herb tea to relieve bronchitis and respiratory congestion, as well as the flu and pneumonia. Eucalyptus can also be used as a steam inhalation to relieve sinus congestion and to facilitate expectoration.

Evening Primrose *(Oenothera biennis)* – Evening primrose has attracted much attention as a medicinal plant, because the oil of the seeds contains high concentrations of gamma-linolenic acid. As a result, evening primrose has demonstrated value in treating conditions like eczema, asthma, rheumatoid arthritis, breast problems and metabolic disorders. The whole plant can be harvested at any time for culinary purposes. The leaves can be enjoyed fresh or steamed. The first year's taproots can also be eaten fresh or boiled like potatoes. The flowers can be added to salads or any other dish as a bright and cheerful garnish. Seeds can be added to breads and biscuits, steamed, or roasted for 15 minutes at 400 degrees F and sprinkled on food.

Eyebright *(Euphrasia officinalis)* – Eyebright has a drying effect and can be used for watery eyes and runny nose. It is a vaso-constrictor and astringent to the nasal and conjunctiva mucous membranes. It brings relief in frequent sneezing bouts. It is also effective for colds, sinus congestion and allergies. As an eye wash, eyebright strengthens the eyes, improves eyesight, and may prevent and reverse cataracts.

False Unicorn *(Chamaelirium luteum)* – This is now an endangered species and as of this writing, no longer available. It is an herb that has been successfully used by midwives to help pregnant women prevent miscarriages. It has safely been used for infertility and to ease morning sickness and nausea during pregnancy. This herb strengthens the female and male reproductive system and may be useful for weakness and congestion of the male and female reproductive organs. It is also indicated for boggy prostate, impotence, infertility, uterine prolapse, ovarian pain, urinary system weakness, and for liver and kidney diseases.

Fennel *(Foeniculu vulgare)* – Fennel improves digestion (especially protein digestion), increases peristalsis, relieves gas, promotes appetite, quiets hiccups, eliminates gout, and dispels worms. It is used with laxatives to prevent cramping. Fennel enriches the quantity and quality of mother's milk, which carries over to the baby to help with colic. It is excellent after radiation and chemotherapy, as it absorbs the toxins. It clears phlegm from the respiratory system, curbs appetite and alleviates hunger pains. Fennel can be used after radiation and chemotherapy to cleanse all the tissues in the body.

Fenugreek *(Trigonella foenum-graecum)* – Fenugreek is a good expectorant for coughs and colds; as a gargle, it can relieve a sore throat. It counteracts catarrh and phlegm, and eliminates uric acid through the lymphatic system. It enriches the quantity and quality of mother's milk. It has also been used as a natural birth control herb. Fenugreek has drawing powers, contains 30% mucilage, which makes it an essential when adding to poultices to treat wounds, inflammation, and other skin problems. Increases breast size.

Feverfew *(Tanacetum parthenium)* – The ancient Greek physician Dioscorides recommended this herbs for all inflammations and hot swellings. Feverfew comes from Latin "febrifugia", which means, "driver out of fevers", and today feverfew is very much under used. It has been used successfully for pain, migraine headaches, chills, fevers, colds, and inflammation from arthritis. Alcohol destroys feverfew's benefits, therefore is should not be made into an extract.

Figwort *(Scrophularia nodosa)* – This herb works on lymph, blood and skin, indicated for chronic conditions such as eczema, psoriasis and acne. It is also effective for lymphatic stagnation, hemorrhoids and cystic breasts.

Fireweed *(Small Flowered Willow)*

Flaxseed *(Linum usitatissimum)* – Flaxseeds are high in Omega-3 fatty acids with their beneficial effect for cardiovascular diseases, to reduce inflammation, allergies, even cancer. Flaxseeds are a great non-habit forming laxative and stool softener.

Flaxseed Tea

Flaxseed tea can be helpful during a gallbladder attack. Mix 1 tbsp organic flaxseeds with 12 oz of purified water in a glass or stainless steel pot. Bring to a boil and simmer for 10 minutes. Strain and sip slowly while the tea is hot/warm.

Flaxseed Spread

1/3 cup hazelnuts or walnuts
¼ cup flaxseeds
¼ cup honey

Grind hazelnuts or walnuts and flaxseeds until they are pulverized. Place in a small glass bowl. Add the honey and mix well. Serve on toast or firm whole-grain cracker, or apple.

Foti *(see He Shou Wu)*

Forsythia *(Forsythia suspense)* – Used in Chinese medicine known as Lian Qiao, this herb is effective against a wide spectrum of bacteria and fungi. Mostly used to treat flus and colds, to reduce fever and boost immunity. It is also helpful for inflammation in the body.

Foxglove *(Digitalis purpurea)* –Foxglove was discovered in the 1700's to stimulate the kidneys to release excess fluid, and a tea brewed from the foxglove leaves was used in treating dropsy, a disease in which water accumulates in the body and causes it to swell up. It is a source of digitalis, important for its stimulating and regulating action on the heart. It is too powerful to use without medical supervision. In small amounts, this herb is known to treat edema associated with congestive heart condition. In large doses, it is a deadly poison, and will likely stop the heart.
Caution: Poison. Do not use!

Fringe Tree *(Chionanthus virginicum)* – Fringe Tree is a cholagogue and antispasmodic, and primarily affects the liver and gallbladder. It is indicated in cases of bilious colic, jaundice, gallstone pain, and non-inflammatory liver problems in a person with yellow sclera, hepatic pain and light gray stools.

Ganoderma/Reishi *(Ganoderma lucidum)* – This fungus (mushroom) is indicated for immune hypo- (cancer, AIDS and chronic fatigue syndrome) or hyper-functioning (lupus, rheumatoid arthritis, crohn's disease, and ankylosing spondylitis. Ganoderma is an active anti-hepatotoxin as well as a cardiotonic, antioxidant and nervine. It is also used for ADD/ADHD (disturbed shen) and for lowering cholesterol levels. It is also used to treat altitude sickness, allergies, insomnia and leukopenia.

Garcinia *(Garcinia cambogia)* – This fruit may be helpful in controlling appetite, thereby reducing weight. Research has shown that garcinia triggers fatty acid oxidation in the liver, preventing excess carbohydrates from turning into fat. It is an appetite suppressant, burning fat via thermogenesis, supplying the body with more energy. Garcinia prevents the formation of fatty tissues.

Gardenia *(Gardenia jasminoides)* – Gardenia (Zhi Zi) flowers are used in Chinese medicine to flavor teas. The fruits are used for fever, high blood pressure, insomnia, hepatitis and for sprains, swellings and bruises. The flowers are a main source of essential oil used in aromatherapy and in the perfume industry. Gardenia is the happiness plant.

Garlic *(Allium sativa)* – Garlic is also known as "Russian penicillin", because of its strong antibiotic, anti-microbial, anti-fungal and anti-parasitic action. It is a general health enhancer, lowers blood pressure and cholesterol. Fresh garlic protects against colon cancer, it is a stimulant, diaphoretic, expectorant and stomachic. Garlic stimulates the lymphatic system to throw off waste materials. Do not use garlic herbal supplements also known as "social garlic", because they are devoid of "allicin" (the sulfur smell), where its medicinal properties lie.

Gayfeather *(Liatris spicata)* – The tuberose roots can be prepared as a soothing tea for kidney ailments or as a gargle for sore throats.

Gentian *(Gentiana lutea)* – Gentian is one of the most bitter tonics. It stimulates appetite and digestive secretions. It supplies abdominal organs with lots of blood, and stimulates adrenaline. Gentian is a famous European alpine herb, recognized in strengthening the body, particularly for weak digestion, absorption, and lack of appetite. It has been used in people suffering from leukemia.

Germander *(Teucrium chamaedrys)* – This herb can be made up into a tea to quiet an upset stomach and to promote appetite. It was once consumed in treating gout.

Ginger *(Zingiber officinale)* – For indigestion and gas pain, motion sickness, nausea, and a general stimulant aiding respiratory congestion and joint pain. Increases absorption of whatever is ingested by 30 %, food, vitamins, etc., even pharmaceutical drugs. A hospital in Israel confirms that when patients ingest ginger for nausea while undergoing chemotherapy treatments, it significantly raised their levels of chemo-drugs in their bloodstreams. Therefore, they simply lowered their drug dosage. Increases HCL. It is an excellent free radical scavenger and anti-oxidant. Today's commercial Ginger Ale does not contain natural ginger. Paul Schulik wrote a book on ginger and states that ginger is "good for everything".
Dried root: internal warming, digestion. Fresh root: external warming, diaphoretic.

Ginkgo *(Ginkgo biloba)* – When looking at a gingko leaf, it looks very similar to our brain. Ginkgo stimulates cerebral circulation and oxygenation, therefore increasing mental energy, mental focus and mental clarity. It improves peripheral circulation, and is a vasodilator. It increases the supply of blood to the body's vital tissues and organs, such as the brain and heart. Gingko may be helpful for tinnitus through increased circulation to the inner ear. Ginkgo also improves eyesight, such as macular degeneration. Ginkgo is a longevity herb.

Ginseng, American *(Panax quiquefolium)* – American Ginseng has long been recognized as being the world's best ginseng. Although it is similar to Asian ginseng, it differs in chemical structure. Asian ginseng is warming, builds energy and heat in the body, where as American ginseng is more neutral in its effects and tends to cool and calm the system. American ginseng reduces fatigue, strengthens adrenal response, enhances reproductive performance, improves liver metabolism and enhances immunity. The Chinese regard American Ginseng as a yin tonic, reducing heat in the digestive and respiratory systems. For this reason it is considered more favorable for individuals with a hotter constitution. American Ginseng has also been used to strengthen the blood (not just for anemia), for exhaustion, especially when exhaustion is due to stress, as well as for sexual weakness.

Ginseng, Korean *(Panax ginseng)* – Korean and Chinese ginsengs are extraordinary herbs to rejuvenate the body, regenerate frayed or overtaxed nerves, and to discourage mood swings and depression. Although panax ginseng has a particular affinity for the male body to build strength and to nourish the reproductive and circulatory systems, it can also be used by women for a short time, about 6 weeks with a 6 months break in between. Women who need to build strength and energy greatly benefit from panax ginseng's grounding and yang (masculine) qualities. Panax ginseng is often available as "white" or "red" ginseng. White ginseng is unprocessed and helpful in assisting digestion and when recovering from an illness. Red ginseng is actually white ginseng that has been cooked and dried. Processing ginseng roots in this way affects the ginsenosides, ginseng's active ingredients, which makes red ginseng more heating and stimulating, good for physical activities and as a sexual tonic.

Ginseng, Siberian *(see Eleuthero)*

Ginseng, Tienchi *(Panax notoginseng)* – This is a lesser known panax ginseng. It is mostly used for injuries and trauma due to its strong haemostatic action for acute conditions. It can be used internally and externally for bleeding, swelling and pain caused by traumatic injuries, even gunshot wounds. Tienchi ginseng is often preferred for younger people and those that are active in sports. It improves the flow of chi, strengthens the heart and improves athletic capacities. For people with heart conditions this is the preferred ginseng, as it does not over stimulate, which can occur with the other ginsengs.

Goat's Rue *(Galega officinalis)* – A lesser known herb used to help reduce blood sugar levels and thus is indicated for diabetes. It is also a powerful galactagogue, stimulating the production and flow of mother's milk. It may also stimulate the development of the mammary glands.

Goji *(see Lycii)*

Goldenrod *(Solidago odorata)* – This gentle and safe herb is one of the best choices for hay fever and allergies, (it slows down histamine release) when the eyes are red and irritated, and there is congestion, sneezing and a runny nose. It also relieves cramping when there is gas. It is a specific for weak kidneys, when the kidneys cannot suck in new blood and process the buildup of waste materials. It can be used for kidney stones or for inflammation/ulceration in the bladder. Goldenrod

152

soothes and tones the urinary tract, and rebuilds/regenerates the urinary system. Goldenrod is for people who lack endurance, or are unable to persevere through difficulties.

Gokshura/Puncture Vine *(Tribulus terrestris)* - Supports the proper functioning of the urinary tract. Gokshura has also been used effectively for nonspecific impotence and to increases sperm production.

Goldenseal *(Hydrastis canadensis)* – Goldenseal is often referred to "the King of the mucous membranes". Goldenseal's effectiveness is due to its primary active component hydrazine. Another constituent is berberine, found also in barberry and Oregon grape root. Goldenseal is a powerful anti-microbial, to combat colds, flu, diarrhea and infections. It can be used topically for skin infections, as an eye wash, as well as for mucous membrane inflammations. Because it has the ability to cleanse mucous membranes, it is an excellent choice for respiratory infections. Goldenseal reduces blood sugar and can relieve stress and anxiety due to high blood sugar levels. It is also being used for female problems, such as inflammation of the vagina, uterus, and urethra. Goldenseal has shown to stimulate macrophages and tumor inhibitors.
Caution: Because goldenseal has a tendency to lower blood sugar, and if this is a problem, use myrrh instead.

Gotu Kola *(Centella asiatica)* – Gotu kola is one of the best herbs to calm, rejuvenate and revitalize the nerves and brain, strengthens memory and intelligence, and improves concentration. In Sri Lanka, gotu kola is a favorite food for elephants. Gotu kola promotes mental clarity. It balances right and left brain, excellent to take in a glass of milk before meditations. Good for emotionally caused depression, especially when accompanied with sluggish digestion, and for treating a nervous breakdown. Gotu kola also improves blood circulation.

Gravel Root/Queen of the Meadow *(Eupatorium purpurea)* – Gravel root is known to break kidney stones and flush sediments from the kidneys, soothing mucosal irritations in the urinary tract, good to use when there is blood in the urine, as well as for fluid retention, and frequent nighttime urination.

Graviola/Soursop *(Annona muricata)* - This is a small evergreen tree from the Amazon Rainforest. Natives have a rich history of using this herb for its profound healing properties – among them, for immune, circulatory and lymphatic support. Graviola has very strong abilities to prevent abnormal cellular division. It is used as a heart tonic, nervine, for colds and flu, even cancer.

Green Tea *(Chamellia sinensis)* - Strong flavonoid content gives this plant antioxidant properties defending the body against free radicals and supporting the immune system. Reduces LDL serum levels and can keep blood sugar levels from rising even though it is a nervous system stimulant containing caffeine.

Grindelia/Gumweed *(Grindelia spp)* – This resinous herb has a toning effect on the lungs and the kidneys. Its stimulating action makes it useful as an antispasmodic expectorant and diuretic, good for asthma, coughs and pneumonia. Grindelia acts to relax smooth muscles and heart muscles. This explains its use in the treatment of asthmatic and bronchial conditions when associated with a rapid heartbeat and nervousness. Because of its relaxing effect on the heart and pulse rate, there may be a reduction in blood pressure. Externally, use the fresh plant as a poultice for dermatitis caused by poison ivy and poison oak, to reduce itching, and to dry up lesions.

Ground Ivy *(Glechoma hederacea)* – Ground ivy is a common plant and is little known for its anti-viral, expectorant, diuretic, diaphoretic and anti-inflammatory properties. It can also remove lead from the body.

Guaiac/Lignum Vitae *(Guaiacum officinale)* – This tree provides constituents that are anti-inflammatory, diuretic and alterative. Used for osteo-arthrititis, rheumatoid arthritis and Lyme's disease.

Guarana *(Paullinia cupana)* – A central nervous stimulant, this plant contains caffeine. It is a mood elevator, aphrodisiac and "be happy" herb.

Guar Gum *(Cyamopsis tetragonoloba)* – Guar gum is a fiber from the seed of guar gum, a dietary water soluble fiber to assist in curbing appetite. It is also being used as a laxative, to treat diarrhea, diabetes, obesity, cholesterol, and to prevent the hardening of the arteries (atherosclerosis). Guar gum is used in the food and cosmetic industries as a thickening agent. Guar gum works by normalizing the moisture content of stool, absorbing excess liquid in diarrhea, and softening the stool in constipation. Caution: Do not use when experiencing colon disorders or gastrointestinal surgery.

Gum Arabic *(see Acacia)*

Gumweed *(see Grindelia)*

Gymnema *(Gymnema sylvestris)* – Gymnema has a molecular structure similar to that of sugar that can block absorption of up to fifty percent of dietary sugar calories. This sugar blocking action works well in cases of diabetes, reducing insulin requirements, and for weight loss in people on high sugar/carbohydrate diets.

Hawthorn *(Crataegus oxycantha)* – Hawthorn is a specific tonic herb for the cardiovascular system bringing micronutrients to the heart, arteries and capillaries. It restores the cardiovascular system, strengthens blood vessels, excellent to use for any type of cardiovascular problem, such as cardiac weakness, mitral valve prolapse, cholesterol, hypo - and hypertension, and fatty degeneration. Hawthorn also acts on connective tissues, supportive in chiropractic treatments, when there is an inability to hold spinal adjustments, as well as for hernias, hemorrhoids, varicose veins, prolapsed organs, and collagen deficiency. Hawthorn berries are for the heart and hawthorn leaf and flower for blood circulation.

Helonias *(see False Unicorn)*

Hen-and-Chicks *(Sempervivum tectorum)* – Freshly pressed leaves and their juice are used externally to soothe skin conditions, including burns, wounds, ulcers, insect bites, sore nipples, inflammations, hemorrhoids, eczema, fungal infections, as well as itchy and burning parts of the skin. Infusions are used internally to treat inflammations of the mucous membranes and has long been used to treat dysentery, diarrhea, worm infestations, and for heavy menstrual bleeding. Gargles of the juice may be used to treat throat inflammations, including tonsillitis and stomatitis (inflammations of the oral cavity. Traditionally, the leaves were chewed to relieve toothache and the juice sniffed to stop nosebleeds.

He Shou Wu/Foti *(Polygonum multiflorum)* – This is a tonifying herb to nourish the kidneys, liver and the blood, and to stimulate liver and bowel function, and to lower cholesterol levels. This legendary oriental "elixir of life" offers fantastic rejuvenative properties. Some believe that Professor Li Chung Yun who lived to the ripe old age of 256 used He Shou Wu.

Hibiscus *(Hibiscus sabdariffa)* – Hibiscus is best known for its beautiful flower, but also for its unique medicinal properties. It improves cardiovascular function, supports healthy cholesterol levels, promotes healthy blood pressure, and supports healthy blood glucose levels. Hibiscus has antioxidant properties to fight cellular damage and to support the immune system. Studies have shown that drinking two cups of hibiscus tea a day for four weeks lowers blood pressure significantly. Anthocyanin is one of the components found in hibiscus flowers, which are known to improve the functioning of blood vessels and to strengthen the protein collagen to give structure to cells and tissues, including blood vessels.

Hing *(see Asafoetida)*

Holy Basil *(see Basil, Holy)*

Honeybush *(Cyclopia intermedia)* – Indigenous to a small mountainous region in Southern Africa, honeybush makes a deliciously sweet tea with many health benefits. Honeybush is caffeine free and rich in anti-oxidants. South African scientific studies have established that honeybush can regulate women's menstrual cycle, prevent breast -, prostate- and uterine cancer, reduce the risk of osteoporosis, contains anti-fungal and anti-viral properties, lowers fat and cholesterol levels, and is anti-depressant, anti-inflammatory and anti-diabetic.

Honeysuckle *(Lonicera japonica)* – Honeysuckle is a powerful anti-bacterial and anti-viral, effective in treating influenza, sore throat, colds, urinary and intestinal infections, and mastitis.

Hops *(Humulus lupulus)* – Hops has long been used for making beer. For gastric spasms due to nervousness, this strong muscle relaxant and sedative herb can be used during times of high anxiety to calm and promote restful sleep. Hops has also been used to decrease the desire for alcohol. It cleanses the liver and increases the flow of bile.
Caution: Do not use during times of depression.

Sleep Inducing Pillow

Fill a pillow with hops, lavender, and flaxseeds.
Sleeping on this pillow may provide you with a non drug-induced sleep, calming nerves and prevent nightmares.

Horehound *(Marrubium vulgare)* – Horehound candies and syrups have been known since Victorian times to soothe a sore throat, to treat lung congestion and coughs. It also sustains healthy vocal cords, for hoarseness, laryngitis and lung congestion. Horehound can be used to treat stomach conditions and to remove obstructions from the liver and the spleen.

Horny Goat Weed *(see Epimedium)*

Horse Chestnut *(Aesculus hippocastanum)* – Horse chestnut is a vago-tonic, to strengthen and tone veins, and to soothe irritated varicose veins. It has been used for leg pain and swelling due to varicose veins and poor circulation in the legs.

Horseradish *(Cochlearia armoracia)* – This culinary root vegetable is best known for its ability to cleanse sinuses and open up air passages. But it can also be used for digestion problems, to increase stomach secretions, as a diuretic, when there is excessive water retention, expectorant, for damp lung problems, asthma, allergic rhinitis, post-nasal drip, and parasites. Externally, horseradish can be applied as a pain relieving compress for neuralgia, pain the in the back of the neck, and for stiffness.

Horsetail/Shavegrass *(Equisitum arvense)* – The botanical name for this herb is derived from Latin meaning "horse bristle", because of the plant's signature. It is high in minerals, especially silica and calcium, and is well known as being a "bone-knitter". Silica allows for calcium absorption and is therefore recommended for brittle fingernails, broken bones, osteoporosis, porous teeth, hair split-ends, to repair damaged bone cartilage, to revitalize the skin, for toning connective tissue, to increase urine production and to shrink inflamed mucosal tissues, particularly the prostate and bladder. Silica found in horsetail also aids circulation. Horsetail is good for the eyes, ear, nose, throat and the glandular system. Externally, use horsetail in a bath to invigorate the body and to increase metabolism. Children are supple and limber because they have large amounts of silica in their body. As we age, the body becomes heavy with too much calcium and therefore we use our ability to become stiff and immobile.

Hydrangea *(Hydrangea arborescens)* – This herb increases the flow of urine and is indicated for urethritis or cystitis. It relieves the pain and eases the passing of urinary stones. Hydrangea can be used for back pain caused by kidney problems. It is also effective for arthritis and rheumatism due to calcium deposits in the body.

Hyssop *(Hyssopus officinalis)* – Hyssop has many uses. It is an anti-viral especially effective for inhibiting herpes and influenza viruses. This fragrant herb is a carminative, emmenagogue and diaphoretic. Hyssop can be used for intestinal viruses, colds, flu, nausea, flatulence and delayed menses. It has also been used for sleeplessness and nervousness.

Indian Gooseberry *(see Amalaki/Amla)*

Indian Pipe *(Monotropa uniflora)* – Indian pipe is helpful in formulas for pain management, its action being similar in effect to nitrous oxide, making one conscious and aware of pain, but distant from it.

Inmortal *(Asclepias asperula)* – Inmortal is a good medicine for asthma, pleurisy and bronchitis, as it stimulates lymph drainage and dilates bronchial tubes. As a mild, reliable cardiac tonic, especially for congestive heart disorders, it relieves pressure on the heart valve. It is also a strong diaphoretic and menses stimulant. In the fall dig out some roots, cut them up into small pieces and dry them. After they are dry use mix ½ teaspoon with one cup of water, bring to a boil, then simmer for 30 minutes. Drink one cup 3 – 4 times a day for respiratory conditions. The root acts as a bronchial dilator, while stimulating lymphatic drainage. In the kitchen, the unopened flower buds can be cooked, just like peas. Young shoots, less than a few inches tall can be eaten as an asparagus substitute. Young seed pods are very appetizing. The seeds are delicious sprouted.

Iporuru *(Alchornea castaneifolia)* – This plant is well-known to the Indigenous people of Peru for soothing aching joints and improving flexibility in movement and range of motion, as well as for recovery after battle and hard work. It is also effective for arthritis pain and inflammation.

Isatis/Woad *(Isatis tinctoria)* – Known to be a potent natural herbal antibiotic, as it kills a broad range of germs. A Chinese herb used for dry and sore throat, heat rash, abscesses, and swelling due to internal heat excess. Isatis has also been used for delirium and fainting spells.

Jamaican Dogwood *(Piscidia erythrina)* – Jamaican dogwood is an anti-depressant herb with uplifting properties, and a good pain reliever. Good to use when someone has pain and cannot go to sleep. It is used especially for painful periods (dysmenorrhea) and facial nerve pain (Bell's palsy, trigeminal neuralgia and TMJ). This tropical bark can also be used for back pain, acute pain and spasms of the bladder, vagina and muscles.
Caution: Dilates pupils.

Jerusalem Artichoke *(Helianthus tuberosus)* – Jerusalem artichoke balances and stabilizes blood sugar levels, reduces sugar cravings and hypoglycemia, improves calcium absorption and has a positive effect on intestinal flora. People in Europe use Jerusalem artichoke for weightloss with great success. It is suggested to eat artichoke one day cooked and the other day raw, and so on, for the best benefit.

Jerusalem Artichoke Salad

Mix 1 cup well-scrubbed and chopped Jerusalem artichokes and 1 cup chopped carrots. Blend 3 Tbsp olive oil, 1 ½ Tbsp lemon juice, 1 – 2 Tbsp fresh tarragon, and 1 Tbsp capers. Mix everything together and serve.

Jerusalem Artichoke, Roasted

Preheat oven to 500 degrees. Scrub and peel 1 lb Jerusalem artichokes and place in a shallow roasting pan. Mix 3 cloves of garlic, chopped, with 2 Tbsp olive oil and drizzle over chokes. Add salt and pepper. Cook for about 20 minutes, tossing once or twice.

Other Jerusalem Artichoke Recipe Ideas

Here are some other ideas you can cook up with Jerusalem artichokes: carrot and artichoke soup, artichokes with rosemary in wine, artichoke mash (like mash potatoes), and artichoke vegetable medley.

Tip: Jerusalem turn brown very quickly after washing and peeling, use lemon juice to prevent this from happening.

Jujube *(Zizyphus jujube)* – This sweet tasting fruit is nutritive, anti-hepatotoxin, a chi tonic and a nervine. Used for weakness, irritability, and to stabilize the nervous system. Chinese Traditional Medicine (TCM) considers this fruit to calm the shen.

Juniper *(Juniperus communis)* – The berry of juniper is a strong diuretic and urinary antiseptic useful in bladder and kidney conditions, especially when chronic. A stimulant to the stomach for stressed out digestive functions, and for deficient hydrochloric acid production. Juniper increases the elimination of metabolic waste (uric acid, gout) and promotes the vital force within.
Caution: Do not use for hot acute urinary inflammation.

Kava Kava *(Piper methysticum)* – This is a remedy for nervousness and insomnia, known as the Figi Island Spit Drink! Kava kava has analgesic and sedative properties, as well as being one of the most powerful muscle relaxants. Influences the senses (touch, smell…). It is a mucous membrane anodyne, reducing pain and sensation in the throat, stomach and urinary tract. Kava is excellent for genitourinary pain and is also useful for fibromyalgia, restless leg syndrome, muscle spasms and insomnia with muscular tension.

Kelp *(laminaria digitata)* – This mineral rich seaweed promotes and strengthens healthy thyroid function, as well as healthy bowels and proper immune function. It contains alginates that help remove heavy metal contaminants from the body, cleansing and soothing the intestines. High in vitamin content, kelp also contains more than two dozen important minerals as well as trace minerals, proteins, carbohydrates and essential fatty acids. Kelp is known to remove radioactive toxins from the body.

Khella *(Amni visnaga)* – A powerful antispasmodic to the small bronchi, this ancient Egyptian medicinal plant is helpful in preventing asthma attacks, especially at night.

Kola Nut *(Cola nitida)* – This strong stimulant herb can prevent fatigue, as it contains more caffeine than coffee beans.
Caution: Do not use extensively if there the adrenals are stressed and exhausted.

Kudzu *(Pueraria lobata)* – Kudzu can be used as a building tonic for convalescence, debility, run down states, and as a heart tonic. Kudzu grows wild throughout the Japanese countryside and the south-eastern United States, where it had been introduced to reduce soil erosion. It escaped cultivation and is now growing over forests in America, literally. Kudzu vines were once used to weave baskets, ropes and cloth. It is the root that is being used for food and medicine. It is rich in starch. In traditional medicine the starch is seen as being anti-emetic, febrifuge, antidotal, thirst relieving, and diaphoretic. It is used to treat alcoholism, colds, diarrhea, dysentery, enteritis, fever, measles, seating, thirst, insect bites, chicken pox, snakebite, typhoid, skin rashes and more. Kudzu starch is seen as a building tonic which makes the body healthier and better able to resist disease, an ideal medicine to help a person recover from illness. Kudzu is highly effective at suppressing alcohol cravings and improving the function of organs affected by ingestion of alcohol. Kudzu can also reduce high blood pressure, elevated blood sugar, as well as to treat migraine headaches and stomach acidity. In addition, Kudzu root has also been used for deafness, torticollis, back spasms, angina pain, and mild congestive heart failure, for sinus congestion, irritable bowel syndrome and diarrhea. The best way to use kudzu starch is to make a hot drink with it. Place two teaspoons of kudzu root starch and a tablespoon of honey or sugar in a cup, add one tablespoon of cold water, mix well, then add little by little one cup of hot water, mix again until smooth. You may add a little ginger, raw or powdered. This drink is excellent for a weak and debilitated person, because it gives quality carbohydrates, which are easily absorbed by the body. One hot cup of kudzu in the morning is wonderful for those experiencing heart problems. Regular use can improve cardiovascular function. Kudzu root starch can be used in the same way as arrowroot, corn starch, gelatin, or flour to thicken sauces and puddings.

Lady's Slipper *(Cypripedium pubescens)* – Lady's slipper calms all stresses, insomnia, tension and anxiety. It has a sedative effect, relieves muscle spasms and makes an effective remedy for recurring headaches. Lady's slipper is good for someone who needs grounding.

Energizing Kudzu Tea

Dissolve 1 tsp kudzu root starch in 1 cup of cold water and add a dash of freshly grated ginger root. Heat it up and bring to a boil, stirring until the tea begins to thicken. Remove from heat and drink warm.

Lady's Mantle *(Alchemilla vulgaris)* - Known as a woman's herb. Lady's mantle is good for balancing the reproductive system, especially for young girls (menarche). Monks collect dew from lady's mantle to make holy water, which cleanses all illnesses. It is useful for women who have a hard time accepting pregnancy and the "mantle" of motherhood. It also tonifies the uterus after childbirth.

Lavender *(Lavendula angustifolia)* – This beautiful flower has cooling and nervine properties, useful for emotional upset, depression and pain. It is tonifying against faintness and palpitations due to a nervous heart. Gets rid of headaches. Lavender also has anti-viral and anti-bacterial properties. Spiritually, it connects to one's higher self.

Lemon Balm *(Melissa officinalis)* – Melissa is a Greek word and means "Bee". Lemon balm strengthens the nervous system, the heart and the stomach area. It loosens harden mucous in the digestive tract and soothes the mucus membranes. As a nervine, it eases digestive tract spasms and is also helpful for nervous tension, depression, migraine, anxiety, as well as heart palpitation and insomnia. The tea brings comfort to women after giving birth, strengthens the emotional heart to prevent postpartum blues. Lemon balm is a good tasting remedy, appropriate for children's colds, stomachaches and headaches. It can also be used on the skin, as a wash or spritzer to eliminate all sorts of skin conditions.

A Well-Known Old European Remedy

The following remedy can be carried in your purse to have on hand while away from home, in case you experience indigestion, anxiety, dizziness, headaches, faintness, or any kind of discomfort. It is known in Europe as a sort of "rescuing" medicine. As a child I use to get carsick. My grandma always brought with her that little brown bottle and she would place a few drops of the medicine on a sugar cube. I would then gladly take her medicine; it tasted good and made me feel well again.

To Make:
Place equal parts of lemon balm and peppermint into a glass jar. Add water and brandy in equal parts to cover the herbs, tighten the lid and place the jar in a warm place or sunny window for approximately 4-6 days. Then strain the liquid and add equal parts of honey or cane sugar. Mix and transfer into a dark bottle.

Lemon Grass *(Cymbopogon citracus)* – This fragrant grass can be made into a tea to treat colds, stomach problems, abdominal cramps, headaches, dizziness and stress. Lemon grass is an excellent blood cleanser, good to add to cleansing formulas.

Lemon Verbena *(Aloysia triphulla)* – Sometimes called vervein, lemon verbena can be beneficial for strengthening the nervous system, easing stress, improving digestion, easing colic, reducing fevers during a cold, and relieving spasms in the digestive track (colon). It can also be used for coughs (expectorant).

Licorice *(Glycerrhiza glabra)* – This is a demulcent and expectorant herb for coughs and respiratory congestion. This sweet herb is an adaptogen, demulcent, expectorant, anti-viral and anti-depressant. Licorice strengthens endocrine function, especially the adrenals, ovaries, Isles of Langerhans and hypothalamus making it useful for chronic fatigue, menopausal symptoms, hypoglycemia and auto-immune disease. Promotes estrogen production; increases energy and improves adrenal function. Has a soothing influence upon gastric mucosa, it's an excellent remedy for peptic and duodenal ulcerations, arthritic symptoms and chronic constipation. Liquefies mucus!
Caution: Do not use in the case of heart conditions, causes water retention and elevate blood pressure!

Ligusticum *(Ligusticum wallichii)* – This plant is related to osha root, helpful for amenorrhea, dysmenorrhea and abdominal pain. In TCM it is used to move blood and Chi and important for "Wind" conditions – sudden headaches, dizziness and itchy skin rashes.

Ligustrum *(Ligustrum lucidum)* - The berries are used as a tonic for yin-deficient kidney and liver. Symptoms include dizziness, spots before the eyes, lower back pain and tinnitus. They also stimulate immune activity especially to increase white blood cell count depleted by chemotherapy or radiation.

Lily of the Valley *(Convallaria majalis)* – This early spring plant with its fragrant white flowers has a similar action as digitalis but is less toxic, to promote regular heart action and to increase blood pressure in hypotensive cases.
Caution: Should be administered by a knowledgeable healthcare practitioner.

Linden *(Tilea spp)* – A tea made from the flowers and leaves is delicious and thirst quenching. The linden tree is large and beautiful, and simply by sitting under it, one is "healed". Many poetries and songs were written in honor of this noble tree. Linden has diaphoretic properties, useful in breaking fevers. It is specifically for a person who has a cold/fever and cannot relax. It is also helpful for nervous tension, stress and insomnia due to its relaxing properties. For the type A person it can prevent the development of arteriosclerosis, hypertension, when associated with nervous condition. Linden can be found in high-end cosmetic, as it softens and calms the skin.

Lipstick Tree *(see Annatto)*

Lobelia *(Lobelia inflata)* – Known as the Indian tobacco, lobelia is a strong bronchial dilator, expectorant, and antispasmodic, used for asthma and any lung congestion, as well as hiccoughs. Lobelia attaches to the same receptor site in the brain which nicotine attaches to, helpful when one wants to quit smoking. Use it in small dosages, because in larger doses, lobelia paralyzes the cerebrospinal centers and will cause nausea and a drop in blood pressure.

Lomatium *(Lomatium dissectum)* – Lomatium is a powerful anti-viral/bacterial for urinary and pulmonary conditions, as well as for treating colds and flu. Lomatium may prove useful for Lyme's disease.
Caution: Do not use long term, may induce wide spread rash and a low-grade fever due to the body's cleansing process!

Lovage *(Levisticum officinale)* – Lovage has a celery scented fragrance and has long been used to flavor fine liquors and digestive bitters. Lovage stimulates a healthy appetite for those who have lost interest in food, promotes strong digestion, relieves a congested liver, relieves water retention, and improves circulation. The French consider lovage to have powerful antitoxic actions against poisons. Lovage has also been used for psoriasis, parasites, and as a vermifuge, especially against tapeworm.

Lycii/Goji *(Lycium chinense)* – In TCM it is used especially to increase circulation to the lower extremities. e.g. cold feet, varicose veins, and peripheral neuropathy. Rich in flavonoid compounds which strengthen vascular integrity. Lycium is also used to strengthen the eyes.

Maca *(Lepidium meyenii)* – Maca is a tuber that has been cultivated for more than 2,000 years at high altitudes in the Andean mountains. Maca is used for energy, longevity and fertility. It has also been widely used by athletes to enhance energy levels and to help build muscle mass and strength. Maca does not contain hormones itself. Instead, it provides a unique set of nutrients that directly fuel the endocrine system and help the glands produce vital hormones in precise dosages predetermined by one's own body.

Magnolia Bark *(Magnolia officinalis)* – In the Chinese system it is known to be effective in relieving pressure, fullness and oppression in the abdominal region. It can also be used for abdominal pain, oppression in the chest, excess phlegm in the respiratory tract, and shortness of breath.

Magnolia Flower *(Magnolia liliflora)* – A Chinese source says that the unopened flower of the magnolia tree "corrects" the energy in the body. It is further said to warm the three burner spaces, lubricate the muscles, benefit the nine body cavities, open up the nose, expel mucous, reduce facial swelling, and promote the growth of hair.

Ma Huang *(Ephedra sinica)* – Ma huang may be beneficial for the temporary relief of hay fever, sinus congestion and allergy induced asthma. Opens air passages due to its antispasmodic action; it is a bronchial dilator. Because of its stimulating action, with extended use, it will deplete the adrenal reserves and leads to problems like nervousness, adrenal exhaustion, hypertension and insomnia. If mahuang is the herb of choice, take with astragalus. Astragalus replenishes the adrenal glands. Caution: Do not use if there is hypertension, cardiac problems, or when taking MAO inhibiting medication.

Maitake *(Grifola frondulosa)* – This mushroom is indicated for hyper immune response (allergies, auto-immune disease) or hypo immune activity (cancer, HIV, etc.) It has been useful in therapy for AIDS, cancer and hypertension. Maitake's liver protecting activity makes it an excellent part of any hepatitis protocol.

Manaca *(Brunfelsia uniflorus, grandiflora)* – Manaca is a blood purifier and helps remove excess body fluid. The root of manaca is said to stimulate the lymphatic system. Herbal healers along the Amazon use a root decoction of manaca to treat arthritis, rheumatism, colds and flu, uterine cramps.

Maravilla *(Mirabilis multiflorum)* – As an appetite suppressant, it relieves hunger pangs by anesthetizing the stomach lining, allowing one to go longer between meals.

Mangosteen *(Garcinia mangostana)* – Mangostein has anti-bacterial, anti-fungal and anti-tumor properties. According to recent laboratory research, mangostein extract may fight against several cancers, including breast, liver and leukemia. It also appears to have anti-histamine and anti-inflammatory properties. Some of the benefits: antioxidant protection against free radicals, maintains immune system health, promotes joint flexibility, provides positive mental support, reduces allergies, and reduces joint inflammation. The way mangostein works is on a cellular level, it enhances the natural state of the cell structure of the body. When the cells function at the optimum, then every process of the body functions better, metabolism, assimilation, elimination and detoxification.

Maral *(Rhaponticum carthamoides)* – This plant can be found growing wild in southern Siberia. Maral root is an adaptogenic herb traditionally used to alleviate fatigue, treat impotence, speed recovery from illness and improve mood in cases of mild depression, improves memory and learning, and increases working capacity of tired skeletal muscles. Research has shown that maral root can significantly increase muscle mass, while decreasing body fat in people who exercise at the same time, while reducing mental and physical fatigue. Aids the body in the synthesis of protein, protect the body from environmental stress, replenish depleted physical and psychical reserves due to hard training and exhaustion. Maral root stimulates and enhances the body's natural steroids, but does not have a long term negative impact on the physiology as many unnatural steroids do. It

increases metabolism, good for people who want to loose weight, because it burns calories at a higher rate. It could be labeled as "energetic enthusiasm".
Caution: It must be taken with a lot of liquids, because it needs to be dissolved in the stomach area and less in the colon area.

Marjoram *(Origanum majorana))* – The name marjoram/oregano has caused confusion over the years because you don't come across simply one oregano or even just a few, but rather a whole genus of herbs, all of which have been called marjoram/oregano, used mostly for culinary purposes. Marjoram, also named sweet marjoram, looks very much like oregano, but is milder and less pungent in taste than oregano. Historically, marjoram has been used to treat anxiety and insomnia. Today, herbalists use the dried leaves with other calming herbs to promote healthy restful sleep, or to make an excellent stuffing for sleep pillows. Marjoram can also be used as a tea for indigestion, coughs, headaches, and to promote menstruation. Marjoram's aroma is uplifting and soothing to the nerves.

Marshmallow *(Althea officinalis)* -- With its demulcent properties it is a wonderful herb for irritated, inflamed mucous membranes, such as bladder, throat, stomach, small and large intestines, vagina, and the lungs. The most soothing of all herbs, it is helpful for painful urination, blood in stool, for dryness and inflammation.

Matarique *(Cacalia decomposita)* – In diabetes it may decrease the amount of insulin necessary; a specific for non-compliance adult onset diabetes, it works on cell membrane permeability to blood sugar.

Meadowsweet *(Filipendula ulmaria)* – Contains aspirin-like properties, which relieve fever and rheumatic pain. Because of its bitter properties this herb is excellent for digestive complaints. It is actually used for excessive gastric acid secretion, hiatal hernia and nausea. Additionally, it may be effective for arthritis pain, headaches, muscle and back pain.

Melilot *(Melillotus spp)* – Known as yellow or white sweet clover, it is an anti-spasmodic, anodyne, anti-inflammatory and diuretic. It is indicated for sharp stabbing pain such as optic neuralgia, sciatica or ovarian neuralgia. The herb also strengthens vascular integrity and reduces capillary leakage for conditions such as edema, varicose veins and trauma injuries.

Melissa *(see Lemon Balm)*

Milk Thistle *(Silybum marianum)* – Milk thistle has the capability of rebuilding the liver after toxic exposure, and of reversing liver damage. Milk thistle also increases bile to help breakdown fat. It is indicated for cirrhosis of

> Milk Thistle can be ground into a powder, which you can add to granola, yogurt, salads, sandwiches, soups, etc.
> Please do not heat milk thistle!

the liver, as well as for nephro-toxicity, psoriasis and Hepatitis A-D. Milk thistle is used in Germany to dispel jaundice. It is also a free radical scavenger.

Mistletoe, European *(Viscum album)* – The European mistletoe is a powerful nervine and cardiac depressant, which acts on the vagus nerve. It can be used as a cardiac tonic and to stimulate circulation, for nervous tachycardia, as well as to reduce high blood pressure and arteriosclerosis. It also strengthens capillary walls. When migraines are due to high blood pressure, the European mistletoe may be helpful. The action of mistletoe occurs via the autonomic nervous system.
Caution: Berries are toxic, do not eat!

Monk's Pepper *(see Chaste Tree Berry)*

Morinda *(Morinda citrifolia)* – Morinda stimulates the nerve endings around the mucous membranes, and is especially good for the eyes. Morinda stimulates the optic nerve and also increases the blood flow to the eye area. Because of the increased blood flow, morinda has a minor effect on the mucous membranes of the mouth and nasal cavities, which may sometimes help with taste, (18 % of population) and smell (27 % of population), and eyesight (around mid 70% of population).

Mormon Tea/Brigham Tea *(Ephedra nevadensis)* – Mormon tea is not as potent as its Chinese relative, but contains enough ephedrine-related alkaloid to make it effective. Mormon tea acts as an energy tonic to strengthen and restore body vitality. It is being used to treat asthma, relieving muscle spasms in the bronchial tubes. Mormon tea has a pronounced diuretic and decongestant effect and was used wherever urinary tract problems occurred.
Caution: Mormon tea contains ephedrine and is contraindicated in cases of heart problems and high blood pressure.

Motherwort *(Leonurus cardiaca)* – This is a nice nervine, for heart palpitations, and when feeling overwhelmed by too many activities. It is a female tonic, as it improves blood flow to the female organs. Motherwort can also be used as a sedative for hysterical complaints, tachycardia, and a nervous pulse. Culpepper says, "…it is calming to the trembling heart…dispelling of melancholic vapors from the heart."

Mugwort *(Artemisia vulgaris)* – This bitter plant is an excellent digestive tonic. It is an effective remedy for parasites and worms. Some herbalists say that it is an excellent nervine for uncontrollable shaking, nervousness, and insomnia. Mugwort can bring on menstrual cycles when mixed with valerian and cramp bark.

Muira Puama *(Ptychopetalum olacoides* – This South American tree is also known as potency wood, as it stimulates libido and pelvic circulation without the adverse responses that sometimes occur with yohimbe.

Mullein Flower *(Verbascum thapsus)* – Topically, mullein flower oil acts as an anti-inflammatory and local anodyne. It has been used for treating earaches and otitis media, as well as sore muscles.

Mullein Leaf *(Verbascum thapsus)* – Demulcent, expectorant and anodyne properties make this herb useful for irritations of the lungs and bowels. Mullein leaf can be added to other respiratory herbs to help with coughs, whooping cough, bleeding lungs, bronchitis, asthma and pleurisy. Use the flowers for sinus congestion and ear pain.

Mullein Root *(Verbascum thapsus)* – Used for various colon conditions, such as colitis, polyps, etc., it also increases digestion and assimilation. Mullein root balances the amino acids in the body and in doing such, increases neuro-peptide activity, which in turn tells the body to work more efficiently. Mullein root balances the inner active processes of the gastro-intestinal system. In the lining of the intestinal tract there is an acid balance that is very intricate, very vital to the assimilation of nutrients etc., which mullein root harmonizes and balances.

Mullein Leaf, Flower, Root *(Verbascum thapsus* – Using the whole plant, leaf, flower and root, mullein increases oxygen supply and assimilation in the circulatory system. There is also increased nutrient assimilation. This combination is almost a life tonic, as it increases life force vitality.

Mulungu *(Erythrina mulungu)* – Indigenous people of Brazil have long used this herb as a natural relaxant. In today's herbal medicine it is considered an excellent remedy to calm agitation, soothe the nervous system and promote healthy sleeping patterns.

Mustard *(Sinapis alba)* – This pungent herb helps promote appetite, and stimulates the stomach mucous membranes, which helps digestion. An infusion stimulates the urinary system and the reproductive system, good to use for delayed menstruation. Has thermogenic properties, (calorie-burning,) excellent to add to a weight loss program. Mustard can be used externally as a plaster for sore and stiff muscles, to loosen them up and carry away the toxins that cause the muscles to tighten.

How To Make Your Own Prepared Mustard

It is easy to make your own prepared mustard. You can make a smooth mustard with powdered mustard, or your can make a crunchy mustard with the whole seeds. Here is my favorite recipe: Fill 1/3 of a pint glass jar with white and brown mustard seeds. Now add tarragon vinegar and fill almost to the top of the jar. Close the jar with a tight lid. Let this sit for a while (about 2 hours), it will swell up. Shake it up a little and place in refrigerator overnight. Next day grind this mush in a food processor to desired consistency. In a refrigerator this mustard will keep for several months.

Myrrh *(Commiphora myrrha)* – Makes an effective anti-bacterial gargle for sores in mouth, gums and throat. Internally, myrrh stimulates white blood cells and is specifically indicated for acute infections of the mucous membranes of the throat, stomach and bowels.

Neem Bark *(Azadiracta indica)* – The bark of the neem tree is a bitter tonic, astringent, vermifuge, anti-parasitic, and anti-viral. Neem can be taken to clear away all foreign and excess tissues, as its astringent action promotes healing.

Neem Leaf *(Azadiracta indica)* – The leaves of the neem tree removes toxins, purifies the blood, neutralizes free radicals in the body, heals ulcers in the urinary passage, as well as for any type of skin disease. Neem is also beneficial for the eyes. Neem can be taken to clear away all foreign and excess tissues, as its astringent action promotes healing.

Nettle Leaf *(Urtica dioica)* – The leaves of the stinging nettle plant neutralizes uric acid, shrinks inflamed tissues, and increases thyroid function. It is also known to bring back natural hair color. It is high in vitamin K and guards against excess bleeding. Nettle leaf is an excellent nutritive, because of its high mineral content, such as calcium, magnesium, as well as iron for the production of red blood cells. Herbalists have long recommended nettle leaf for allergies, as it contains natural antihistamine properties. For this purpose, it is best to use in capsule form.

Nettle Root *(Urtica dioica)* – The root of the stinging nettle has a strong action on the kidneys because of its diuretic properties. It is being used for the relief of benign prostatic hyperplasia (BPH), as it shrinks the prostate gland. It is a tonic, astringent, anti-diarrheal, and can strengthen the immune system, as well as the lymphatic system.

Nettle Seed *(Urtica dioica)* – The seed of the stinging nettle can be used to improve renal function, to increase excretion of waste. Nettle seeds have also been utilized for goiter, tuberculosis, and malarial fevers.

Nopal/Prickly Pear Cactus *(Opuntia spp.)* – Effective in lowering blood sugar in cases of juvenile-onset diabetes and adult-onset diabetes, and particularly where chronic hyperglycemia prevails. It can also be used as a diuretic, anti-inflammatory, and for toothache and canker sores.

Nutmeg *(Myristica fragrans)* – Nutmeg stimulates digestion and increases absorption of nutrients in the small intestine. This is an excellent herb for "coldness", be it physical, mental or emotional. Nutmeg increases circulation and warmth in the lower parts of the body.
Caution: Large doses may cause double vision and even coma!

A Healthy Drink For The Whole Endocrine System

This highly nutritious drink feeds the whole endocrine system, is a great body energizer and mood elevator. Although it takes 2 days to get it ready, there is little to do. Well worth the wait, and it is absolutely delicious.

Sprout four tbsp of oats by soaking overnight in water, then allow to sprout for about 1 ½ days. Put into blender with one cup of water, whiz for 30 seconds, add 2/3 cup more of water, blend another 30 seconds, then strain. Place into the blender the oat milk, six whole raw almonds, one tsp vanilla extract, a dash of nutmeg, one tbsp whey powder, and either one banana or apple. Blend for about 30 seconds. Enjoy!

Oats *(Avena sativa)* – Every part of this plant strengthens and nourishes the nervous system. Used for nervous exhaustion, anxiety, impaired sleep patterns, and weak libido. Also, it reduces withdrawal effects from nicotine and caffeine. Oats contains calcium and magnesium, which are essential nutrients for the nervous tissues. It soothes the frayed feeling brought on by "burning the candle at both ends."

Olive *(Olea europaea)* – This is a popular herb used in Europe for hypertension, impaired circulation, diabetes, and as a diuretic. Its effects on high blood pressure are slow acting but definite and long lasting. Olive leaf is also anti-viral. Perhaps it is no wonder that people living in the Mediterranean, surrounded by olive trees, do not have high blood pressure. Their daily diet includes an abundance of olive oil, olives, as well as olive leaves.

Onion *(Allium cepa)* – Since ancient times, onions have been used in cooking, as well as a medicine. Onions have decongestant and anti-bacterial properties. My grand-mother always said, onions pull the disease out of the body. For years she was ridiculed over this statement. But today, researchers have proven that when an onion is cut open and left in a sick room, it will absorb a person's illness, as well as bringing the person back to good health. Amazing!

How To Make An Onion Pack

Here is an old and time tested remedy for a sore throat, cough, or respiratory congestion, even for an earache. Cut up an onion into small pieces. Place into a frying pan with 1 tablespoon of olive oil. Fry for about 1 – 2 minutes, just enough to heat up the onion. Place onto a towel or paper towel and make a pouch, so that the onions cannot slip out. Apply to affected area, secure with a towel or bandage, and leave it on for several hours or overnight. The onions will turn black as they absorb the illness.

CAUTION: Before applying the onion pack to the affected area, make sure it is not too hot, or it will burn the skin. This is especially true for children, as they are more sensitive.

Oregano *(Origanonum vulgare)* – The name oregano has caused confusion over the years because you don't come across simply one oregano or even just a few, but rather a whole genus of herbs, all of which have been called oregano because of their culinary use. Oregano and marjoram look very much alike, and they are in the same genus. Oregano is also called wild oregano, because it grows wild in the mountains of Greece. Derived from Greek *oros,* meaning mountain, and *ganos,* meaning joy, "Joy if the mountain". Sweet marjoram is less pungent and usually grows in people's garden. Herbalists have made infusion of the leaves of oregano for indigestion, coughs, headaches, and to promote menstruation. Oregano has been describes as a tonic and stimulant.

Orange Peel *(Citrus spp)* – The peels of oranges are a great digestive aid, as it stimulates hydrochloric acid production. Orange peels also reduce gas and nausea.

Oregon Grape *(Mahonia nervosa)* – A good digestive bitter, liver tonic and cholagogue used to increase digestion and absorption especially of fats and oils. It is indicated for dyspepsia, jaundice, elevated bilirubin levels and poor bile formation. Oregon grape is also anti-bacterial/anti-fungal/anti-viral, therefore, it is indicated also for urinary tract infections, strep- and staph infections, intestinal viruses and skin conditions, such as psoriasis and acne. It contains berberine, which is the active constituent in goldenseal. Hence, oregon grape can be used in place of the more expensive goldenseal. Oregon grape can also be used for hangovers, poor protein digestion, and for a sluggish gastrointestinal system. It liberates iron stored in the liver and therefore is helpful for anemia. This bitter herb can also stimulate a sluggish thyroid gland.

Osmanthus *(Osmanthus)* – Osmantus tea is not well known in the western world, but according to Traditional Chinese medicine osmanthus tea improves complexion if used on a daily basis. It has an antioxidant effect in the body, additionally, it has the ability to inhibit melanin formation, leading to a lighter skin tone. This beautiful flower may prevent cancer, diabetes, and kidney disease. Osmathus can be added to other teas as a flavoring agent.

Osha *(Ligusticum porteri)* - A most important medicinal plant used by Native Americans as an anti-bacterial expectorant and bronchial dilator, and for bronchial irritations, congestion or coughs that are dry. Osha has anti-viral and immune stimulating properties. Mild antihistamine activity makes it useful for rhinitis, head colds and allergies. Also known as bear root, because it is the bear's first food eaten after coming out of hibernation. Navajo's tie a small osha root to their children's shoe laces to ward off snakes. It is also placed in Native American homes for protection. A very sacred herb, indeed.

Pansy *(Viola tricolor)* – Pansy is a child's remedy to reduce a fever. It contains methylsalicylates, which decreases inflammation. Pansy is pain relieving, a natural herbal aspirin, and a gentle sedative. Pansy infused oil can be used for skin problems, particularly eczema of the scalp and scabby skin complaints. Because it is so gentle, it can be used to ease cradle cap, diaper rash and eczema in infants.

Paprika *(Capsicum annum)* – Paprika is a mild pepper used in cooking. Gives a beautiful color and enhances flavors.

Parsley Leaf and Root *(Petroselinum crispum)* – Not just a common nutritious culinary herb, parsley is also known for its medicinal qualities. It can be used for edema, bedwetting, frequent urination, gas, infant colic (via breast milk) and bilious colic. It is high in chlorophyll, and it is a wonderful breath-freshener.

Partridge Berry/Squaw Vine *(Mitchella repens)* – This is a great female herb, as it tonifies the uterus by increasing muscle tone and circulation, good for a prolapsed uterus. Use in the last two weeks of pregnancy to prepare for childbirth, as well as for an afterbirth tonic. Men can also use partridge berry for benign prostatic hyperplasia.

Passion Flower *(Passiflora incarnata)* – A sedative, antispasmodic and nerve sedative used for insomnia, nervous headache, neuralgia, muscular/nerve pain, facial tics, pain and stiffness in the neck, mild depression, and for pelvic and spasmodic pain.

It is a specific herb for people who cannot go to sleep because of mental chatter or worry. Herbalists have also recommended passion flower for teething in children,

Pata de Vaca/Cowfoot *(Bauhinia forficate)* – Pata de vaca is also called cowfoot because of the shape of its leaf. It has been used in South America to balance glucose levels and to cleanse the body. Pata de vaca leaves and tea bags are a common item on pharmacy shelves in South America, and normally a standard infusion is drunk after each meal to help balance sugar levels. Used also for elephantiasis and snakebites, and for skin problems, including those of a syphilitic nature.

Pau d'Arco *(Tabebuia impetiginosa)* – Has been used in South America as an immune tonic, anti-microbial, anti-fungal, anti-inflammatory and astringent. The herb's activity on candida overgrowth is variable.

Pellitory of the Wall *(Parietaria diffusa)* – Used for kidney stones and urinary calculi, it is a demulcent and diuretic herb.

Pennyroyal *(Mentha pulegium)* – As an anti-spasmodic, it is useful in flatulent colic, painful menses, abdominal cramping, and to break a fever. It is also known as a uterine stimulant for delayed menstruation.

Peony *(Paeonia lactiflorae)* – In Traditional Chinese System this herb is a blood tonic and an overall cleansing herb. It can be used for conditions in the body due to toxic blood. It is added to formulas to help the body relax and reduce tension.

Peppermint *(Mentha piperita)* – Peppermint is one of the oldest household remedies. It is a time tested carminative used for nausea, gas, stomach and intestinal colic, and as a pleasant flavoring agent. Peppermint tones and relaxes stomach muscles, stimulating the flow of stomach digestive fluids. Peppermint energizes the body by oxygenating the bloodstream. It can be used instead of coffee to energize the body.

Periwinkle *(Vinca minor)* – Periwinkle has been used all over the world for a variety of conditions. It has been used for various cancers, high blood pressure, nervous disorders, and as a sugar balancing agent in diabetics. It delivers more oxygen to the brain than any known substance. It also stimulates vascular and cerebral circulation, appropriate for cerebral insufficiency, "yin" migraines, for impaired memory and cognitive function. It is especially effective with ginkgo and gotu kola.

Persimmon Leaf *(Diospyros spp)* – Although persimmon leaves have long been used as a herbal remedy in China, it is becoming more popular in the USA. The leaves of the persimmon tree steeped as a tea can be used for allergies, because it stops histamine release, as well as for irritability and rapid pulse, which can be the symptoms of to allergies. Persimmons leaves can be an effective weight loss remedy, by raising the body's metabolism. Research has shown that it can lower lipid levels, and regulate blood pressure. It can also relieve constipation and atherosclerosis. Persimmons tea protects the body from carcinogens. There are numerous nutritional benefits, containing high amounts of vitamin C, choline and essential amino acids.

Peruvian Bark *(see Cinchona)*

Pine Tree *(Pinus spp)* – Pine tips and pine needles contain high amounts of vitamin C and are useful for colds, flu, and respiratory ailments. The bark is high in flavonoids, which enhances the vital function of vitamin C. The resin/sap can be applied to wounds for its antiseptic properties. The entire pine tree is edible. Pine buds, pollen, young pine cones (before they become hard), pine nuts, and the inner bark are all edible. Do you know how to tell the red pine tree from the white pine tree? Red pines have clusters of three needles, and "red" has three letters in it. White pines have clusters of five needles, and "white" has five letters in it. Pretty nice way to remember.

Pine Needle Tea

Gather a handful of fresh young pine needles. Wash thoroughly to remove dust and insects. Cut with scissors into ¼ inch length pieces. Bruise the needles to enhance the flavor and place into a cup. Boil 8 – 10 oz of water, and pour over the needles. Let it steep covered for about 20 minutes. You can also boil the needles for about 5 minutes for a stronger tea. You may sweeten your tea with a little honey

Pipsissewa *(Chimaphila umbellata)* – Stimulates removal of waste in the kidneys and flushes the urinary tract. A non-irritating antiseptic diuretic used for chronic genito-urinary infections. It can also be used as an alterative for gouty arthritis, gout and rheumatic pain.

Plantain *(Plantago major)* – Being high in chlorophyll and mucilaginous properties, it is an excellent wound healer, for abrasions, rashes and insect bites. Internally, it is healing to GI tract inflammations from stomach and duodenal ulcers, gastritis, to dysentery and ulcerative colitis. Plantain is also useful for healing mucous membranes of bladder and vagina, and for dental pain.

Pleurisy Root *(Asclepias tuberosa)* – Good for dry coughs and congestion, as it will re-moisten the lungs, making expectoration easier. Use with vitamin C to see the best result. Pleurisy is helpful when there is a tight chest and where breathing is difficult and painful, due to intercostals muscle congestion. It is successful for pleurisy, pneumonia, pericarditis, and bronchitis. Expels mucus, slows rapid pulse and reduces respiratory pain.

Poke Root *(Phytolacca americana)* – For lymphatic swellings, it is an excellent alterative and lymphatic stimulant to clear up an over acid bloodstream. Topically, massage poke root infused oil to increase lymphatic drainage. It has been used for cystic breasts, mastitis and calcium deposits in the milk ducts, also for hard and swollen lymph nodes
Caution: Use conservatively!

Poleo Mint *(Mentha arvensis)* – Poleo is stronger than peppermint as a diaphoretic to stimulate sweating. This plant works well with elder to break a fever; it is also useful as a relaxant for colics and stomachaches.

Poplar Bud *(see Balm of Gilead)*

Poppy Seeds *(Papaver somniferum)* – In America, the field poppy is regarded as a weed, and only a limited amount of the petals are used. It is cultivated in several parts of Germany for the sake of its seeds, which are not only used in cakes, but from which an excellent oil is made, used as a substitute for olive oil. It is a sedative, for pain, insomnia, and anxiety.
Caution: Do not take when going for a drug test!

Poppy, White *(Papaver somniferum)* – Opium, and its two principal alkaloids, morphine and codeine, are extracted from poppy heads before they have ripened. When the petals have fallen from the flowers, incisions are made in the wall of the unripe capsules. The exuded juice is collected by scraping, then wrapped in poppy leaves and further dried in the sun. Opium is a valuable medicine in relieving pain; it is also a sedative, expectorant, and diaphoretic. The word opium is derived from the Greek "opos", meaning juice.
Caution: It is considered poisonous and is illegal.

Prickly Ash *(Xanthoxylum americanum)* – For poor blood circulation, such as cold extremities, varicose veins, it is a stimulating tonic. Used as a carminative it increases digestive juices, warms the stomach and promotes appetite. It is usually added to formulas to increase their potency.

Prickly Pear *(see Nopal)*

Psyllium *(Plantago psyllium)* – Used in a proper manner, psyllium is an excellent cleanser for the intestines and colon. It lubricates, moistens and heals the intestinal tract.
Caution: Drink lots of water with it!

Pulsatilla *(Pulsatilla patens)* – A sedative herb to produce a restful sleep, it may also be used for emotional fragility and exaggeration.

Puncture Vine *(see Gokshura)*

Purslane *(Portulaca sativa)* – This succulent plant, with its minute yellow flower that blooms before midday, is perhaps one of the most nutritious greens in your garden. Purslane has more beta-carotene than spinach, as well as high levels of vitamin C, calcium, magnesium, potassium, iron, protein, thiamine, riboflavin, niacin, alpha linolenic acid, a type of omega – 3 fatty acid, and much, much more. Historically, many Native American tribes have used purslane for food and medicine. European cultures used it as a remedy for arthritis and inflammation. Chinese herbalists found similar benefits, using it for healthy circulatory and respiratory function. In Russia, people dry it for winter. In Mexico it is called verdolaga and is a favorite in omelets, rolled into tortillas, or added into soups and stews. In many cultures, purslane was used as a cosmetic, to cleanse, heal and tighten the skin. It is very similar to aloe vera. To make a skin cleanser, juice one cup of purslane and add it to one cup of distilled water. Wash your face, then apply the purslane tea. Wait for 3 minutes before rinsing it off. You may find that this refreshing treatment for your skin can smooth out a few wrinkles.

Pygeum Bark *(Prunus africana)* – Pygeum is a South African herb and used for congested, enlarged and inflamed prostate accompanied by diminished urine flow, and an increase frequency of urination, especially at night. It is effective in the treatment of benign prostate hyperplasia or prostate inflammation, and for long-standing, chronic prostate problems. Pygeum works by blocking the entry and breakdown of cholesterol in the prostate, which encourages prostaglandins that reveal an anti-inflammatory action.

Quassia *(Picranea excelsa)* – Intensely bitter, this herb stimulates digestion by increasing hydrochloric acid production, bile secretion, small intestine and pancreatic enzyme secretion. It increases absorption and elimination. As an amoebocide, it can be used to treat giardia, dysentery, pinworms, leaky gut syndrome and intestinal worms.

Quebra Pedra *(see Chanca piedra)*

Queen of the Meadow *(see Gravel root)*

Red Clover *(Trifolium pratense)* – This is the best blood cleanser. It is an anti-oxidant with specialized flavonoids that promote healthy cell proliferation and help the immune system suppress harmful bacteria and other invasive microbes. It supports the kidneys as well as the urinary system. It is also used for bronchitis and for expelling phlegm and mucus from the respiratory tract. Red clover has traditionally been known by herbalists for its ability to dissolve tumors. Good for clearing the skin of blemishes, for canker sores, etc., as well as for eliminating gout. Helps discharge nitrogen from the body. When there is nervous energy due to mineral deficiencies and heavy metal toxicity, drink one cup at bedtime. If someone is having difficulties in getting pregnant, red clover affects the hormonal level; it relaxes the body. Red clover is a blood thinner.

Red Currant Juice *(Ribes rubrum)* – Used similarly to black currant juice, although less effective. Red currant juice is especially cooling, refreshing and thirst-relieving, generally preferred during the summer months. Drink black currant in the winter and red currant in the summer.

Red Raspberry *(Rubus idaeus)* – The leaves of the raspberry bush are rich in minerals as well as astringent properties. Raspberry is a tonic to smooth muscle tissues, especially for the uterus and large intestine. It is a pregnancy tonic useful to reduce morning sickness, miscarriage and post partum bleeding. It can be taken throughout the pregnancy with good results. It builds tissue to the extent that it prevents tearing of the cervix of the uterus during birth, as well as in preventing hemorrhaging during childbirth. The contractions of the uterine muscles are regulated during delivery and it also reduces false labor pains. Raspberry leaves are high in iron and enrich early colostrums found in mother's milk. It also prepares breasts for pure milk supply for the nursing infant by cleansing and purifying the blood. Raspberry is also indicated for menorrhagia. Raspberry tea can also be made into a tea to give to children for colds, fevers, stomach aches, to ease colics, and to slow diarrhea.

Red Root *(Ceanothus americanus)* – Red root is useful for overactive mucosa and chronic catarrh. It is also indicated for lymphatic congestion and tonsillitis. Used in a formula with milk thistle and fringe tree, this herb has shown to be effective for treating acute pancreatitis.

Rehmannia *(Rehmannia glutinosa)* – Cooked rehmannia is a blood tonic useful for deficient blood and when the skin is pale, for insomnia, dizziness, irregular menses and palpitations. The processed root is also a kidney yin tonic and helps reduce allergic response. When it is taken in its raw form, it will extract heat from the blood and body, excellent to use for high fever, irritability, constipation and chronic throat pain.

Reishi Mushroom *(Ganoderma lucidum)* – Reishi is a immune modulator. It normalizes high blood pressure and decreases the effect stress has on the cardiovascular system; improves the flow of blood to the head, it enhances memory and promotes overall vitality and longevity. It also helps chronic allergies, frequent colds, and compromised immune conditions.

Rhodiola *(Rhodiola rosea)* – Rhodiola is a cooling adaptogenic herb. It increases physical endurance, enhances immune and sexual function, and has antioxidant properties.

Rhubarb *(Rheum palmatum)* – The root of the rhubarb plant is an appetite stimulant and digestive bitter tonic in small doses; in large doses it is a laxative/purgative.

Rockrose *(Cistus ladanifer)* – Rockrose is for gastro-duodenal anxiety, insomnia, gastritis, and ulcers. Externally it can be used for inflammations osteoarticulares, muscular mialgias, and neuralgias.
Caution: The oleoresin is neurotoxic, hepatoxic and nefrotoxic, therefore, oral administration is not recommended.

Rooibos *(Aspalathus linearis)* – The only place to find rooibos is in the Cedergerg region of the Western Cape of South Africa. This small leguminous shrub has needle like leaves and fine stems with tiny yellow flowers. Dried in the sun, rooibos undergoes oxidation and is processed like traditional tea. Rooibos is caffeine-free and rich in anti-oxidants. Anti-oxidants eliminate the oxidation of free radicals associated with the aging process. Japanese researchers have shown that rooibos tea exhibits anti-mutagenic properties and retards the growth of certain tumors. It has a soothing effect on the central nervous system and can be used by people who are suffering from irritability, headaches, disturbed sleeping patterns, insomnia, nervous tension and mild depression or hypertension. Rooibos can be used for various stomach and digestive complaints, nausea, vomiting, heartburn, stomach ulcers and constipation. With its anti-spasmodic properties, drinking rooibos can help relieve stomach cramps and colic in infants. Because rooibos contains very little tannin, it does not impair the absorption of iron and protein into the body. Rooibos benefits the management of allergies, hay fever, asthma. For skin problems such as eczema or acne apply directly to affected areas.

Rosehip *(Rosa canina)* – Rosehips are the fruit of the rose bush. When the blossoms are left on the plant, seed pods develop, turning a deeply orange or red in the fall. Rosehips can be enjoyed fresh or can be dried for future use. Besides being delicious, they are incredibly rich in nutrients. Rosehips are reported to have up to 60 percent more vitamin C than lemon or oranges. In addition, they contain vitamin B, E, K, pectin, beta-carotene, bio-flavonoids and minerals. As a result, rosehips exert a strong antioxidant effect, protecting against colds and flues, shielding the immune system and various organs and tissues from oxidative stress. Rosehips' high pectin content, a dietary fiber, is recognized to improve blood cholesterol, blood pressure, digestive efficiency, heart health and overall wellness. Clinically proven to promote fullness and suppress hunger cravings, rosehips may be helpful for healthy weight management. If you are prone to urinary tract infections, you might be interested to know that some people drink rosehip tea to prevent recurrences. Studies have also shown that rosehips can help prevent the development of kidney stones. Additional studies have proven rosehips to be helpful to the circulatory system, respiratory system, the thymus gland, and as a blood cleanser. Other health benefits include lowering abnormal body heat, relieving thirst, healing of internal hemorrhaging, aid for dysentery, strengthen the stomach, prevent and help relief chest infections and coughs, cleanse the kidney and bladder, prevent fluid retention, assist with gout and rheumatic conditions, as well as nourishing the skin. As a gentle stimulant it allows healthy bowel movements. Rosehips are extremely alkaline and can restore the natural acid/alkaline balance of the body. You may also want to know that recently rosehips have been recognized in easing headaches and dizziness.

Rosehip Jam Made Easy

Place 2 oz seedless rosehips into a bowl. Add enough apple cider to cover. Let stand overnight. Enjoy for breakfast or anytime. To make a superb dessert I add a little heavy cream to my rosehip jam. Y- u -m-m-y!

Thirst Quenching Tea

Take a pinch of each of the following to make a delicious tea, either hot or cold, rosehips, mint and linden. Pour 8 oz of hot water of this mix and let it steep for 20 minutes. Sweeten lightly and add a little lemon juice, if desired.

Rosemary *(Rosmarinus officinale)* – Rosemary strengthens memory, stimulates capillary circulation bringing more blood to the cells. A carminative, nervine, and cholagogue traditionally used in Europe for gas, nausea, liver headaches, arteriosclerosis, biliousness, depression and mental fatigue. Rosemary is also a powerful antioxidant. It strengthens the heart, stimulates blood circulation, tones the blood vessels, invigorates, and increases awareness. Rosemary is a helpful herb for the convalescent and fatigued person, for low blood pressure and for the one who lacks dynamism. A good mouthwash and hair rinse.

Rue *(Ruta graveolens)* – Has antispasmodic, emmenagogue and carminative properties. Externally, it can be applied to bruises, ganglions, sprains and sore muscles. Planting rue in your garden can keep cats away, because they do not like the odor. You can make pouches with dried rue and place them in areas where you don't want your cats to go to, such as furnitures. One lady told me it keeps her cat off the couch.
Caution: Uterine stimulant; abortive.

Safflower *(Carthamus tinctorius)* – A tea made from safflowers can be helpful for delayed menstruation, congested and stagnant blood, poor circulation, and blood clots. It reduces lactic acid build up, lowers cholesterol, dissolves uric acid and kidney stones, removes phlegm from the system and improves digestive function. It can also be used in cooking as a substitute for the more costly saffron.

Saffron *(Crocus sativus)* – Saffron is a pricey herb. The dried stigmas in the crocus flower are used to make saffron spice. It takes approximately 75'000 saffron blossoms to produce one pound of saffron spice. Saffron is used medicinally for asthma, cough, whooping cough, and to loosen phlegm. It has been used for insomnia, atherosclerosis, and cancer. It is beneficial for the digestive organs, gallbladder and liver. It supports blood sugar and fat metabolism, improves circulation, regulates the heart and liver, and promotes energy. Saffron has also been used for emotional problems, for example depression, shock and fright. Men have used saffron to prevent early orgasm. It is an aphrodisiac for both women and men.

Sage *(Salvia officinalis)* – Since ancient times, sage was known as mankind's savior. The Latin name "salvia" means "savior". It strengthens memory and promotes wisdom. Sage is an astringent herb helpful for hot flashes, or when feeling hot. For people who sweat a lot, sage can reduce perspiration. It is also for mental exhaustion, as it strengthens concentration, and improves memory. Sage is high in minerals. It can also be used for a weak digestion. Externally, sage can be used for skin eruptions, insect bites, stops bleeding wounds, and as a mouthwash, especially for canker sores.

Saint John's Wort *(Hypericum perforatum)* – St. John's Wort rebuilds a damaged nervous system and can be used for neuralgia, agitation, anxiety and depression. It is a mild immune stimulant and anti-viral, a specific for shingles. St. John' Wort can be used internally and externally for nerve pain, such as migratory and shooting pains, nerve injuries, sciatica, neuralgia, and rheumatic pain. It is also anti-inflammatory and anti-spasmodic. St. John's Wort promotes healing of damaged nerves. St. John's Wort is beneficial in wound healing, when the wound is putrid. It cleanses the dirt out of septic wounds, without damaging healthy tissues.

Sangre de Drago *(Jatropha dioica)* – Blood of the dragon is a red tree sap, a cousin of the poinsettia, and can be used for mouth sores, inflamed gums, surface wounds, and to promote a strong and healthy stomach lining and intestinal wall. In addition, nearly 90% of sangre de drago's dry weight is proanthocyandins, one of the most powerful natural antioxidants.

Sanicle *(Sanicula europaea)* – Sanicle relieves mucus congestion in the chest, stomach and intestines. Use as a gargle for mouth and throat inflammation. Externally use as an antiseptic and for cleansing of open wounds.

Sarsaparilla *(Smilax officinalis)* – Sarsaparilla increases the production of testosterone, progesterone, and cortisone. It is used in hormone balancing formulas. Sarsaparilla serves as a precursor for hormone production, useful for bodybuilding. Sarsaparilla is a blood purifier and has been used for skin conditions that are red, hot and inflamed, such as psoriasis and psoriatic arthritis. It is an excellent antidote for poisons. Sarsaparilla stimulates breathing when there is congestion in the lungs. It is also appropriate for arthritis, gout, bursitis, colitis, rheumatoid arthritis and inflammation of connective tissue. It also increases metabolism.

Sassafras *(Sassafras officinalis)* – Sassafras stimulates liver action, which clears toxins from the body, therefore, it is an excellent herb for all internally caused skin disorders such as acne, eczema and psoriasis. It is good to use for inflammatory skin diseases and arthritic conditions, rheumatism, gout, and to relief itching from poison ivy and poison oak. It thins the blood in the summer, thickens it during winter.

Saw Palmetto *(Serenoa repens)* – Saw palmetto is indicated for benign prostatic hyperplasia and cystitis. As an adaptogen, it is especially useful for older, depleted people. It strengthens kidney, lung and reproductive chi. Saw Palmetto is also used as a urinary antiseptic and in cases of low sperm count. Saw palmetto helps electrolyte balances in the body, heightens the absorption of saline into the body, into the organs and the cells. It increases the production of testosterone in the body.

Schisandra *(Schisandra chinensis)* – Schisandra is a powerful adaptogen, which regulates bodily functions and enables the body handle stress. It is also helpful for lung weakness, asthma, coughs, and night sweats. It strengthens hypothalamic/adrenal function and normalizes the nervous system and the activity of the immune system. As a non-habit forming stimulant and anti-hepatotoxin, schisandra enhances athletic performances and stimulates metabolism. Schisandra strengthens the tissues and retains body energy, calms the body, and is helpful in treating forgetfulness. To improve digestion of fatty foods, schisandra helps split fat in the food to fatty acids and glycerin, as well as cleansing the liver and increasing the production of bile. Schisandra decreases fatigue, increases blood circulation, and lowers blood pressure. It astringes the *jing* – the vital essence – and it is rich in anti-inflammatory flavonoids. Schisandra promotes long life. It increases the energy in the brain, muscles, liver, kidney, glands, nerves, and eyes. All in all, schisandra balances all bodily functions, and normalizes all the systems of the body.

Self-Heal *(Prunella vulgaris)* – Self-heal is for liver fire rising symptoms (red eyes, headaches, dizziness), to clear heat and dissolve nodules. Used for swollen glands and lipomas (growth of fat cells under the skin), as it is a lymphatic tonic.

Senna *(Cassia acutifolia)* – Senna is a highly addictive laxative, which irritates the lining of the large intestine, causing fast evacuation of stool. Take with ginger to avoid griping pains. Due to its cathartic and vermifuge qualities, senna can well be used in parasite cleansing programs.

Shavegrass *(see Horsetail)*

Shepherd's Purse *(Capsella bursa-pastoris)* – Shepard's purse is a hemostatic astringent. It can stop gastrointestinal and uterine bleeding. It is also a diuretic. Shepard's purse acts in a regulatory and equilibrating manner on both the heart and blood pressure, when too low or too high. It is also useful as an astringent and diuretic indicated for cloudy, foul-smelling urine, urinary tract infections and diarrhea.

Shiitake *(Lentinula edodes)* – This mushroom has been used both as a food and medicine. Known to lower cholesterol levels, inhibit viral growth, reduce bronchial inflammation, and to protect the liver from environmental toxins. In Japan it is used as a dietary aid for cancer.

Siberian Ginseng *(see Eleuthero)*

Skullcap *(Scutellaria lateriflora)* – Skullcap works on the central nervous system. It can rebuild nerve endings in the brain. Skullcap is indicated for nervous exhaustion, tremors, palsies, trigeminal neuralgia and the tremors of Parkinson's disease. It is also helpful with alcohol and drug withdrawal. As its name suggest, skullcap can be used for any problems related to the skull and head.

Skunk Cabbage *(Symplocarpus foetidus)* – Skunk cabbage is a powerful anodyne and antispasmodic. It is effective in treating spasms of the lungs, diaphragm and back muscles. Add lobelia, skullcap and black haw for a heightened effect.

Slippery Elm *(Ulmus fulva)* – Slippery elm is a wonderful mucilaginous herb, good for nausea, as it stays down when all else fails. It gives strength, because it is highly nutritive. It is soothing to mucous membranes and is excellent for ulcers. Externally, it can be made into a drawing ointment for splinters and boils.

Small Flowered Willow/Fireweed *(Epilobium angustifolia)* – Also known as fireweed, this herb has inflammation-inhibiting and healing effect on acute and chronic inflammation of the prostate gland. Woman can use this herb too, for chronic irritation in the bladder or acute inflammation of the bladder and urethra. Small flowered willow increases urine production (diuretic). It can also be used for diarrhea and associated cramping.

Soapwort *(see Aritha)*

Solomon's Seal *(Polygonatum biflorum)* – Solomon's seal moisturizes the lungs and is indicated for dry coughs with sticky and hard to expectorate mucus. It can also be used for pain in the joints and tendons.

Spearmint *(Mentha spicata)* – Spearmint has similar healing properties as peppermint, but is less stimulating. Because it is milder than peppermint, it is better for children's complaints. It is good for stomach problems, as it increase the circulation in the stomach, soothing the stomach and intestines. Spearmint is excellent in treating morning sickness or vomiting in pregnancy. It is gentle and effective for colic in babies.

Spikenard *(Aralia recemosa)* – Spikenard is a diaphoretic and expectorant herb. It is used for colds and flu with wheezing coughs and irritation of the mucous membranes, with tough stringy mucus, chronic pneumonia and bronchitis. Spikenard is also an emmenagogue and oxytocic used with blue cohosh to stimulate productive contractions in labor.

Spilanthes *(Spilanthes acmella)* – This tropical plant is known for its strong anti-bacterial properties, as well as immune stimulating compounds. Spilanthes is effective against blood parasites, and may possibly be effective against Lyme's disease. Spilanthes also inhibits candida albicans due to its sialagogue (saliva stimulating) effect; it stimulates the parotid glands and the interrelated lymphatic system. By moving the lymphatic fluids, the body will defend itself against disease and assist in the ousting of toxic metabolic waste. Spilanthes is also known as toothache plant, as it can be applied to mouth, throat, teeth and gums, to tone the gums and prevent tooth decay. Add 5 drops of spilanthes extract to a small amount of water and rinse your mouth thoroughly, especially mornings and evenings after brushing teeth. Spilanthes increases blood circulation to the oral mucosa, stimulating salivation.

Squaw Vine *(see Partridge Berry)*

Star Anise *(see Anise, Star)*

Stevia *(Stevia rebaudiana)* – Stevia is a natural sweetener, 50 times sweeter than sugar. It does not upset blood sugar levels, therefore it is safe for diabetics.

Stillingia *(Stillingia sylvatica)* – Stillingia is a powerful alterative, best used in small doses to stimulate eliminatory functions of liver, lymph and kidneys. It is indicated for croup, and spasmodic and irritated cough with mucous membrane tissues that are red and dry.

Stone Root *(Collonsonia canadensis)* – Stone root is used primarily to dissolve kidney stones, and sometimes for gallbladder stones. It is also used for pelvic and venous congestion, for example in treating hemorrhoids and varicose veins.

Storksbill *(Erodium cicutarium)* – Storksbill is a mild uterine hemostat; it can be used after childbirth to cut down on postpartum bleeding and to prevent secondary infections. It is a mild urinary tract astringent, acidifies the urine to normal, to prevent and treat urinary tract infections.

Strawberry Leaf *(Fragaria vesca)* – Strawberry leaf is used in a similar way as red raspberry leaf.

Suma *(Pfaffia paniculata)* – Suma is also called Brazilian ginseng (not to be confused with the Oriental ginseng), and is being used to increase energy, strengthen the immune system, fortify hormones, especially estrogen, regulate blood sugar, and to reduce tumors and cancers. Native Brazilians know suma as "para todo", which means "for everything", including in treating leukemia, Hodgkin's disease, diabetes, chronic fatigue syndrome, and Epstein-Barr. It is an anti-oxidant and beneficial for the heart and to lower high cholesterol. With its adaptogenic properties, suma helps the body adapt to internal and external stressors.

Sweet Annie *(Artemisia annua)* – Sweet annie is indicated for heat in the blood, e.g. nosebleeds, and rashes with bleeding under the skin.

Sweet Flag *(see Calamus)*

Tarragon *(Artemisia dracunculus)* – Tarragon is a cooking herb, but also has medicinal properties. It has been used to treat digestion problems, poor appetite, water retention, and to promote menstruation. Tarragon is high in potassium

Teasel *(Dipsacus japonicus)* – Teasel is astringent, styptic, anti-inflammatory and anti-spasmodic, and can be used internally and topically for lower back pain, stiff joints and trauma injuries. It can also be used for threatened miscarriage. Teasel has also been used for Lyme's disease, fibromyalgia, and chronic fatigue.

Thuja *(Thuja spp.)* – Thuja is a strong anti-viral, diuretic, emmenagogue and expectorant and used particularly for bronchitis. Thuja is also effective when burned in a sick room.

Thyme *(Thymus vulgaris)* – This fragrant herb is not only used in cooking but also for healing. Thyme has been used for nervous condition and depression, to heal wounds, to relieve asthmatic attacks and other respiratory problems, and to calm stomach cramps and gastro-intestinal complaints. Thyme is a powerful germicide and used in mouthwashes and toothpastes, such as Listerine. It is used as a general tonic with antiseptic properties to fight infection, fungal infections, and skin parasites, such as scabies, crabs and lice. Thyme removes mucus from the head, lungs and respiratory passages, very helpful for people with early morning cough fits, or shortness of breath. It strengthens the lungs, and clears the voice. Many famous singers drink thyme tea before singing.

Toadflax *(Linaria vulgaris)* – Toadflax is for chronic liver irritations and hepatitis flare-ups; useful for people who work around industrial solvents, such as painters and mechanics.

Tulsi *(see Basil, Holy)*

Turkey Rhubarb *(see Rhubarb)*

Una de Gato *(see Cat's Claw)*

Usnea *(Usnea barbata)* – Usnea is also named old man's beard, and is a lichen that grows and hangs in strands from pine and oak trees, and sometimes other trees. It is an effective urinary and respiratory antibiotic. Usnea is indicated for spastic colon, strep throat, bronchitis, pleurisy, pneumonia and cystitis. It has also been prescribed for the treatment of pneumonia, tuberculosis, lupus, internal infections, strep, staph, trichomonas and other infected wounds.

Uva Ursi/Bearberry *(Arctostaphylos uva-ursi)* – Uva ursi is a kidney herb and has long been used for all sorts of urinary problems. Uva ursi's main constituent is a glycoside called arbutin, which produces an antiseptic effect on the urinary mucous membrane. It also contains allantoin, which spurs the healing of wounds. Uva ursi strengthens the urinary system, balances the pH of urine that is high in acid, and treats incontinence. For womb problems after childbirth uva ursi is an excellent postpartum remedy to prevent infections. Native American use uva ursi mixed with tobacco to create the smoking mixture called "kinnikinnick".

Valerian Root *(Valeriana officinalis)* – Valerian is high in calcium and magnesium, and widely known as a sedative and anti-spasmodic. It is a strong nervous system sedative, and used for anxiety, irritability, depression, hypochondria, and insomnia due to excessive worry. It is also a mild pain reliever. When valerian is combined with nervines such as skullcap, lemon balm or oats, it is very effective for insomnia, anxiety, nervousness, nervous digestive system, and for headaches due to stress. Valerian slows down the heartbeat while increasing its general force.

Valerian Leaf and Flower *(Valeriana officinalis)* – Culpepper joins with many old writers and recommends to use the whole plant, leaf, flower, and root. He praises this herb to increase longevity with its many comforting virtues. The root's sharp odor is often referred to the smell of dirty socks. The flower on the other hand exudes a beautiful fragrance. The leaves taste delicious and can be added to salads. In the garden, valerian leaf and flowers can be added to the compost pile to attract friendly worms. To protect the garden from frost, work valerian leaves and flowers into the soil. In Germany, a compost tea is made with valerian flowers and sprayed on plants, to improve flowering time and plant growth. During Mother Mary's ascension, (August 15th) valerian leaves have been burned with other herbs for protection.

Violet *(Viola odorata)* – Violet leaves and flowers have been used to dissolve hard lumps and tumors in the body. It is good for internal ulcers, pimples, and swollen glands. Violet can be added to formulas to treat a dry cough. Violet relieves severe headaches by relieving pressure in the head.

Virginia Snakeroot *(Aristolochia serpentaria)* – Virginia snakeroot can be used for digestive tract weaknesses, especially when there is constipation in the elderly. It warms up the center of the body and increases appetite, stimulates metabolism, as well as blood circulation in the extremities. It is also an immune system stimulant, increasing white blood cells.

Watercress *(Nasturtium officinale)* – Watercress is a rich source of nutrients, such as carotenoids, minerals, vitamins A and C, chlorophyll, as well as anti-oxidants and anti-bacterial properties. It has traditionally been used for its detoxifying and restorative properties. It contains indoles, which deactivate and eliminate excess estrogen from the body. Watercress is a cholagogue, stimulating liver and gallbladder function and activity. It is used for stagnant liver chi, biliousness and poor fat metabolism.

White Ash *(Fraxinus americana)* – White ash bark has diuretic, anti-inflammatory, bitter, and anodyne properties. It can be used for uterine atony (lack of muscle tone), arthritis, gouty arthritis and bursitis.

White Oak Bark *(Quercus alba)* – White oak bark is extremely astringent and can be used for diarrhea and can stop internal bleeding. Externally, it can be applied to varicose veins, swollen glands, tumors, goiter, and for lymphatic swellings. It can tighten the tissues around a loose tooth.

White Willow *(Salix alba)* – White willow contains salicin, an aspirin-like chemical (blood thinner), used for reducing fevers and to relieve pain caused by arthritis, bursitis, back pain, sciatica, and headaches. With its astringent properties it can reduce inflammation as well. White willow does not make the stomach bleed like the pharmaceutical drug aspirin, because it also contains a mucilaginous property, which is released in the stomach before its other constituent salicylic acid. White willow is effective for diarrhea with intestinal spasms. A tea made with white willow is excellent for urethra and bladder irritability, as it acts as an analgesic on those tissues. With its high magnesium content it helps calm the nerves.

Wild Carrot *(Daucus carota)* – Wild carrot is also named Queen Ann's Lace. aromatic digestive herb, when there is gas, bloating, and deficient hydrochloric acid production. Wild carrot is also useful for upper respiratory congestion.

Wild Cherry Bark *(Prunus spp.)* – Wild cherry bark makes a good syrup for hot, dry cough, mild bronchitis and asthma in children and adults. It calms respiratory nerves and cough reflex. Wild cherry bark moisturizes lungs, loosens phlegm, and is cooling and soothing.

Wild Ginger *(Asarum canadense)* – Wild ginger is a digestive remedy for gas, nausea, and as a stimulating diaphoretic for colds and flu.

Wild Lettuce *(Lactuca spp)* – History says that the Roman Emperor Augustus had a statue built for the physician who prescribed wild lettuce to him. Wild lettuce is a mild sedative, antispasmodic and anodyne. It can be used along with other sedative herbs for insomnia, anxiety and nervous headaches. Wild lettuce is also useful for spasmodic coughs and smoker's cough. Wild lettuce is also known as poor man's opium.

Wild Yam *(Dioscorea villosa)* – Wild yam is an anti-spasmodic and hormone precursor. Whenever both the liver and the reproductive system are implicated as the cause of hormonal imbalances, wild yam has the capabilities of regulating hormone production. (Caffeine can cause hormonal imbalances). Because wild yam has an overall effect on liver health it can lower blood cholesterol and blood pressure. Some of its properties indirectly assist the liver increase its efficiency and reducing stress, relaxing the stomach muscles and the whole abdominal area. It acts as a sedative on the nerves governing these areas. As a hormone precursor, wild yam provides building blocks needed in the production of progesterone, estrogen and cortisone. Wild yam has been used by Native American women during pregnancy to tone the uterus, prevent miscarriage, as well as for birth control. Pharmaceutical companies have used wild yam in the production of contraceptives, but today, wild yam is synthesized in laboratories to manufacture contraceptives. Wild yam is used for biliary colic, gallstone pains, menstrual cramps, arthritic and rheumatic pains, abdominal and intestinal cramps. It can also be used for chronic problems associated with gas and flatulence. Wild yam is one of the best remedies to remove catarrh from the lungs, and when combined with other cleansing herbs it can remove waste from the system, relieving stiff and sore joints. For people who get easily agitated, wild yam can be soothing to the nerves.

Witch Hazel *(Hamamalis virginica)* – Witch hazel is known for its astringent properties and can be applied to varicose veins, hemorrhoids, sprains, wounds, swelling, and bleeding gums. Internally, (not the commercial product) witch hazel may control diarrhea.

Reduce A Fever With Witch Hazel

For fevers in children and adults, witch hazel can be applied as compresses to cool the body down. When my children were little I used the following gentle and comforting treatment to reduce their fevers. I'd sit at their bedside and kept them warm and covered with blankets. I would then uncover one arm, gently wipe the whole arm with a sponge or cotton ball soaked in witch hazel, cover the arm back again, then continue with the other arm and then the legs in the same fashion. The fever would come down within a short time. Placing a cloth soaked in witch hazel on the forehead keeps the head cool during a fever.

Woad *(see Isatis)*

Wood Betony *(Pedicularis groenlandica)* – Wood betony is a nervine, anti-spasmodic and anodyne. It is indicated for sore muscles, spasm or trauma. It relaxes the skeletal muscles, decreases muscular pain and relaxes muscle spasm. It can also be used in formulas for stress headaches, anxiety, torticollis and for fibromyalgia.

Woodruff *(Asperula odorata)* – This small and adorable plant is also known as sweet woodruff, and has an agreeable odor when dried. This is due to its high coumarin presence. It is known for its antispasmodic, calmative and mood elevating properties, as well as for regulating the activity of the heart. In Germany, it is steeped into Rhine wine to make a delicious drink known as Maibowle, drank on the first day of May.

Cooling Mead Wine

Mead is a sweet honey wine infused with herbs. Some time ago people referred to the full moon in June as the "mead" moon or "honeymoon", hence the popular vacation a bride and groom take after their wedding. To make your own version of mead wine gently heat 16 oz of white grape juice, 8 oz of honey and ½ cup of sweet woodruff leaves until the honey dissolves. Let cool and place in refrigerator for about one hour. When ready to serve pour 2 oz of honeyed juice, 2 oz of white wine (if desired) and 4 oz of soda water into a tall glass. Decorate with sweet woodruff leaves on top and serve.

Wormwood *(Artemisia absinthum)* – Wormwood is an intensely bitter tasting herb that was used since ancient times to stimulate digestion, absorption and elimination. Wormwood increases bile secretion, pancreatic and small intestine enzyme production and hydrochloric acid secretion. Wormwood is best known for its anti-parasitic and vermifuge action, especially when combined with black walnut and clove.

Yarrow *(Achillea millefolium)* – Yarrow is a diaphoretic herb and used for colds, flu, and fevers. It is good for chills and constant nasal drip. Yarrow can also be used as a tonic for a prolapsed uterus or rectum, colitis and diarrhea. Externally, yarrow is useful as a topical anti-inflammatory and for sore muscles, scaly skin, and arthritis. Yarrow can stop bleeding relatively quickly.

Yellowdock *(Rumex crispus)* – Yellowdock is indicated for chronic skin problems, for example psoriasis, skin itch, eczema and acne, especially with excessive oily secretions. It is used for liver and gallbladder insufficiency, jaundice, poor iron absorption/storage and constipation. Yellowdock stimulates bile secretion and can be helpful for constipation, as well as for poor fat digestion. Yellowdock tightens varicose veins, cleanses the lymphatic system, and builds physical endurance. It also tones and nourishes the entire glandular system, especially the pineal gland. Yellowdock increases thyroid function,

Yellow Root *(Xanthorrhiza simplicissima)* – Yellow Root can be used as a digestive bitter and as a liver tonic. Originally used by the Cherokee and early European settlers as an anti-fungal and anti-bacterial. Yellow root, is sometimes referred to as goldenseal because of its similar properties, may have antimicrobial, anti-bacterial, and antiviral properties. This herb dates back to the Native American tribes who used yellow root as a remedy for digestive disorders such as gastritis, eye infections such as conjunctivitis, gonorrhea, canker sores, urinary tract infections and skin issues. According to the University of Maryland Medical Center, yellow root has become one of the most popular herbs in the United States; however, there is minuscule evidence that supports any of the claims made about this herb.

Yerba Mansa *(Anemopsis californica)* – Yerba mansa is very similar in its actions and results to goldenseal. It is known to help with rheumatoid arthritis, inflamed hemorrhoids, cystitis, appendicitis, bleeding gums, and at the onset of allergies.

Yerba Mate *(Aquifoliaceae paraguariensis)* – Yerba mate is used throughout the world to reduce appetite, invigorate the body, and reduce fatigue. It is also known to be a diuretic, tonic, nervous system stimulant and to cleanse the body. Yerba mate's tonic effect on the body helps to regulate sleep cycles and reduce fatigue. It is recommended for arthritis, headache, hemorrhoids, fluid retention, obesity, fatigue, stress, constipation, allergies, and hay fever. It cleanses the blood, tones the nervous system, slows down aging, stimulates the mind, controls the appetite, stimulates the production of cortisone, and is believed to enhance the healing powers of other herbs.

Yerba Santa *(Eriodictyon californicum)* – Yerba santa means "sacred herb" and is an excellent respiratory herb to treat coughs, damp bronchitis, damp asthma, and discharge from the nose. It is an old remedy for tuberculosis. Yerba santa is an expectorant, which means it expels mucus from the lungs and the respiratory system. It also contains antispasmodic and anti-fungal properties. Yerba santa is an old remedy for tuberculosis. This herb increases the secretion of body fluids, such as saliva, and is useful when there is dryness in the body. It loosens "things" that have hardened in the body. Yerba santa can be added to herbal formulas to increase their effectiveness.

Yohimbe *(Pausinystalia johimbe)* – Yohimbe is an aphrodisiac for both male and female, as it increases sexual potency and sperm count. It increases testosterone production. Yohimbe dilates blood vessels of the skin and mucous membranes, increasing blood circulation to the skin and sex organs. At the same time it lowers blood pressure. Take Yohimbe with fruits or fruit juices for the safest and best results.
Caution: Do not use when there is high or low blood pressure or heart problems.

Yucca *(Yucca spp.)* – Yucca contains steroidal saponins (a soap like material) including sarsapogenin, a potential cortisone precursor; used internally and externally for slow healing ulcers, skin eruptions, and joint inflammation. Yucca does not penetrate the bloodstream, but acts only on the intestinal flora, regulating and balancing the bacterial colonies in the colon.

By stimulating friendly flora and inhibiting unfriendly bacteria, the amount of toxins absorbed into the body are decreased, therefore lowering the build-up of toxins in the joints and elsewhere, seemingly related to degenerative diseases like arthritis. Yucca tea applied to the soil will help hold water longer, crucial for us living in the desert. A customer told me, when he was working for the Santa Fe railroad company in the hot desert of the southwest, he would drink yucca tea to help him stay hydrated. As well, Native American firefighters drink yucca tea to stay hydrated during long hours of fighting large fires. Yucca's soap like properties can be used as shampoo and soap, and is still being used today by Native Americans.

Zhi Zi *(see Gardenia)*

Will is the Root,

Knowledge is the Stem and Leaves,

and Feeling is the Flower

- Sterling -

HERBAL FIRST AID KIT FOR RADIATION PROTECTION

Aloe Vera Gel: Tissue damage from x-ray exposure or other radiation burns.
Astragalus Root: Rebuilds and protects the immune system. Can be taken daily.
Bach "Rescue Remedy": A combination of flower essences that can quickly soothe anxiety, fear, stress, sadness & cleanse the "Emotional" damage. 4 drops on the tongue or in water, as often as needed throughout the day. Works well on humans and our animal friends.
Barberry: Ancient Egyptian's mixed the berries with fennel seeds for protection against the plaque. Contains properties effective against a wide variety of bacteria, viruses & fungus.
Bee Pollen: Immune fighter & radiation protection
Cats Claw: Radiation & immune system
Charcoal Caps: Acts like a magnet for anything toxic.
Echinacea Root: Fight chemical toxic poisoning & immune system
Garlic: Protect cells from free radical & radiation damage. Anti-septic & anti-biotic
Ginseng: Panax American, Korean,
Pseudoginseng (Tienchi): Radiation protection.
Siberian Ginseng (Eleutherococcus): Radiation protection. Great stress tonic.
Ginkgo: Protects against DNA damage, radiation emits free radicals, which in large quantities can cause chromosome damage, birth defects & cancer.
Horseradish: Inhibits DNA damages.
Irish Moss: Radiation poisoning.
Kelp: Radiation poisoning
Miso Soup: Has a neutralizing effect on Radiation
Milk Thistle: Antioxidant. Will act to inhibit free radical scavengers. Radiation protection.
Pau D' Arco: Immune system. Radiation effects.
Schizandra: Protects against free radical damage. Radiation protection.
Seaweed: Has a neutralizing effect Spirulina (Blue-green algae): Helps lesson the affects of toxic poisoning, radiation, and chemical toxins. Natural
Vitamin C: Amalaki & Rosehips: Increases production of interferon

HERBAL SAFETY GUIDELINES

Based on the American Herbal Products Association Botanical Safety Index, these guidelines are provided to create meaningful safety classifications for botanicals. Botanicals should always be used in a rational and informed manner. Illness or negative reactions can occur from excessive consumption, individual sensitivities and allergic reactions. Seek qualified expert advice before using a botanical with which you are unfamiliar.

Acerola Berry Extract
Keep out of the reach of children

Acidophilus Powder
Keep out of the reach of children

Agar Agar Powder
Taking this product without adequate fluid may cause it to swell and block your throat or esophagus and may cause choking. Do not take this product if you have difficulty in swallowing. If you experience chest pain, vomiting, or difficulty in swallowing or breathing after taking this product, seek immediate medical attention.

Aloes
Do not use this product if you have abdominal pain or diarrhea. Consult a health care provider prior to use if you are pregnant or nursing a baby. Discontinue use in the event of diarrhea or watery stools. Do not exceed recommended dose. Not for long-term use.

Angelica Root
Not to be used during pregnancy. Avoid prolonged exposure to sunlight.

Arnica Flowers
For external use only. Can cause allergic dermatitis with extended use or in sensitive persons. Not to be used on open wounds or broken skin.

Ashwagandha Root
Not to be used during pregnancy. May potentiate the effects of barbiturates.

Barberry Root Bark
Not to be used during pregnancy.

Black Cohosh Root
Not to be used during pregnancy or while nursing.

Black Walnut Hulls
Not recommended for long-term use.

Bladderwrack
Not to be used during pregnancy or while nursing, or by persons with hyperthyroidism. Not recommended for long-term use.

Blessed Thistle Herb
Not to be used during pregnancy.

Bloodroot Root
Not to be used during pregnancy. May cause nausea and vomiting. Do not exceed recommended dosage.

Blue Cohosh Root
Not to be used during pregnancy.

Boldo Leaf
Not to be used by persons with gallstones, serious liver conditions or obstruction of the bile duct. Consult your physician before using this product.

Borage
Not recommended for long-term use. Not to be used during pregnancy or while nursing.

Buckthorn Aged Bark
Do not use this herb if you have abdominal pain or diarrhea. Consult a health care provider prior to use if you are pregnant or nursing a baby. Discontinue use in the event of diarrhea or watery stools. Do not exceed recommended dose. Not for long-term use.

Calamus Root
Not to be used during pregnancy. To be used only under the supervision of an expert qualified in the appropriate use of this herb.

California Poppy
Not to be used during pregnancy. May potentiate pharmaceutical MAO inhibitors.

Camphor Granules
Keep out of reach of children. In case of ingestion contact a poison control center immediately. For external use only if properly diluted.

Cascara Sagrada Aged Bark
Do not use this product if you have abdominal pain or diarrhea. Consult a health care provider prior to use if you are pregnant or nursing a baby. Discontinue use in the event of diarrhea or watery stools. Do not exceed recommended dose. Not for long-term use.

Catnip Leaf & Flower

Not to be used during pregnancy.

Cayenne

Avoid contact with eyes or open wounds.

Chamomile Flowers, Roman

Not to be used during pregnancy.

Chaparral Leaf

Seek advice from a health care practitioner before use if you have any history of liver disease. Discontinue use if nausea, fever, fatigue or jaundice occur (e.g. dark urine or yellow discoloration of the eyes).

Chaste Tree Berries

Not to be used during pregnancy. May counteract the effectiveness of birth control pills.

Coltsfoot Leaf

For external use only. Do not apply to broken or abraded skin. Not to be used during pregnancy or while nursing. Avoid excessive or long-term use.

Comfrey Leaf

For external use only. Do not apply to broken or abraded skin. Not to be used during pregnancy or while nursing. Not recommended for long-term use.

Devil's Claw Root

Not recommended for use by persons with gastric or duodenal ulcers.

Dong Quai Root

Not to be used during pregnancy.

Elecampane Root

Not to be used during pregnancy or while nursing. Large doses may cause vomiting, diarrhea, spasms, and symptoms of paralysis.

Ephedra (Ma Huang)

Seek advice from a health care practitioner prior to use if you are pregnant or nursing, or if you have high blood pressure, heart or thyroid disease, diabetes, difficulty in urination due to prostate enlargement or if taking an MAO inhibitor or any other prescription drug. Reduce or discontinue use if nervousness, tremor, sleeplessness, loss of appetite or nausea occur. Not intended for persons under 18 years of age. Keep out of reach of children.

Eucalyptus Leaf

Not to be used by persons with inflammatory diseases of the gastro-intestinal and bile ducts and severe diseases of the liver. Do not use eucalyptus preparations on areas of the face and especially the nose in infants and young children.

Feverfew Flowering Tops
Not to be used during pregnancy.
Feverfew Leaf
Not to be used during pregnancy.
Flax Seed
This herb should be ingested with at least 6 oz. of liquid. Not for use by persons with bowel obstruction.
Garlic Capsule
Not to be used while nursing.
Gentian Root
Not to be used by persons with gastric or duodenal ulcers or when gastric irritation or inflammation is present. Consult a health care practitioner prior to use if you are pregnant or suffering from high blood pressure.
Ginger Root
Not to be used in excess during pregnancy.
Ginkgo Leaf
May potentiate pharmaceutical MAO inhibitors.
Goldenseal
Not to be used during pregnancy.
Guar Gum
Taking this herb without adequate fluid may cause it to swell and block your throat or esophagus and may cause choking. Do not take this herb if you have difficulty in swallowing. If you experience chest pain, vomiting, or difficulty in swallowing or breathing after taking this herb, seek immediate medical attention.
Guggal
Do not take Guggulu while experiencing acute kidney infections and rashes; avoid eating sour foods, exhaustion, sun exposure, alcohol, and anger, when taking this herb.
Henna Leaf Red Powder
For external use only.
Hop Flowers (Sweet)
Not recommended for use by persons suffering from depression.
Horehound Herb
Not to be used during pregnancy.
Horsetail (Shavegrass)
Equisetum arvense should not be used by persons with cardiac or renal dysfunction. Not recommended for long-term use.

Hydrangea Root

Use with caution. Do no exceed recommended dose. Avoid long-term use.

Hyssop Herb

Not to be used during pregnancy.

Juniper Berries

Not to be used for more than four to six weeks in succession. Persons with inflammatory kidney disease should not use this herb. Not to be used during pregnancy.

Kava Kava Root

Not for use by persons under the age of 18. If pregnant, nursing or taking a prescription drug, consult a health care practitioner prior to use. Do not exceed recommended dose. Excessive consumption may impair ability to drive or operate heavy equipment. Not recommended for consumption with alcoholic beverages.

Kola Nuts

Not to be used during pregnancy. Not to be used by persons with hypertension or gastric or duodenal ulcers. Not recommended for excessive or long-term use.

Lemongrass

Not to be used during pregnancy.

Licorice Root

Not for prolonged or excessive use except under the supervision of a qualified health practitioner. Prolonged use may cause potassium depletion and sodium retention resulting in symptoms of hypertension, edema, headache, and vertigo. Not for use by persons with hypertension, hypokalemia, edema, cirrhosis, or the liver and cholestatic liver disorders, and diabetes. Not to be used during pregnancy or while nursing.

Lobelia Herb

Not to be used during pregnancy. Do not exceed recommended dose. May cause nausea and vomiting.

Lomatium Root

Not to be used during pregnancy. When used internally this product may cause a rash. Discontinue use if rash occurs.

Lovage Root

Not to be used during pregnancy or by persons with impaired or inflamed kidneys.

Lycii Berries (Gou Qi Zi)

Not to be used during pregnancy.

Menthol Crystals

Keep out of reach of children. In case of ingestion contact a poison control center immediately. For external use only if properly diluted.

Mistletoe Herb
Not for use by persons with protein hypersensitivity and chronic-progressive infections such as tuberculosis and AIDS. Do not exceed recommended dosage.

Motherwort Herb
Not to be used during pregnancy.

Mugwort
Not to be used during pregnancy.

Nutmeg
In large amounts may cause dizziness, stomach pains, rapid pulse, nausea, anxiety, liver pain, double vision and coma.

Oregon Grape Root
Not to be used during pregnancy.

Osha Root
Not to be used during pregnancy

Parsley Root
Not to be used during pregnancy or by persons with inflammatory kidney disease.

Pennyroyal, European Herb
Not to be used during pregnancy.

Periwinkle Herb
Not for use by persons with low blood pressure or constipation.

Pleurisy Root
Not to be used during pregnancy. May cause nausea and vomiting.

Poke Root
To be used only under the supervision of an expert qualified in the appropriate use of this herb.

Prickly Ash Bark
Not to be used during pregnancy.

Psyllium Seed Husk
Taking this herb without adequate fluid may cause it to swell and block your throat or esophagus and may cause choking. Do not take this herb if you have difficulty in swallowing. If you experience chest pain, vomiting, or difficulty in swallowing or breathing after taking this herb, seek immediate medical attention.

Queen of the Meadow
For external use only. Do not apply to broken or abraded skin. Not to be used during pregnancy or while nursing. Not recommended for long-term use.

Red Clover Blossoms
Not to be used during pregnancy.
Rehmannia Root Steamed (Shu Di Huang)
Not for use by persons with diarrhea and indigestion.
Rhubarb Root
Do not use this product if you have abdominal pain or diarrhea. Consult a health care provider prior to use if you are pregnant or nursing a baby. Discontinue use in the event of diarrhea or watery stools. Do not exceed recommended dose. Not for long-term use.
Rosemary leaf
Not to be used during pregnancy
Rue Herb Powder
Not to be used during pregnancy. Not for use by persons with poor kidney function. Avoid prolonged exposure to sunlight.
Safflower Petals
Not to be used during pregnancy or by persons with hemorrhagic diseases or peptic ulcers. Ingestion of this herb may prolong blood coagulation time.
Saint John's Wort Herb
May potentiate pharmaceutical MAO inhibitors. Avoid prolonged exposure to sunlight when taking this herb.
Sandalwood Yellow, Indian
Not for use by persons with diseases of the parenchyma of the kidney. Do not use for more than six weeks in succession without consulting a physician.
Sarsaparilla Root
Not recommended for use by persons taking blood-thinning agents.
Sassafras Root Bark
Use with caution. Avoid excessive or long-term use.
Senna leaf
Do not use this herb if you have abdominal pain or diarrhea. Consult a health care provider prior to use if you are pregnant or nursing a baby. Discontinue use in the event of diarrhea or watery stools. Do not exceed recommended dose. Not for long-term use.
Senna Pods
Do not use this herb if you have abdominal pain or diarrhea. Consult a health care provider prior to use if you are pregnant or nursing a baby. Discontinue use in the event of diarrhea or watery stools. Do not exceed recommended dose.
Sheep Sorrel Herb
Not recommended for use by persons with a history of kidney stones.

Shepherd's Purse
Not to be used during pregnancy or by persons with a history of kidney stones.

Spikenard Root
Not to be used during pregnancy.

Tansy Herb
Not to be used during pregnancy. To be used only under the supervision of an expert qualified in the appropriate use of this substance.

Tonka Beans
Use as an aromatic fixative in potpourris or other crafts. Not for internal use.

Uva Ursi leaf
Not to be used during pregnancy. Not to be used by persons with kidney disorders, irritated digestive conditions or in conjunction with conditions or remedies that produce acidic urine. Not for prolonged use unless consulting a health care practitioner.

Vitamin C Powder
Keep out of the reach of children

Wheat Grass Powder
Keep out of the reach of children

White Oak Bark
Avoid application to extensively damaged skin.

Wild Cherry Bark
Use with caution. Do not exceed recommended dose. Not recommended for long-term use.

Wormwood. Herb
Use with caution. Not to be used during pregnancy or while nursing. Do not exceed recommended dose. Not recommended for long-term use.

Yarrow Flowers
Not to be used during pregnancy. Consult a health care provider prior to external use if you suffer from allergies related to the Asteraceae family.

Yellow dock Root
Not recommended for use by persons with a history of kidney stones.

Yohimbe Bark
Contraindicated in existing liver and kidney diseases and in chronic inflammation of the sexual organs or prostate gland. Not recommended for excessive or long-term use. May potentiate pharmaceutical MAO inhibitors.

WHAT IS A PEPPER?

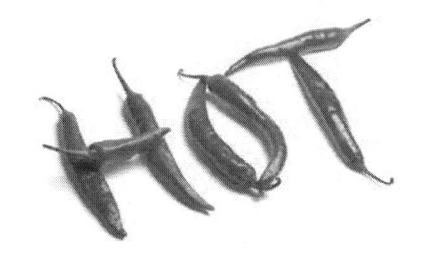

Green, Black and White Peppercorns

Green, black and white peppercorns are the fruits of a tropical vine, *Piper nigrum*, a species completly different from the capsicum peppers, (bell pepper, cayenne, chili pepper). The most spicy of this group is the black peppercorn, picked when unripe, and then dried. If instead of being dried, the unripe berries are freeze-dried or submerged in brine, it becomes the kinder, gentler green peppercorn. When the same berry is left to ripen on the vine, and then is shorn of its outer skin the mild white peppercorn is born.

Pink Peppercorns

Pink peppercorns are berries from a South American tree, *Schinus terebinthifolius*. The pink peppercorns adds mild pungency and stunning color to food.

Szechuan Pepper

Szechuan pepper is also known as *fagara* and *anise pepper*. This aromatic dried berry from the prickly ash tree has a hot woody flavor and is one of the ingredients of Chinese five spice powder, and is commonly used in Asian fish dishes. Dry-roasting it before use heightens the flavor.

Cubeb Pepper

Cubeb pepper is also known as *Piper cubeba*. This pepper like spice was extremely popular in the middle Ages. Now, it is still being used in Egypt and other countries in the Middle East.

Grains of Paradise

Grains of paradise are also known as *Aframomum melegueta*, discovered by Portugal in the 15th century, it became an inexpensive substitute for pepper.

200

Chili Pepper

Chili pepper is from the *Capsicum* family and can be as small as a pea or as large as an eggplant, in hues of cream, yellow, orange and green. Their pungency ranges from sweet to flaming hot. All peppers contain capsaicin. Their heat is determined by the amount of capsaicin they contain and is measured in HU = Heat Units on a scale from 0 – 1,500,000 HU. Ghost pepper and Trinidad Scorpion are the hottest pepper and usually come with a warning.

Chipotle

When fresh jalapenos are smoke-dried, the resulting withered peppers with a hot smoky flavor are called Chipotle.

Paprika

Paprika is the mildest of peppers. It adds beautiful color to dishes.

Five Spice Powder

Five Spice blend is used throughout China and Vietnam to flavor many dishes.

7 star anise pods
1 tbsp fennel seeds
1 tbsp Szechuan pepper
2 tsp cloves
2 tbsp cinnamon cut in small pieces

Combine all ingredients in a spice grinder and grind to a powder.

Seven Spice Seasoning
(Shichimi Togarashi)

Use this popular blend in soups, vegetables, quinoa, grains, or with noodles.

1 tbsp white sesame seeds
1 tbsp minced tangerine zest
½ tbsp Szechuan pepper
½ tsp ground cayenne
1 tsp poppy seeds
1 tsp black sesame seeds
One 2-inch square Japanese seaweed (Nori) finely chopped

Combine all ingredients in a spice grinder or food processor and grind coarsely.

Chai Tea

Just what you need when you wake up in the morning, without the caffeine.

1 cup loose honeybush
3 tbsp dried ginger small pieces
1 tbsp dried cinnamon samll pieces
2 tsp cloves whole
1 pinch cardamom seeds
1-2 vanilla beans cut into 1/4 inches
1 pinch coriander seeds
1/4 tsp dried nutmeg
Mix all ingredients and use 1 tsp to make one cup.

Curry Powder

1st Ingredients
2 tbsp cumin seeds
1 tbsp allspice berries
1 tsp anise seeds
1 tbsp coriander seeds
1 tsp cloves
1 tsp mustard seeds
1 tsp poppy seeds

2nd Ingredients
2 tbsp turmeric ground
½ tsp cinnamon ground
1 tbsp ginger ground
1 tsp fenugreek ground

Combine first seven ingredients in a small skillet over low heat. Dry-roast for two minutes or until the mustard seeds start popping. Let cool, transfer to a spice grinder and blend to a fine powder. Add the last four ingredients and blend to mix.

Harissa

Harissa is a spice blend and used in Algerian, Moroccon and Tunisian. Use it whenever you crave a spicy dish.

3 large dried chili peppers, seeded and stemmed
1 tsp mint, dried - 1 tbsp olive oil - 1 tbsp coriander seeds
1 tbsp caraway seeds - 8 garlic cloves – 1 tsp cumin seeds

Soak chilies and mint in 1/3 cup of hot water for about 30 minutes. Transfer the chilies and mint to a food processor and add remaining ingredients. Blend to a smooth paste.

Herbes de Provence

This is a French herbal seasoning blend from the south of France (Provence). Combine all ingredients and add to dishes for a Mediterranean flavor.

2 tsp thyme, dried	1 tsp savory, dried
2 tsp basil, dried	½ tsp fennels, ground
1 tsp marjoram, dried	½ tsp lavender, dried
1 tsp rosemary, dried	

Annatto Paste

Use this flavorful and colorful paste in any dishes to add beautiful color and taste.

1 tbsp olive oil
½ cup annatto seeds
1 cup fresh orange juice
¼ cup fresh lemon juice
1 ½ tsp dried oregano
1 tsp allspice
1 tsp cumin
2 garlic cloves, unpeeled
¼ tsp cayenne
½ tsp salt

Heat the oilive oil in a skillet until hot. Add annatto seeds and sauté stirring constantly for about 5 minutes. Transfer to a bowl and add the orange and lemon juice. Let this soak for about 3 hours. Combine oregano, allspice and cumin in a skillet and dry-roast for 2 minutes. Transfer to a bowl. Do the same with the garlic until it is slightly darkened, then cool and peel. Drain the annatto and transfer to a food processor. Add the roasted spices, garlic, cayenne and salt and blend to a paste.

Chimichurri

This Argentinian recipe is a deliciously spiced parsley sauce and traditionally used on grilled meats, but is also wonderful on vegetables and in soups.

½ cup olive oil
5 tbsp red balsamic vinegar
5 garlic cloves, minced
½ cup onion, chopped
½ cup parsley, chopped
1 tbsp oregano, dried
1 tsp black pepper
¼ tsp hot red pepper
Peruvian salt to taste

Combine the oil and vinegar in a bowl and mix. Stir in the rest of the ingredients. Let stand for 3 hours before serving.

Hawaj

This aromatic, earthy Yemenite recipe is delicious in soups or cooked vegetables.

2 tbsp black pepper
2 tbsp caraway seeds
2 tsp cardamom
2 tsp turmeric
1 tsp coriander seeds
1 tsp saffron threads

Grind in a food processor.

Za'atar

Za'atar is used as a seasoning spread on breads or in dips.

½ cup sesame seeds
5 tbsp thyme crumbled
2 tbsp marjoram crumbled
2 tbsp sumac crumbled

Dry-roast sesame seeds in a skillet over low heat for 2 minutes. Cool, and add the remaining ingredient and mix well. Add 2 tbsp ground pistachios to vary the recipe.

Salad Dressing

This is a health-enhancing and delicious salad dressing. Prepare it fresh whenever you are having a salad.

1 garlic clove, minced
½ tsp parsley, chopped
¼ tsp ginger, powdered
¼ tsp onion, powdered
dash horseradish, powdered
dash cayenne, powdered

Mix ingredients with 3 tbsp olive oil and 1 ½ tbsp freshly pressed lemon juice.

HYDROSOLS

Hydrosols or hydrolates, are pure, water-based solutions created when essential oils are steam distilled. A hydrosol is a potent, yet subtle form of medicine that can be ingested as well as applied directly to the skin, unlike most pure essential oils. In fact, hydrosols are considered the homeopathic version of aromatherapy, and as such are ideal for use with children, pregnant women, animals, and those with fragile immune systems.

Hydrosols from flowers are called Flower Waters or Flower Hydrosols. Hydrosols from herbs are called Herbal Hydrosols. They are about 20-30 times more concentrated in herbal strength then herb teas. Use one teaspoon hydrosol for each cup of water. If you add one drop of essential oil to the diluted hydrosol water you have a powerful herbal/aromatherapy tea.

The Many Uses of Hydrosols

<u>For Beauty and Skin Care</u>: Spritz undiluted hydrosol on face, hair, nails and body. Add to your homemade beauty products. Add one to two cups to your bath water.

<u>For Pets</u>: Add to their drinking water, spritz their coat and beddings.

<u>For your laundry</u>: Add to the last rinse cycle, soak a small cloth and add to your dryer, spray on clothing during ironing.

<u>For your Home</u>: Hydrosols are safe for your Feng Shui fountains, diluted or undiluted. Spritz around to freshen a room.

<u>For Healing</u>: Spray Lavender on burns, cucumber to cool the skin, clary Sage for hot flashes, chamomile for diaper rash, etc.

<u>In the Kitchen</u>: Add undiluted to your soups, stocks, salad dressings, baking, etc.

<u>Beverages</u>: Add one teaspoon to 6 to 8 oz of water. Add a splash to a glass of wine or champagne. Make hydrosol ice cubes!

<u>Travel</u>: Make your own wipes for traveling or at home.

Store hydrosols in your refrigerator. Since hydrosols are distillates, they are pure and do not contain any bacterias. If you handle your hydrosols in a clean way, they can last for about one year. "Old" hydrosols can be added to your bath water.

Individual Hydrosols

Angelica
(Angelica archangelica)
Angelica hydrosol is sedative, grounding and calms the nerves, useful during times of high stress and states of anxiety. For mental chatter add one teaspoon to one cup of water and sip very slowly. A mild digestive, angelica hydrosol has warming properties and can be used to improve appetite and to tone digestive system.

Birch Yellow
(Betula alleghaniensis)
Yellow birch hydrosol is known to break kidney and bladder stones. It may also be helpful for gout and rheumatic complaints. Birch is a counter-irritant, good for muscular aches and strains. It can be inhaled for hypertension. Good as a mouth wash.

Chamomile, German/Blue
(Matricaria recutita)
German/blue chamomile hydrosol is cooling and soothing. It is the hydrosol of choice for irritated skin, rashes, acne, burns, etc. It also makes a wonderful healing spray for sunburn, when it hurts too much to touch. One study shows that German chamomile was 60% as effective as a topical corticosteroid cream. Try blending it with some green or white clay for a healing facial masque. *Suzanne Catty recommends it for internal use (both as a beverage or a douche) for candida, thrush, and vaginal infections, as well as for digestive spasms. German chamomile is instantly anxiolytic. Drink it or mist it on when stressed before exams, presentations, or major events to calm and center.

Chamomile, Roman
(Anthemis nobilis)
Roman chamomile hydrosol is soothing and relaxing for various skin conditions, such as dry, flaky, itchy skin, rashes, acne, eczema, etc. Mucus membranes, for example of the mouth, gums, respiratory tract, anal and genital areas, may safely be treated with this gentle and soothing anti-inflammatory. Some herbalists recommend Roman chamomile hydrosol internally for intestinal cramps and spasms as well as for urinary tract infections. Use it as a sitz bath to soothe and heal hemorrhoids. Make natural antiseptic diaper wipes or wet paper towels. Use it to soothe 'sandpapery' eyelids. A compress of Roman chamomile hydrosol on the forehead gently eases a migraine.

Clary Sage
(Salvia sclarea)
Clary sage hydrosol is a "woman's choice" hydrosol, used for menstrual cramps, bloating, water retention, moodiness and other signs of PMS. For menopausal symptoms, mix with sage hydrosol. Clary sage hydrosol mixed with rose hydrosol, misted on the face, gives the skin a moist, dewy glow. Clary sage has aphrodisiac, euphoric and antidepressant properties. *Suzanne Catty says that it makes a good beverage for those giving up the alcohol habit, calming the symptoms of withdrawal. Clary sage hydrosol is good to use for emotional traumas and heartache.

Cornflower/Batchelor's Button
(Centuria cyanus)
Cornflower hydrosol has cooling and relaxing properties. Use it as a toner for delicate, dry or mature skin. For hot flashes spritz it on your face and feel the cooling effect. Spray on bruises to speed up healing. As an eye compress, cornflower soothes irritated eyes. Good for computer eyes!

Cucumber
(Cucumis sativus)
Cleopatra used cucumber juice to preserve her skin! Cucumber hydrosol is very cooling and soothing to the skin. A mild astringent, aids in removing dead skin cells, alleviates inflammations and irritants.

Echinacea
(Echinacea purpurea)
Echinacea hydrosol has immune boosting properties. This hydrosol is still being researched.

Frankincense
(Boswellia carteri)
Frankincense hydrosol is great for the skin, due to its rejuvenating and anti-aging properties. Internally, frankincense is diuretic and very drying. You may combine with sandalwood hydrosol to treat urinary and reproductive system problems.

Bird Bath
Birds love water, especially here in the hot Arizonan desert. Leave a birdbath out for your birds at all times and add no more than 10% hydrosol to 90% water. Watch them enjoy it! Even your caged birds will love it.

Geranium
(Pelargonium graveolens)
Geranium hydrosol is balancing and adaptogenic for oily, dry, acneic, and sensitive skin. To combat dry and rough skin on elbows, knees, even for calluses on hands or feet, use as compresses daily for several weeks. Use it neat as a make-up remover. Geranium is a humectant, attracting moisture to and holding it in the skin. Anti-inflammatory and very cooling, geranium hydrosol calms sunburns, rashes, insect bites, and any topical conditions where heat is present. It is also effective for broken capillaries, coupe rose, rosacea, and other skin conditions with redness. Geranium hydrosol eases PMS symptoms, menopausal conditions, and hormone related moodiness. A feel good Hydrosol; it balances male and female energy.

Ginger
(Zingiber officinalis)
Ginger is known to help with digestion and circulation. Just add a splash to some fizzy water and a little honey, and you have a delicious ginger drink. Drink it with your meals to improve digestion and absorption.

Goldenrod
(Solidago Canadensis)
Taken internally, goldenrod is a strong diuretic and cleanser to the entire hepato-renal system without having the "squeezing" effects of juniper or cypress. It prevents and treats kidney stones. Because of its astringent and relaxing properties it may be useful in treating stress or diet-related "runs" in both people and animals. Topically, use it as a compress for fluid retention, and uric acid in the joints and tissue. Add it to the bath to soothe rheumatic and arthritic pain. This hydrosol is a strong anti-inflammatory and moderate antispasmodic for sore muscles, stiff neck, tendonitis, and repetitive strain injuries. Goldenrod hydrosol balances high as well as low blood pressure. Goldenrod carries the intense vibrations of heat and sun. It opens the solar plexus and diaphragm, bringing calmness to that area. It is wonderful in energetic healing for the emotions and the heart and for helping to release old anger.

Greenland Moss
(Ledum groenlandicum)
Greenland moss is often called Labrador tea in Canada. Greenland moss is said to be a powerful detoxifier and a support to both the liver and the immune system, and may be beneficial during recuperation time after a major illness. It also stimulates lymphatic circulation.

Immortelle
(Helichrysum italicum)

Immortelle hydrosol has anti-inflammatory and cicatrisant properties helpful in treating bruises, swelling, and other tissue damages. Immortelle can be used after surgery, as it speeds the healing of wounds from incisions and needles, reducing swelling and bruising, and also to assist the liver detoxify the anesthetic. In skin care, use immortelle hydrosol for sensitive, mature or congested skin, and for scars. Use as a mouthwash after dental work. For gingivitis or receding gums, use one tablespoon with water as a mouthwash two times daily for six months. Internal use of this hydrosol can speed recovery after a long illness. For liver problems use in combination with milk thistle, artichoke and other bitter herbs. It is soothing to the emotional heart.

Elecampane
(Inula graveolens)

Elecampane hydrosol is a powerful mucolytic and can be used for thrush, vaginitis, and leucorrhea. Elecampane hydrosol is effective for any kind of respiratory condition, chronic or acute. In skin care, use it for congested and acne skin. To clean pores, mix with an appropriate exfoliant or clay.

Kewda
(Pandanus odoritissimus)

Kewda hydrosol has a delicate floral scent and can be used to flavor foods, particularly sweet rice dishes. Raises low blood pressure and assists digestion.

Lavender
(Lavendula angustifolia)

Lavender hydrosol is an "all purpose" hydrosol. It is gentle, balancing for all skin types, cooling in summer's heat, soothing sunburns, as well as healing skin irritations from bug bites and stings. It gently tones oily, dry and mature skin, cleansing gently and safely. Lavender hydrosol is relaxing and revitalizing. *Suzanne Catty says to spray the skin both before and after shaving or hair removal to reduce inflammation, get a closer shave, and prevent ingrown hairs. It can ease stress and reduce mental fatigue. Children love lavender hydrosol and it can be used to calm cranky moods, sprayed on a pillow for a restful night's sleep, and to clean cuts and scrapes, "to kiss and make it better". Lavender hydrosol is an "adaptor," adapting itself to your body and your psyche's needs, soothing or revitalizing as needed. Good for jet lag. It is a wonderful addition to creams and lotions.

Lemon Verbena
(Lippia citriodora)
Lemon verbena hydrosol has a wonderful refreshing lemony aroma. Use it as a facial spray for all skin types to revitalize and balance. On tiring trips it can be sprayed on the face to stimulate and keep the driver alert. This is a great hydrosol to use as a cooling and tasty tonic drink (1 teaspoon per cup of water or soda water with a bit of sugar and poured over ice cubes).

Linden Blossom
(Tillia europea)
Linden hydrosol is very calming during stressful times. It is good to use for exhaustion, when the body wants to stop, but the mind keeps whirring. Linden hydrosol has an anti-depressant effect, relieving anxiety, easing insomnia, and is somewhat euphoric. It can be taken as a tonic drink. In hot weather, linden hydrosol cools the body and soul. It is perfect as a baby spray, or you may add a few drops to baby's water. Spray on pillow before bedtime to induce prophetic dreams and promote lucid dreaming. This hydrosol is very soothing to the skin, and works well in treating puffy and devitalized skin.

Mastic
(Pistacia lentiscus)
Mastic hydrosol is known to be effective for venous and prostatic congestion.

Melissa/Lemon Balm
(Melissa officianalis)
Melissa hydrosol has a refreshing, revitalizing lemon like scent, and is known for its anti-viral effects. As a preventative, add a teaspoon of the hydrosol to bottled water every day during the flu and virus season. Use as a compress to help ease the symptoms of shingles. Melissa hydrosol is often recommended to settle upset stomachs, nausea and indigestion. The gentleness of melissa hydrosol makes it a great toner/astringent for oily skin, as well as being a good antioxidant and anti-inflammatory. Apply undiluted melissa hydrosol to herpes sores six to ten times a day, and take one-half tablespoon internally at each application. Melissa is both uplifting and anti-depressant, as well as being relaxing! It is more calming to the body than the mind. It is also helpful for times of emotional crisis. Studies have shown positive results for attention deficit hyperactivity disorders (ADHD). For children with ADHD and ADD use 1 oz of melissa hydrosol in 32 oz of water and have them drink it throughout the day. For adults, double the quantity of hydrosol (2 oz per 32 oz of water).

Neroli/Orange Blossoms
(Citrus aurantium)
Neroli hydrosol is toning, astringent and delicious. Neroli hydrosol is mildly sedative without causing sleepiness. It stops caffeine jitters and is good to use during stressful times. Neroli hydrosol is supportive when quitting a habit or addiction, such as smoking. It is uplifting and has aphrodisiac properties. Neroli hydrosol is quite effective for children with ADD and ADHD and can be used topically and internally for this purpose. It is an old European remedy for colicky and cranky babies.

Oregano
(Origanum vulgare)
Oregano hydrosol is safer to use than the essential oil, good for people with delicate systems and who are too fragile in handling essential oil treatments. There is no risk of damaging the mucus membranes. Oregano hydrosol makes a good mouthwash or gargle for canker sores, mouth sores, gum and tooth infections, and a sore throat. Oregano hydrosol has been traditionally used as a daily beverage to aid digestion and as a general health tonic. Oregano hydrosol can be used in a sitz bath or douche for vaginitis, candidiasis, pruritus, and similar conditions. Add to enema water or in colonics, particularly as part of an anti- parasite treatment. *Susanne Catty recommends combining oregano hydrosol with bay laurel hydrosol in treating lymphatic infections or immune system weakness, or to bolster the system during allergy season. Mix oregano hydrosol with an appropriate clay and use as a mask on acne skin, for an anti-bacterial effect. Good for animals too, as a wound-cleanser, if a cut or injury becomes infected.

Peppermint
(Mentha piperita)
Peppermint hydrosol is known for its digestive, anti-inflammatory, and mind-stimulating properties. People with Crohn's disease, colitis, or irritable bowel syndrome should try it, as it has provided significant relief to a number of people suffering from these conditions. Peppermint hydrosol is an effective digestive tract cleanser, having mild anti-bacterial and anti-fermentative properties and can be combined with other hydrosols, such as chamomile, basil or rosemary. Peppermint hydrosol is also a great mouthwash and breath freshener. When used topically for its mild antiseptic effect, it can gently ease the itch of rashes and stings. Peppermint hydrosol is soothing after shaving, easing razor burn. Peppermint hydrosol can be used in hydrotherapy treatments for stiff muscles, aches and pains, and for sprains and strains. Add it to hot water it will have a cooling effect, added to cold water it will have a heating effect. Peppermint is also helpful in combating a hangover, since it both settles the stomach and energizes. A good coffee substitute when you need a quick energy lift. Added to cold water, Peppermint hydrosol is the ultimate thirst quencher.

Rosemary
(Rosmarinus officinalis)

Rosemary hydrosol is helpful for treating the respiratory system. It also has a strengthening and toning effect on the reproductive system. *Susanne Catty says to use it internally for three weeks to clear mucus from the digestive tract, improve liver function and digestion, and to clear the skin. Rosemary brightens the complexion, as it decongests clogged pores, bringing impurities to the surface. It is also excellent and refreshing used in a toner. Mist on damp hair to promote healthy, shiny hair. It also acts as a reconstructor for chemically over-treated or damaged hair.

Rose
(Rosa damascena)

Rose hydrosol is a hormone balancer for all ages. Because of its balancing effect on the endocrine system, it is highly recommended for PMS, cramps and moodiness. Excellent as an alternative to hormone replacement therapy in postmenopausal women, combined with other essential oil, herbs or other naturopathic treatments. Rose hydrosol treats the autonomic nervous system and makes you "feel good". I use rose hydrosol to moisturize my dry eyes. I either make an eye compress or I put two drops of rose hydrosol in each eye. It cools my eyes, removes redness and burning sensations. *(Caution: make sure to use rose hydrosol and not rose essential oil added to water. Read the label).* Rose hydrosol is suitable for all ages and skin types. It is a humectant especially suitable for dry, mature, sensitive and devitalized skin. Added to the final hair rinse water will give the hair a lingering fragrance. For a sensuous bedroom aroma try spraying the sheets with it. Rose hydrosol has a special affinity with the heart, letting you love yourself. But, true emotional healing and opening of the heart makes you more vulnerable and fragile in the short term. Get support from your loved ones when seeking to heal these emotional, heart-centered parts of your being. Rose hydrosol can be added to desserts, beverages, or a glass of champagne. *(Caution: rose hydrosol has a cleansing effect, use small quantities to avoid loose stool).* I always have a small rose hydrosol spray bottle in my car. While traveling I spritz some on my face, hands and arms for a physically and emotionally cooling effect.

St. John's Wort
(Hypericum perforatum)

St. John's Wort hydrosol is a mood elevator, and very effective in cases of seasonal affective disorder (SAD). It has anti-depressant and mild euphoriant properties. Saint John's Wort hydrosol is wonderfully healing on the skin, softens and clarifies the complexion, giving a dewy glow after a week or two of daily use. Combine with helichrysum for scar treatments.

Sage, White
(Salvia apiana)
White sage hydrosol has a very powerful energy field, and is extraordinary in dispersing negative energy (after an argument, etc.), when misted through the air. Smudging with white sage is used in Native American rituals for emotional healing and protection. If you are in a place where the smoke of white sage is not appropriate, or even forbidden, you can use the hydrosol. White sage hydrosol cleanses crystals and other healing tools. Apply by anointing the chakras and energy points of the body. Increases good energy!
Caution: Not recommended for internal use.

Sandalwood
(Santalum album)
Sandalwood hydrosol is slightly astringent, cooling and very calming to the skin. It is great for mature and troubled skin, as it contains anti-inflammatory properties. Sandalwood hydrosol has a wonderful rich scent and is known to preserve the skin and promotes healing. Spray on sore throats for a cooling effect. It has shown to be effective for recurring bladder infections and cystitis.

Witch Hazel
(Hamamelis virginiana)
Witch hazel hydrosol is made from the leaves and twigs. We are not referring to witch hazel USP that you pick up at your local pharmacy. That one has between 14 and 30% alcohol added to it. Witch hazel is one of the most important anti-aging and anti-oxidant hydrosol. It reduces redness, rashes and scaly skin and acts as an anti-inflammatory. In the summer, it is great to calm bites and stings. It is famous in shrinking varicose veins and hemorrhoids. It has a long history of traditional and alternative medicine uses, specifically for the treatment of hemorrhoids, burns and fevers. It is known as a soothing skin freshener, astringent, pore tightening and anti-inflammatory. Relieves itching, and soothes skin irritations. When my children were little, I used witch hazel hydrosol to reduce their high fever. Firstly, keep your child comfortable, relaxed, warm and covered with a natural fiber blanket. Secondly, to cool the hot and feverish little head, place a cloth or thick paper towel soaked with witch hazel hydrosol on the child's forehead *(Please, do not cover the eyes, it is scary for a child)*. Thirdly, uncover one arm and lightly wipe the entire arm with a witch hazel soaked cotton ball. Cover that arm up again. Uncover the other arm and repeat. Uncover one leg and repeat, then uncover the other leg and repeat. Do not uncover or wipe the torso. Lastly, tell your child, "I love you very much". Within ½ hour my children would be fast a sleep and the fever reduced to almost normal.

Yarrow
(Achillea millefolium)
Yarrow hydrosol helps reduce fever and eases aches and pains associated with flus and colds. It is a good digestive aid and improves digestion (especially fatty foods), increases elimination, calms gastric spasms, and can quickly relieve indigestion and heartburn caused by overindulgence. Yarrow hydrosol stabilizes body fluids and gets rid of excess water without being overly diuretic. Use it as a compress for fluid in joints and for rheumatic pain or on any other part of the body where fluids have accumulated. Yarrow hydrosol is mildly anti-bacterial and antiseptic, good for acne skin conditions, and as an anti-inflammatory to heal damaged skin from sun and wind. Yarrow hydrosol's astringent and styptic properties can be used to clean wounds and stop bleeding. Yarrow promotes mental calm and peace.

Ylang Ylang
(Cananga odorata)
Ylang Ylang hydrosol is known for its aphrodisiac properties. It relieves anxiety and nervous exhaustion.

Zdravetz
(Geranium macrorrhizum)
Zdravetz hydrosol is made from Bulgarian's wild geranium. It has adrenal balancing properties. Most of all it is being used in men's perfumes for its musty and musky green scent.

Hydrosol Compresses for the Eyes

1 oz. rose hydrosol	2 oz distilled water	dry eyes
1 oz. chamomile hydrosol	2 oz distilled water	sore or tired eyes
1 oz. lavender hydrosol	2 oz distilled water	conjunctivitis
¼ oz cucumber hydrosol	2 oz distilled water	puffiness under eyes

You may also use these hydrosols undiluted for eye compresses.

* Suzanne Catty is a well-known Canadian researcher and advocate of hydrosols. She is the author of Hydrosols, The Next Aromatherapy.

INCENSE

Incense burning has been part of rituals and ceremonies for thousands of years. Though its use in the Far East has never waned, the practice was largely overlooked in the West until recently. Now that its healing properties have been rediscovered, many people utilize these aromatic substances to cleanse the atmosphere, to reduce stress, to renew energy, even to help insomnia or to stimulate creativity.

In the study of aromas much progress is being made. A professor of psychiatry at Yale has found that people exposed to certain pleasant scents show less stress, as measured by blood pressure, heart rate and muscle tension. Further scientific studies have been researching why the sense of smell is so very powerful. The human olfactory system is still somewhat a mystery to modern science, although there are certain commonly accepted theories. One common belief is that nerve cells of the nose transmit a scent directly to the limbic system, the primal part of the human brain. In doing so, the sense of smell circumvents the thought process entirely, and makes us feel the response to stimuli before we think it! This may explain why the sense of smell is so emotionally charged.

By selecting the proper incense and combination of ingredients, we can shape the emotional experience through the limbic system, and perhaps awaken latent energies within. So relax and enjoy the subtle scents. See where your mind goes freely!

According to the Ayurvedic medicine, specific body types benefit more from certain kinds of incense.

Vata (Air) does best with sandalwood, myrrh, frankincense, almond, musk, basil and camphor.

Pitta (Fire) does best with rose, saffron, jasmine, gardenia, geranium and other such flowers,

Kapha (Water) does best with resins such as myrrh, frankincense, camphor, pine and herbs like cedar, sage and basil.

Incense Herbs

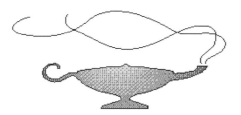

Benzoin
(Styrax benzoin)
Benzoin is a wonderful incense, with a sweet and sensuous scent. It is extremely balancing, while also comforting to the mind. This may be the reason that it has been used for centuries in incense, perfume and potpourri. Used medicinally, it calms nervous disorders such as depression, stress and PMS. It is also commonly used to treat respiratory disorders such as asthma and bronchitis.

Breuzinho
(Burseraceas, Protium sp)
Breuzinho is a very unique resin taken from an Amazonian rainforest tree. The resin is saturated with pollen from all the flowering plants of the South American rain forest. Some Amazonian healers use breuzinho to catalyze and to strengthen their different herbal formulas. When inhaled, breuzinho acts directly on the central nervous system. It is indicated for nervous instability, calming down anxiety and anguish, and to help reduce stress symptoms. Good for asthma and other respiratory system obstruction. It can also be used as an excellent complement for practices of slow and centered physical exercises, such as yoga, body relaxation, meditation and others. Breuzinho promotes serenity and a healthy environment.

Camphor
(Cinnamonum camphora)
Camphor awakens *prana* (the vital life force), opens the chakras, and to brings spiritual clarity. You can burn it or sprinkle it in a room to clear unwanted emotional residues, creating a wholesome meditation environment. Medicinally, camphor smoke is used for respiratory difficulties, muscular pain and as an immune system builder. It is useful for asthmatic attacks, as it is a strong bronchial dilator.

Cedar Tips/White Cedar
(Thuja occidentalis)
White cedar pieces were found by archeologists in charcoal vessels in Tutankhamen's tomb. Cedar is good for outside incense burning, as it creates a lot of smoke.

Cedar Leaf
(Cedrus deodar, libani, atlantica, descurrens)
Cedar is good to use when praying. Cedar smoke has been used to create a bridge between heaven and earth, and for speaking with the Creator. Osiris, the Egyptian God of Heaven is identified with cedar and therefore the cedar tree is called the "heavenly tree". Cedar symbolizes abundance and spiritual strength, and can help during times of overwhelm.

Comfrey
(Symphytum spp.)
Comfrey smoke, as a smudge or in a candle, releases worries and cares. It detoxifies the mind and the emotions of negativity. Comfrey has a calming and soothing effect on body, mind and emotions, taking away the highs and lows. It can be mixed with sweetgrass and white sage.

Copal
(Bursera microphylla)
Copal is either a golden, black, or white resin whose sacred smoke carries messages to the spirit world. Its spirit inspires divine insights and allows you to see life more clearly. The ancient Mayans used copal as a spiritual cleanser. Copal has properties that positively influence the immune system, preserving and protecting the integrity of an individual from external elements. Copal incense could be used in your sacred ceremony of thankfulness, and to clear the mind.

Dragon's Blood
(Daemomorops draco)
Dragon' blood resin is taken from the fruits of a palm tree from the marshy regions of Southeast Asia. It is usually burnt with other substances since it creates a very strong black smoke. It is a very powerful negativity dispeller.

Fir
(Abies spp)
Fir is for grounding, harmony, compassion, and for freeing blockages. Problems that appear to be the result from physical blockages, such as feelings of heaviness in the legs or slow intestinal movements, may actually be caused by blockages in the energy bodies. The fluidity of fir helps to promote the smooth flow of energy

Frankincese/Olibanum
(Boswellia carteri)
Frankincense is the most universal of all incenses and has been used in every culture. The name derives from *frank,* an old French word meaning pure or free and the Latin *incensum*, to smoke. Frankincense induces feelings of emotional stability, enlightenment, protection, courage, introspection and inspiration. It evokes the Divine, warms the heart, clears the mind, and enables spirit to soar; its thick white smoke is a wonderful cleanser of bacteria and viruses that are often present when many people gather.

Juniper
(Juniperus spp.)
Juniper needles create a sweet, warm fragrance. Juniper smoke helps to clear away feelings of fear, failure and stagnation. Fresh or dried leaves are tossed onto the hot rocks in the purifying sweat lodge ceremony. Medicine men brush away the disease with a burning/smoking juniper twig on patients recovering from illness. Use the smoke of juniper and pray for its assistance in overcoming worry and defeatism.

Myrrh
(Commiphora myrrha)
Myrrh's deep fragrance has always been seen as a sacred substance connecting heaven and earth. In ancient Egypt, myrrh was used during funerals and in embalming, and was thought to accompany the soul on its journey to the spirit world. The smoke of myrrh can be used to cleanse the aura. Burned as incense, myrrh strengthens the link between our crown and base chakras. Its fragrance evokes tranquility, calms the nervous system, and eases sorrow and grief by helping to heal the wounds caused by feelings of loss and rejection. Myrrh has very strong anti-bacterial and anti-microbial properties enabling the purification of an area.

Palo Santo
(Burserea graveolens)
Palo santo is also known as holy wood, used by the indigenous people of the Amazon for its medicinal properties and fragrance. Palo santo is used for purification and meditation, and to increase energy flow in the body. It can be burned to ward off bad energies, misfortune, and calamity. As an incense, the wood can be lit and it will burn a few seconds to a minute, filling a space with its sweet warm fragrance.

Patchouli
(Pogostemon cablin)
Patchouli smoke is invigorating, assisting one into action. It encourages farsightedness, astuteness and liberation from boundaries.

Pinion Resin
(Pinus spp.)
Pinion resin smoke encourages trust, direction, perseverance and mindfulness. Pinion resin dredges hidden impurities from the depths of the system.

Sandalwood
(Santalum album)
For centuries, the scent of sandalwood has filled Buddhist and Hindu temples throughout Asia to aid holy men with their prayers, meditations, and other spiritual practices. Sandalwood is good to burn before meditations, quieting us so that we can hear and connect with the infinite wisdom. The smoke from the sandalwood tree brings serenity, harmony, peace, wisdom and sensitivity.

Sweet Grass/Seneca Grass
(Heirochloe odorata)
Sweet grass has a vanilla-like fragrance, and is sacred to the Native Americans. Sweet grass' sacred protective smoke is said to carry prayers and wishes to the heavens to be heard. Used in ceremonies, sweet grass has purifying properties and encourages positive energies to be drawn to the sacred space. (Use white sage first to cleanse the atmosphere).

White Sage
(Salvia apiana)
White sage has long been used by Native Americans to smudge places, people and objects, as well as to heal and cleanse away negativity, and any bad feelings or thoughts. White sage is a symbol of cleanliness and purity. Burning white sage supports the path to wisdom, brings mental clarity and emotional balance.

Yerba Santa
(Eriodictyon californicum)
Yerba Santa may be burned as an incense to create a sanctuary conducive for healing. It is excellent for respiratory problems. The smoke brings up old and degenerate issues, memories of previously experienced illnesses, fears, and untruths, to the surface, where they eventually disappear.

Holy Smokes
Place a small amount of the following combination on a charcoal: frankincense, myrrh, dragon's blood and copal, in equal parts. Feel how this smoke invokes a sense of sacredness.

How To Use Charcoal

When using self-igniting charcoal use a container, such as an incense burner or ashtray, because sparks will jump around while burning incense. Put some sand in the burner under the charcoal, because the charcoal gets very hot and will break glass or ruin your table top if using a metal burner. You may break the charcoal in halves or thirds or whatever size you wish to use. Ignite your charcoal piece with a match, set it on the sand and let it finish heating clear through, about two minutes. This burns out all the smells that are not incense. Place your incense of choice on the charcoal, enjoy its fragrance and observe its influence on your moods.

How To Use Smudge

Native American healers have always smudged (burned specific plants) to purify a space of toxic energy, feelings and thoughts, to create a fragrant atmosphere that attracts healing and helping powers. For smudging, you will need the following items that represent the four elements, water, earth, air and fire. A shell (abalone shell is best) to burn the herbs in. The abalone shell represents the element of water and the herbs the element of earth. You will also need matches or a lighter, and a feather or fan of feathers. The feather represents the element of air. The element of fire is introduced when you light the herbs. Wave the smoke over your body with the feather, not forgetting the arms and legs. After you have smudged yourself you can smudge other people or places. When you are done, let the ashes cool down and give them back to the Earth with care.

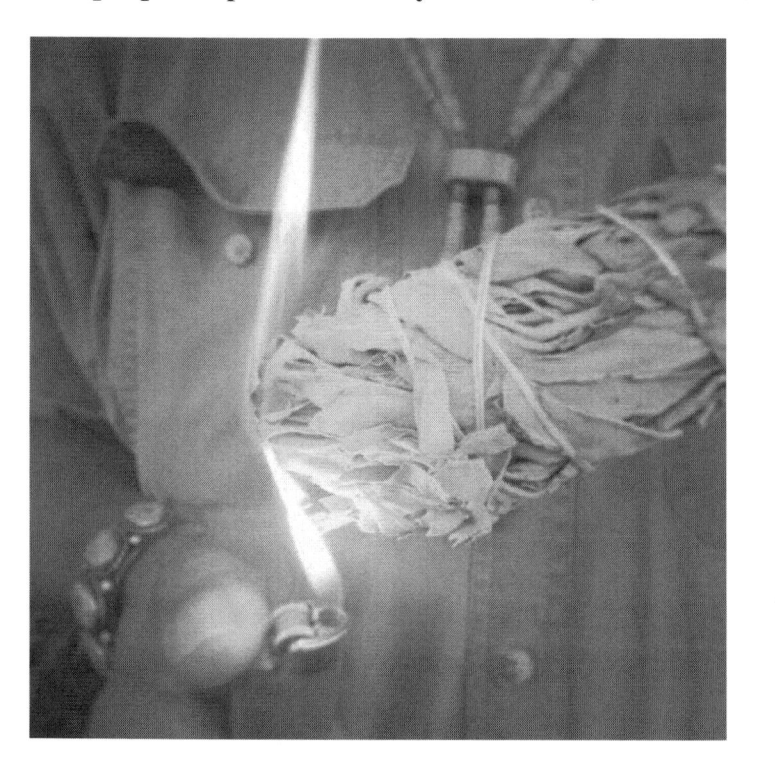
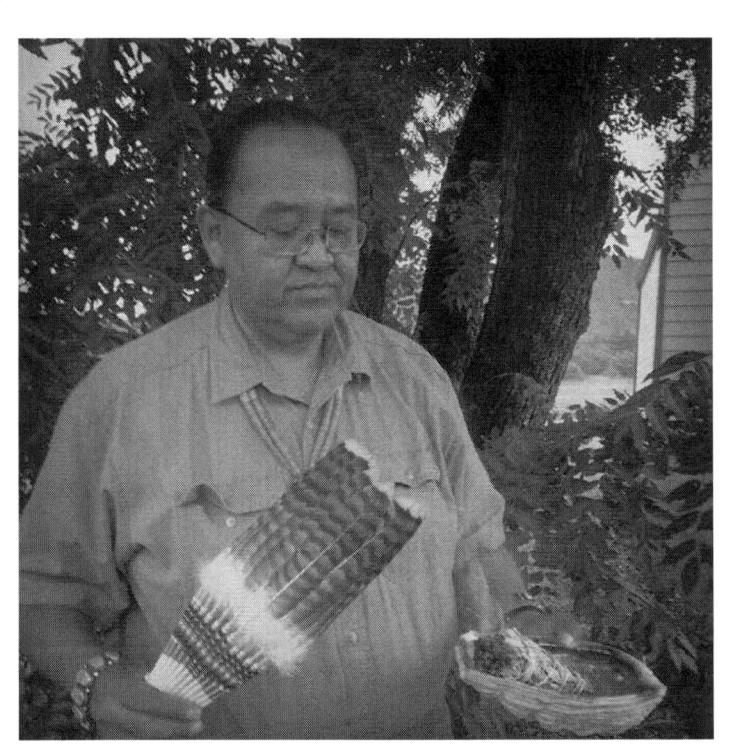

INFUSED OILS

Infused oils, or herbal oils, are simply herbs infused in oil. Infused oils can be used externally for massages, skin treatments, healing ointments, dressings for wounds and burns, and occasionally for enemas and douches. Some infused oils can be used internally, for example, garlic infused in olive oil is excellent in salads.

Alkanet Infused Oil
(Alkanna tinctoria infused in grapeseed oil)
Alkanet infused oil is a natural colorant and sunscreen.

Arnica Infused Oil
(Arnica montana infused in extra virgin olive oil))
Arnica infused oil is excellent to use on bruises and sprains, as it encourages healthy re-absorption of blood clots. Arnica infused oil reduces pain, swelling, and inflammation after injuries.
Caution: Do not use when the skin is broken! Do not used internally!

Bloodroot Infused Oil
(Sanguinaria canadensis infused extra virgin olive oil)
Bloodroot infused oil has been used historically for the treatment of various skin cancers, and also for sores, warts, eczema, and other dermal & epidermal problems.

Bhringaraj Infused Oil
(Eclipta alba infused in certified organic sesame seed oil)
Bhringaraj infused oil is a traditional oil used in India to promote hair growth and prevent premature graying.

Calendula Infused Oils
(Calendula officinalis infused in extra virgin olive oil)
Calendula flower infused oil has been used externally for slow healing wounds, bed sores, bruises, cuts, scratches, varicose or broken veins, eczema, gum inflammation, inflammatory eruptions such as measles, chicken pox, hemorrhoids, persistent ulcers and burns, and as a strong anti-fungal such as athlete's foot and nail fungus calendula infused oil is also beneficial for diaper rash and can be gently applied to baby's bottom to promote tissue repair.

Carrot Infused Oil
(Daucus carota infused in soybean oil)
Carrot infused oil is rich in vitamins and beta carotene. It is a tonic to the skin and assists in the healing and formation of scar tissues. Soothing for itchy skin, and other skin conditions.
Caution: The macerated oil is sometimes confused with the essential oil, which is obtained by steam distillation of carrot seed.

Chamomile Infused Oil
(Matricaria chamomilla infused in extra virgin olive oil)
Chamomile infused oil has shown to inhibit inflammation and has been used to treat dermatitis and other minor skin irritations. In one study it was found that chamomile was nearly as effective as hydrocortisone.

Chaparral Infused Oil
(Larrea tridentate infused in extra virgin olive oil)
Chaparral infused oil activates the skin to detoxify. It is excellent for acidic conditions, such as acne, as it discourages the spread of bacteria. Chaparral infused oil can be used as a body poultice in case of lymphatic congestion, or for hemorrhoids. Chaparral infused oil releases cellular memory.

Chickweed Infused Oil
(Stellaria media infused in extra virgin olive oil)
Chickweed infused oil is useful for sores, abscesses, skin irritations and rashes. Chickweed contains saponins, which exert an anti-inflammatory action similar to cortisone.

Comfrey Leaf Infused Oil
(Symphytum officinale infused in extra virgin olive oil))
Comfrey infused oil has mucilaginous, astringent and toning properties, rich in allantoin (an agent which promotes cell proliferation), with impressive wound and bone healing properties, both internally and externally. Use it as a poultice for bone knitting and fractures and as a compress or poultice for cuts, burns and varicose veins. It is said to regenerate aging tissues.

Dandelion Flower Infused Oil
(Taraxacum officinalis infused in extra virgin olive oil)
Dandelion flower infused oil may help regulate the acid balances in the cell structure. When you have an acid balance, the cells are more conducive to the absorption of nutrients, to build new and healthier cells. It is a cancer preventative as it nourishes and promotes healthy cells, inhibiting malformation of cells. Individuals who have a history of genetic cancer, family trait of cancer (genetic karma) may use dandelion flower infused oil to reduce the manifestation of cancer. Healthy cells are more efficient at absorbing nutrients and detoxifying the body. Good for rashes, cuts, sores etc., enhancing the cellular structure, therefore the healing process.

Hawthorn Infused Oil
(Crataegus oxycantha infused in extra virgin olive oil)
Hawthorn infused oil is a cardiovascular tonic. It also affects the connective tissues and can be applied for collagen deficiencies. Hawthorn is also know to increase qualities of love.

Mugwort Infused Oil
(Artemisia vulgaris infused in extra virgin olive oil)
Mugwort infused oil is for people whose feet are constantly cold - even when in a warm place. This may be a sign of poor blood circulation. Mugwort infused oil increases blood circulation and energetic flow within the various meridian pathways of the body, similar to the "moxa" treatments of oriental acupuncture. Apply mugwort oil to areas of the body, which are blue in color or cold to the touch, such as varicose veins.

Mullein Flower Infused Oil
(Verbascum thapsus infused in extra virgin olive oil)
Mullein flower infused oil is very effective for ear infections and pain, when the eardrum is not perforated. Mullein flowers infused oil is known to reduce pain and swelling in the glands and joints. Traditionally, it was also used as an anti-aging and rejuvenating facial oil and applied to reverse skin thinning, reduce flaking and itching.

Neem Leaf Infused Oil

(Azadirachta indica infused in organic sesame seed oil)

Neem leaf infused oil is known to have powerful anti-bacterial and anti-fungal properties for pitta-related skin inflammations. Neem is usually infused in a base of sesame seed oil.

Nettle Leaf Infused Oil

(Urtica dioica infused in extra virgin olive oil)

Nettle leaf infused oil helps stimulate the skin, improves circulation and is helpful for arthritis. Nettle leaf infused oil can be used in hair preparations to stimulate hair growth and improve the condition of the scalp. Nettle leaf infused oil is rich in minerals and plant hormones.

Plantain Infused Oil

(Plantago major infused in extra virgin olive oil)

Plantain infused oil helps relieve skin and scalp irritations, and reduces inflammation. Plantain infused oil is traditionally used to nourish and treat sensitive, irritated skin and scalp, helps restore injured or tired skin, and for continuous anti-aging treatments.

Quince Infused Oil

(Pyrus cydonia)

Quince infused oil is used in high quality cosmetics for dry skin, and skin that is dry from external influences, such as dry air. Quince infused oil is good for rashes, but not allergic rashes. In a bath, it is deeply relaxing. May also help with hemorrhoids.

Ratanjot Infused Oil

(Onosma echioide infused in Grape seed oil)

Ratanjot infused oil is widely used in countries such as India as a cooking additive and natural dye. Ratanjot infused oil has been used in India for skin eruption, rheumatism and palpitation of the heart.

Red Clover Infused Oil

(Trifolium pratense infused in extra virgin olive oil)

Red clover infused oil can be applied externally for various skin conditions such as psoriasis, eczema, scaly, cancerous growth, dry skin and acne. Red clover infused oil helps alleviate nervousness and stress-related symptoms.

Seaweed Infused Oil
(Palmaria palmate, Laminaria digitata, Postelsia palmaeformis, Chondrus crispus infused in extra virgin olive oil)
Seaweed infused oil contains dulse, kelp, sea palm, and Irish moss. Seaweed infused oil is highly nutritive and can be used as a body oil. It's extraordinarily soothing, calming, detoxifying, and normalizing effect on the skin gives you a feeling of well-being and relaxation.

St. John's Wort Infused Oil
(Hypericum perforatum infused in extra virgin olive oil)
The flower petals are macerated in virgin olive oil to produce beautiful red St. John's Wort infused oil. St. John's Wort infused oil is known to promote the healing of various nerve damages, especially on the extremities, such as fingers, toes, tail bone, etc. This oil is known to rebuild nerve structures and can be applied topically for nerve pain after injury or trauma, back injury and for other conditions such as skin cancers, varicose veins, scrapes and burns.
Caution: May cause photosensitivity.

Wild Yam Infused Oil
(Dioscorea villosa infused in extra virgin olive oil)
Wild Yam infused oil is widely used without side effects for menstrual distress, miscarriage, infertility, menopause and endometriosis. Wild yam infused oil regulates hormonal action, balancing the ratio of progesterone to estrogen. American herbalists have long used wild yam for painful menstruation, ovarian pain, cramps and problems in childbirth. Wild yam infused oil is effective in reducing hot flashes. Wild yam has also been used for gallbladder pain, to lower cholesterol and blood pressure.

Yerba Santa Infused Oil
(Eriodictyon californicum infused in extra virgin olive oil)
Yerba santa infused oil is useful primarily as a bronchial dilator in treating upper respiratory ailments such as asthma, pneumonia and coughs. Yerba santa infused oil also opens the sinuses, and increases the secretions of body fluids, i.e. saliva. I have a friend whose husband had a very bad cough and refused to take cough remedies. Every night before bed she would massage his chest with yerba santa infused oil. He, and she, were able to sleep all night without coughing. Oils penetrate through the skin deep into the internal organs, such as the lungs.

Violet Infused Oil *(Viola tricolor infused in extra virgin olive oil)*
Violet infused oil can be used for skin problems, particularly eczema of the scalp and scabby skin complaints. Because it is so gentle, it can be used to ease cradle cap, diaper rash and eczema in infants. Its high concentration of the flavonoid rutin, violet infused oil has been traditionally used to strengthen capillary walls.

MINERALS

Calcium "The Great Builder"
Calcium is essential for healthy nerve, brain and structural function. With a sufficient amount of calcium in the body, new tissues and cells remain strong and vital. The greatest amount of calcium is found in seeds, such as sesame, sunflower and pumpkin, as well as in almonds, figs, dark greens, oats, rice, barley, carrots, seaweed. Herbal sources of calcium include oats, horsetail, skullcap, hawthorn berry, gotu kola and stinging nettles.

Magnesium "The Great Relaxer"
Magnesium found in plants is considered to be the finest relaxer, tranquilizer and laxative in nature. Magnesium brings relaxation to an agitated nervous system, soothing irritated tissues and cells associated with nerve function. It also relieves constipation and irritation in the bowel resulting from an over-stressed physiology. The greatest amount of magnesium is found in orange and yellow foods, such as carrots, yellow squash, sweet potato, yellow corn, black mission figs, and raw goat's milk. Herbal sources of magnesium include gotu kola, skullcap, horsetail, alfalfa, nettles, hawthorn berry and oat seeds.

Sodium "The Youth Element"
Sodium in it's naturally occurring form is considered to bring youthfulness to the bodies tissues. Sodium is essential for healthy digestion, capillaries and arteries. It is necessary for maintaining flexibility and mobility in the joints. Without proper sodium the joints would stiffen and calcify prematurely, and the lining of the stomach would not secrete the necessary enzymes for healthy digestion. The sun is considered the sodium star, so all fruits and vegetables which ripened in the sun contain ample amounts of sodium. Other significant sources of sodium include seaweeds such as kelp, dulse and nori, as well as black mission figs, whey, celery and raw goat's milk. Herbal sources of sodium include alfalfa, chlorella, spirulina, stinging nettles and raspberry leaf.

Potassium "The Great Alkalizer"
Potassium neutralizes acidity in the body, which has built up from eating unsuitable foods, as well as from an incorrect metabolism. It alkalizes blood chemistry. Potassium, when in balance, prevents the growth of cysts, fibroids and other benign growths. Without potassium balance, the nervous system may become agitated; thoughts become disturbed and the entire

psycho-physiological balance is upset. All fresh fruits and vegetables contain ample amounts of potassium, especially figs, celery, dandelion greens and other dark green leafy vegetables. Herbal sources of potassium are found in stinging nettles, dandelion, alfalfa, seaweed, parsley, chickweed and cilantro.

Phosphorus "The Light Bearer"

Phosphorus feeds the brain and nerve cells, as well as the bones. Brain and nerve phosphorus is obtained largely through animal derivatives and single cell algae, while bone phosphorus can be obtained through seeds and nuts. Without adequate phosphorus one may feel dull and lethargic and may lack radiance. One's bones may be deficient and early structural disorders may arise. A vegetarian must maintain spiritual and emotional balance in order to hold adequate phosphorus in the system. Sources of phosphorus derived from fish and poultry, seeds, spirulina, chlorella, nuts and whole grains can adequately keep balance in the physiology.

Silicon "The Magnetic Element"

Silicon feeds the nerve cells, nerve sheath, hair, nails, skin, eyes, teeth, brain cells and tissues. Silica brings magnetism to the nerves, brings radiance to the skin, luster to the hair, builds strong teeth and nails, and brings balance to the emotional system. A person lacking silica is tense, irritable, rough, lacks luster, and appears cold and difficult to get to know, and generally feels on edge much of the time. While a person who is rich in silica will sparkle, radiate joy and harmony, express dynamism in personality, attract others, show luster in hair, eyes, teeth and nails, and generally be very magnetic. People are naturally drawn to silica rich people. Without adequate silica one remains lonely and feels depleted. Silica is found in the outer husk of whole grains, seeds and nuts. Herbal sources of silica include horsetail, wild oats, dandelion leaf, onions, alfalfa and nettles.

Iron "The Frisky Horse Element"

Iron builds vigor and stamina, gives strength and virility. Without adequate iron the blood becomes depleted and one feels weak, anemic and frail. Iron from inorganic sources may not be absorbed well into the tissues and can cause constipation, yeast overgrowth and lead to autointoxication. Iron attracts oxygen into the constitution and gives mental energy and clarity of mind. Naturally occurring sources of iron are found in figs, raisins, dark leafy vegetables, black cherries, chlorella, spirulina, nettles, dandelion leaf, raspberry leaf, alfalfa, chickweed, parsley, red clover. Herbal iron tonics inclusive of the herbs are best assimilated when gentian root is added to the formula.

Iodine "The Emotional Metabolizer Element"

Iodine is the element which feeds the thyroid gland and maintains metabolic and emotional balance throughout the body. Without adequate iodine the thyroid gland may dysfunction and lead to metabolic changes. Every emotion we experience is processed through the thyroid gland. Without adequate iodine emotional instability may arise and the nervous system may feel distraught. Ample sources of iodine are found in seaweeds such as kelp, dulse and nori, as well as onions and black walnut hulls and nuts.

MOXIBUSTION

Moxibustion, or moxa for short, is a technique used in traditional Chinese medicine in which a stick of burning mugwort, *(Artemesia vulgaris),* is placed over an inflamed or affected area on the body. The purpose is to stimulate and strengthen the blood flow and energy, or *chi,* of the body. Moxibustion is used for people who have a cold or stagnant condition. The moxa stick is burned to warm up the blood and chi that are not circulating well. The warmth of moxa penetrates deep into the body, without burning the skin. Moxibustion is used to treat pain and inflammations. For example, if treating a person with tendonitis, the moxa stick is burned over the elbow area. It is also very effective for menstrual cramps, where the stick is waved over the abdominal area. Burn moxa over the belly button for unstoppable diarrhea. Moxibustion is particularly known for its ability to turn breech presentation babies into a normal head-down position that is considered safer during childbirth.

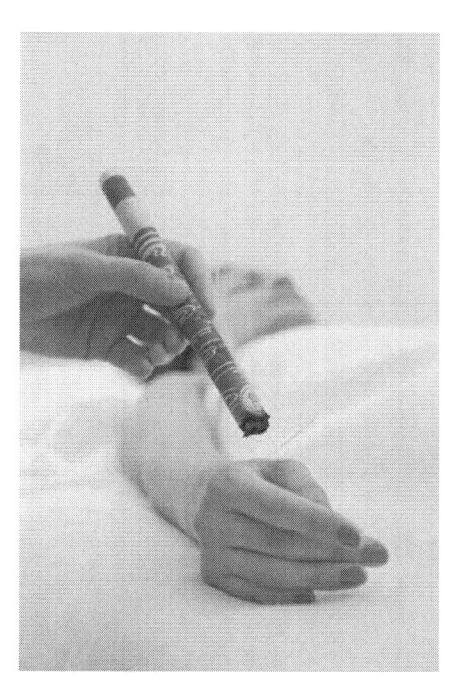

MEDICINAL MUSHROOMS AND FUNGI

Cordyceps (Cordyceps sinensis)
Common name: Caterpillar Fungus
Chinese name: Dong Chong Xia Cao

anti-tumor
blood pressure
cardiovascular
Cholesterol
immune enhancer
kidney tonic
liver tonic
sexual potentiator
lungs/respiratory
stress

Enokitake (Flammulina velutipes)
Common name: Golden Needle Mushroom
Japanese name: Enokitake

anti-tumor
immune enhancer

Lion's Mane (Hericium erinceus)
Common name: Lion's Mane
Japanese name: Yamabushitake

cardiovascular
nerve tonic
lungs/respiratory

Maitake (Grifola frondosa)
Common name: Hen of the Woods
Japanese name: Maitake

anti-tumor
anti-viral
blood pressure
diabetes
immune enhancer

Delicious Mushroom Recipe

You will need:
1 small onion, chopped
1 garlic, chopped
1 tablespoon butter or olive oil
4 oz fresh or reconstituted* mushrooms
A little cream or half-and-half
salt, pepper, nutmeg

Sauté onion and garlic in the butter for 2 minutes, add mushrooms, and sauté together until all liquid has evaporated. Add cream and spices and lightly warm. Serve and enjoy.

*How to reconstitute dried mushrooms: Pour hot water over mushrooms and let stand for at least one hour, or overnight.

Reishi (Ganoderma lucidum)
Chinese name: Ling Chi
Japanese name: Reishi

anti-inflammatory
anti-tumor
anti-viral
blood pressure
cardiovascular
immune enhancer
kidney tonic
lungs/respiratory
stress

Royal Sun Agaricus (Agaricus blazei)
Common name: Royal Sun Agaricus
Japanese name: Himematsutake

anti-tumor
immune enhancer

Shiitake (Lentinula edodes)
Chinese name: Xiang Gu
Japanes name: Shiitake

anti-tumor
anti-viral
blood pressure
cholesterol
immune enhancer
kidney tonic

Yun Zhi (Trametes versicolor)
Common name: Turkey Tail
Chinese name: Yun Zhi

anti-tumor
anti-viral
kidney tonic
liver tonic

NETI POT (NASAL RINSE)

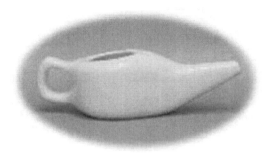

Benefits of Nasal Rinse

- Removes mucus and pollution from the nasal passages and sinuses
- Helps prevent respiratory tract diseases
- Helps with eyesight
- Daily use relieves allergies, colds and sinusitis
- Cooling and soothing to the mind
- Beneficial in the treatment of headaches and migraines
- Alleviates anxiety, anger and depression
- Removes drowsiness, making the head and sense organs feel light and smooth

Instruction for Nose Washing

1. Boil some water (it helps to sterilize the water, so that you don't introduce something nasty into your sinuses)
2. Pour the boiling water in the neti pot (pour it while it's boiling to help clean the Neti Pot itself).
3. Drop in some grains of salt for ph balance
4. Let the water cool to where it is slightly warm. Hot water is irritating and dangerous. Cool water is not soothing.
5. Have a big bowl in one hand.
6. Using your other hand put the Neti Pot up to one nostril.
7. Tilt your head slightly, aiming the other nostril down a bit.
8. Relax. (This is the hardest part to explain.) If you are calm, the water flows right through. But if you aren't, it just won't flow. The first time it may take some time before any water goes through. It seems to have something to do with that reflex where you can't swallow and breathe at the same time. If you keep breathing out your mouth, relaxed, the water should gently flow through the nose on its own. There's no forcing it.
9. Throat lozenges can help with irritation caused by dribbles down the throat.

When you are all done, put your head down in a sink and blow out any water through your nose. Beware that there is water in parts you're not aware of: It can come trickling out at any moment in the next 15 minutes after using a Neti Pot. One helpful way to get rid of some of this is to take a washcloth, pinch it over your nose, and throw your head back. A gurgle of water will drain out of your sinuses and into your throat. Now blow your nose again.

PLANT CONSTITUENTS SOLVENT GUIDE

It is very important to know which solvent to use to liberate the desired healing and nutritive properties from plants to make effective medicines. Here is a guideline:

Water
Gums (softens)
Sugars
Proteins/Enzymes
Vitamins (some)
Tannins
Glycosides
Saponins
Bitter compounds
Starch
Polysaccharides (hot)
Pectins
Alkaloids (some)

Alcohol 50-70%
Alkaloids
Salts
Glucosides
Sugars
Vitamins
Enzymes
Tannins (some)
Bitter compounds
Saponins

Absolute Alcohol
Alkaloids
Glycosides
Volatile oils
Waxes
Resins
Fats
Tannins (some)
Balsam
Sugars
Vitamins

Vinegar
Sugars
Tannins
Glycosides
Bitter compounds

Glycerin
Sugars
Enzymes (dilute)
Glucosides
Bitter compounds
Saponins (dilute)
Tannins

Lipids
Wax (when heated)
Volatile oils
Camphors
Vitamins (some)

NATURAL PRESERVATIVES

Grapefruit Seed Extract
(Citrus grandis and Glycerin)
Grapefruit seed extract (GSE) is a natural antioxidant and natural preservative with anti-bacterial properties. It is extracted from grapefruit seed and pulp and then blended with pure vegetable glycerin to make it non-irritating to the skin and mucous membranes. Use GSE at .5 to 1 % to preserve home made cosmetics, or 2 % to create anti-bacterial creams, salves, rinses and soaps. Add 3 – 6 drops per gallon of water as a disinfectant for drinking water. To prevent Parvo and other infectious diseases add grape seed extract to pet water, 1 drop to 8 oz of water. Also, GSE can be used on horses, sprayed on huffs to prevent thrush and other bacteria. GSE has a shelf life of approximately 7- 9 years.

Rosemary Oil Extract
(Rosmarinus officinalis)
Rosemary oil extract (ROE) is a natural preservative with anti-microbial properties and can be added to creams, lotions and oils to prevent oxidation. Add 0.1 % to 0.5% of undiluted ROE to preserve your homemade products.
Caution: Do not confuse with rosemary essential oil!

Vitamin E
(D-alpha tocopherol)
Vitamin E is an essential fat-soluble vitamin composed of eight naturally occurring compounds (the fractions are called alpha, delta, epsilon, eta, gamma and zeta tocopherol, and four other substances called tocotrienols). While each of these compounds exhibits different biological activities, alpha tocopherol has the highest biological activity and is the most widely available form of vitamin E. The potency of vitamin E oil is measured by its alpha tocopherol content. A 200IU/g vitamin E contains 200 units of alpha tocopherol per gram of oil and the rest of it is an unspecified amount of the beta, delta, epsilon etc. components.

SALTS

Facts about Salts

Sodium is a necessary mineral and considered to bring youthfulness to the body's tissues. Sodium is indispensable for healthy digestion, capillaries and arteries, and to help maintain flexibility and mobility in the joints. Without proper sodium, the joints would stiffen and calcify prematurely, and the lining of the stomach would not secrete the necessary enzymes for healthy digestion. Sodium has the ability to dissolve calcium deposits around the joints, arteries, capillaries and muscles, allowing the bloodstream to carry them out of the body. Sodium is crucial for maintaining the health of every cell in the human system. If we had no sodium, we'd cease to exist. The FDA's maximum recommended daily quantity of sodium is 2,400 milligrams.

But...

Commercial table salt used in our food is the furthest thing from ideal. During the refining process of table salt, natural sea salt or rock salt is stripped of more than 60 trace minerals and essential macronutrients. Commercial refined salt is not only stripped of all its minerals, besides sodium and chloride, but it also is heated at such high temperatures that the chemical structure of salt changes. In addition, it is chemically cleaned and bleached and treated with anti-caking agents, which prevent salts from mixing with water in the salt container. Unfortunately, the anti-caking agents perform the same function in the human body, this means, refined salt does not dissolve and combine with the water and fluids present in our system. Instead, it builds up in the body and leaves deposits in organs and tissues, causing severe health problems such as high blood pressure, fluid retention and kidney problems. Two of the most common anti-caking agents used in the mass production of salt are sodium alumino-silicate and alumino-calcium silicate. These are both sources of aluminum, a toxic metal that has been implicated in the development of Alzheimer's disease and that certainly does not belong in a healthy diet. To make matters worse, the aluminum used in salt production leaves a bitter taste in salt, so manufacturers usually add sugar in the form of dextrose to hide the taste of the aluminum.

To learn more about the benefits of salt and why it is the most misunderstood nutrient, please read the book "Salt, Your Way To Health" by David Brownstein, MD.

Individual Salts

Alaea Sea Salt *(see Hawaiian Red Sea salt)*

Black Salt

Black salt is actually pinkish in color. Black salt is mined in India and has a pungent, sulfur-like odor. According to ayurveda black salt is a carminative, aperient, tonic and stomachic, useful in flatulence, colic, dyspepsia, indigestion, bowel complaints, etc.

Celtic Salt

Celtic salt is a high mineral sea salt harvested near the coast of northwestern France. The method used for gathering these nutritional salts follows a 2,000 year-old Celtic tradition and is supported by modern quality control standards. Farmers channel ocean water, rich in a wide variety of minerals into a series of clay-lined ponds. The wind and sun evaporate the ocean water, leaving a mineral-rich brine. The salt farmer briskly stimulates this live mixture, and dazzling salt crystals form. The Celtic salt is then gathered by hand using wooden tools. This harvesting method preserves the vital balance of the minerals found in Celtic salt.

Dead Sea Salt/Masada Salt

Dead Sea salt has the highest contents of natural minerals. It contains potassium, magnesium & bromide. Potassium helps regulate the moisture level of the skin, magnesium helps promote healing and bromide has a soothing relaxing effect. They revitalize and help draw the toxins from the skin. Because it increases circulation it moves trapped fluid from joints reducing stiffness and pain. Dead Sea salt is well known for its ability to relieve aches & pains, reduce stiffness & relax muscles. It also relieves skin problems such as acne, eczema & psoriasis.

Dead Sea Water

Dead Sea water is rich in magnesium and can be used in place of water in creams, lotions, skin treatments, facials, hair wraps & body wraps.

Dendritic Salt

Dentritic salt is a fine grain salt, which has been crystallized to provide more surface area and irregular surfaces. This is desirable when making scented bath salts because the increased surface area helps retain the fragrance, requires fewer pigments and reduces clumping. Combine with medium grain salts if you like the chunky look. This natural salt absorbs essential oils and fragrance oils twice as efficiently as other salts used in bath mixes. It's specially formulated to prevent caking, add flow ability and keeps the scent in your salts longer. Use 1 cup of dentritic salt to every 20 cups of other salts used. Not for internal use.

Epsom Salt

Epsom salt (magnesium sulfate) is named for the mineral rich waters of Epsom, England, where it has been known since the 17th century. But did you know that it is more than just a purgative. Epsom salts added to a bath promotes perspiration and draws acidic wastes - mainly uric acid - through the pores of the skin. This helps to relieve pain. It is also very beneficial as a stress reducer and can even ward off a cold or the flu if used at the onset of symptoms. You can also feed Epsom salts to your plants, vegetables, and lawn for greener grass and big, healthy vegetables.

Hawaiian Red Sea Salt

Hawaiian red sea salt, or alaea sea salt, is a natural, non-processed salt, and is rich in minerals from the sea and volcanic red clay (which is high in iron oxide) from the earth. It is considered to be a sacred salt because it originates from both the sea and the earth. Alaea salt was traditionally used to cleanse and bless homes and belongings and was also used in healing rituals. It is said to have curative properties when used for sore throats, wounds, body aches, muscles sprains, gum infections, cold sores, etc. It is believed to draw toxins from overworked muscle tissues. This is a beautiful naturally colored salt for detoxifying bath salts and salt scrubs. It can also be used to speckle other white sea salts.

Masada Salt *(see Dead Sea salt)*

Mineral Salt

Mineral salt is also known as rock salt and is mined in Utah. It is less heating and is believed to not cause water retention or aggravate pitta.

Rock Salt *(see Mineral salt)*

Sea Salt, Pink

Pink sea salt is from a pollutant-free ancient seabed in the western United States. This salt is not altered with coloring, anti-caking additives or bleaching, and is not kiln dried. The minerals in this ancient seabed are captured within the crystallization of the salt and they're not removed, which is why the salt is colored. Pink sea salt is the best tasting salt you will ever eat. Its glistening color crystals represent the minerals your body needs, including calcium potassium, sulphur, magnesium, iron, phosphorous, iodine, manganese, copper, zinc and over 50 other trace minerals.

Sea Salt, White

Sea salt, which many times still smells of the ocean, contains many minerals that are necessary in our everyday diet. When used in the bath or in scrubs, they are great for detoxifying and removing dead skin.

Solar Salt

Solar salt is produced by solar evaporation of seawater from the Great Salt Lake. The salt crystals are refined by washing with clean saturated brine to remove surface impurities, drained of excess moisture, dried and screened to size. Contains no anti-caking or free-flowing additives or conditioners. Should be stored in a dry, covered area at humidity below 75%.

Beautifying Salt Glow

2 cups Dead Sea salt
3 teaspoon honey
6 drops tangerine essential oil
6 drops pink grapefruit essential oil
6 drops red mandarin essential oil

Run the water into the bathtub, (don't make the water too hot or you will get sleepy and not refreshed). In a small bowl mix the oils and honey into the Dead Sea salt. Step into the bath water. Take a handful of the salt mixture and scrub down your body. Let the mixture fall into the tub. Repeat this process until your entire body is "glowing". Soak for 20 minutes to refresh and rejuvenate.

SWEETENERS

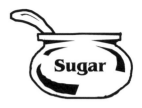

The sweet taste after a meal helps fermentation and aids digestion. Ayurveda recommends having food with a sweet taste at both the beginning and the end of each meal. There are a lot of sweeteners to choose from, and they vary in degrees of processing and nutrition. Organic sweeteners have the added benefit of being grown and processed in a way that is not only healthier for us but for the environment as well. However, refined white sugar has been stripped of its nutrients and should be avoided, because the heat released by white sugar can – in excessive amounts – damage the liver. In addition, the body burns up nutrients to digest white sugar, especially calcium, which adversely affects the teeth and bones. White sugar also negatively impacts the nervous system by stripping calcium from the myelin sheath, producing nervous disorders.

Dandelion Flower Sweetener

Take dandelion flowers, just barely cover with water, and bring to a boil, for approx. 15 minutes. Cool and strain. Add an equal amount of turbinado sugar and cook to a honey consistency.

Cream of Wheat with Jaggery

Delicious! Gives strength, stamina and vigor to the elderly. In a non-stick pan, dry-roast 1 cup of cream of wheat over low heat, stirring constantly. When the color changes, add one tablespoon of butter (or ghee) and cook for 2 more minutes. Add 3 cups of water and bring to a boil. Reduce the heat and stir in ½ cup of jaggery. Cook for 3 minutes and remove from heat. Stir in ½ cup of almond butter and ½ cup of powdered coconut. Allow to cool. Stir in one teaspoon of powdered cardamom seed. Stir and serve while still warm, with a sprinkle of black pepper.

Agave Sweetened Apple Compote

Peel and slice 8 apples. Add cinnamon and nutmeg to taste, and one cup agave sweetener. Simmer for a few minutes until tender. Enjoy this sweet nectar without guilt, either by itself, on toast, mixed in muesli, or other cereal. I like it on top of plain macaroni pasta.

Agave Sweetener

Agave sweetener is a natural fructose sweetener extracted from the agave plant. Indigenous people of Mexico gather the sweet juice, aguamiel, from various species of agave. Agave has a glycemic index of 11, absorbs slowly into the bloodstream, avoiding the "rush" often associated with refined sugar. Agave sweetener is 50% sweeter than sugar, yet with fewer calories, and is sodium free.

Barbados Molasses

Barbados molasses is one of the first products created in the sugar-making process. It is lighter and sweeter than blackstrap molasses, and is an excellent choice when blackstrap is too strong or not sweet enough.

Barley Malt

Barley malt is made by fermenting grains. The fermenting bacteria convert the grain starches into simple and complex sugars.

Blackstrap Molasses

Blackstrap molasses is the final product produced in the sugar-making process. As the final product, blackstrap molasses contains more vitamins, minerals, and trace elements (iron, potassium, calcium and magnesium) found naturally in the sugar cane plant, making it more nutritious than most other sweeteners. Molasses builds blood, muscles, heart, and can be eaten during times of debility, pregnancy and postpartum.

Brown Sugar

Brown sugar is actually white sugar with syrup added to make it look brown. Not so good!

Date

Date "sugar" is made by pulverizing dried dates. It is not "refined" like sugar, and therefore, contains the nutrients and minerals found in dates. Also, date sugar contains fiber.

Demerara Sugar

Demerara sugar is a crunchy, medium grain, golden brown sugar, rich in natural sugarcane molasses. It is by far one of the healthiest sugars to consume because it contains 11 calories per tsp. as compared to 16 calories per tsp. of refined white sugar. It also contains good amounts of calcium, phosphorus, iron and potassium, which are only found in trace amounts in refined white sugar. A great natural sugar for sugar body scrubs.

Fructose

Fructose is a natural sugar found in plants and fruits, but generally is highly refined and made from cornstarch. It is low or devoid in nutrients. For some people there are disadvantages when consuming large amounts of fructose: increased LDL cholesterol levels, uric-acid levels in the blood, and triglyceride levels. However, it is absorbed more slowly in the gastro-intestinal tract than glucose, producing only a slight insulin response, resulting in smaller fluctuations in blood-sugar levels.

Honey

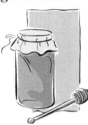

Honeybees make honey from the nectar of flowering plants. Honey flavors vary depending upon the plants from which the nectar is derived. Honey is sweeter than sugar and has more calories than white sugar. Raw honey has medicinal benefits, contains enzymes, minerals and B-complex vitamins.

Jaggery

Jaggery is also known as gool or goodh in India. Jaggery is an Indian raw, natural sugar containing vitamins and minerals. This sugar is golden brown in color, tastes somewhat like molasses, and looks like lumpy turbinado sugar. Jaggery has healing properties and can be used for difficult, painful or burning urine, anemia, debility, and for rejuvenation.

Maple Sugar

Maple Sugar is one of the best natural sugars. Maple sugar is nutritive and demulcent. Maple syrup is good for cough and fever.

Rice Syrup

Rice syrup is a sweetener, prepared by culturing rice with enzymes to break down the starches, straining off the liquid, and cooking it to the desired consistency. Brown rice syrup contains 50% soluble complex carbohydrates, which take from two to three hours to be digested resulting in a steady supply of energy. This syrup can be evaporated to form a rice syrup powder.

Stevia

Stevia is native to Paraguay. It is a small green plant bearing leaves, which have a delicious, refreshing, and sweet taste, 30 times sweeter than sugar. People in Paraguay have long been using stevia leaves to sweeten bitter teas and as a sweet treat. Stevia does not add sugar to the bloodstream, therefore can be used by diabetics.

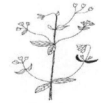

Stevia

Sucanat

Sucanat is the only sugar cane product of its kind, and is made by blending together the two products that typical sugar processing separates - sugar and molasses. The initial pressing of the sugar cane plant contains all of the elements of both sugar and molasses. Through the sugar making process, these two products are separated. All of the nutritional benefits of the sugar cane plant remain with the molasses leaving sugar as "empty calories." In making Sucanat, molasses and sugar are blended together creating a dry sweetener, containing vitamins, minerals and trace elements of the sugar cane plant and a lower sucrose level than refined white and brown sugar. (Another delicious version of Sucanat is <u>Sucanat with Honey</u>).

Turbinado

Turbinado sugar or evaporated cane juice, sometimes referred to as "unrefined sugar", is made from sugar cane juice that is released by pressing sugar cane stalks. It is different from refined sugar in that it is typically 50% less processed and therefore contains more molasses than refined sugar. It is a perfect mineral rich sweetener. Cane sugar builds body tissues, increases urination, and is considered an aphrodisiac. It can also be used in your cosmetics. The natural golden color gives your sugar scrub a more natural look than regular white refined sugar.

Substitution Chart

Sweeteners	Equivalent to 1 Cup of White Sugar
Sucanat	1 cup
Unrefined sugar	1 cup
Date Sugar	1 cup
Barley malt	1 1/2 cups reduce liquids by 1-2 Tbs.
Brown rice syrup	1 1/2 cups reduce liquids by 1-2 Tbs.
Brown rice syrup	1 cup
Fructose	1/2 to 2/3 cup
Molasses	1/2 to 3/4 cup
Concentrated fruit juices	varies
Honey	1/2 cup reduce liquid by 1/2 cup & temperature by 25 F
Stevia	1 Tablespoon

VEGETABLE, NUT & SEED CARRIER OILS

Vegetable carrier oils are un-perfumed oils extracted from kernels, nuts, seeds, fruits and other organic materials. Vegetable carrier oils are used in aromatherapy when adding pure essential oils, or in making cosmetics and toiletries. In aromatherapy, they carry essential oils into the body. But, vegetable carrier oils are more than just vehicles for essential oils and such, as they have health-giving qualities of their own. Vegetable carrier oils should be cold pressed to ensure that the vitamins, minerals and therapeutic fatty acids are not destroyed. In the 'cold' pressing process, excessive heat is avoided in order to minimize changes to the natural characteristics of the oil. Traditionally, there are several methods of cold pressing. In one, the raw material (seeds, nuts, kernels and fruits) is simply pressed with a hydraulic press and the oil is squeezed out. This process is only used for soft oily seeds and plant material such as olive, sesame and sunflower. Harder nuts or seeds require more force. The nuts or seeds are placed in a horizontal press with an enormous 'screw'. As this turns, the oil is squeezed out and drips into a trough below.

- **When combining essential oils with carrier oil, blend 12-30 drops of the essential oils into one ounce (30 ml) of the chosen carrier oil.**

- **Some carrier oils are edible.**

- **Store your carrier oils in the refrigerator to extend their shelve life.**

Individual Vegetable, Nut & Seed Carrier Oils

Aloe Vera Oil
(Aloe barbadensis and Glycine Soja)
Aloe vera is moisturizing and cooling, incredibly useful for any type of burn, including sunburn and X-ray burns. Aloe vera can also be used for cuts, bruises, bug bites, dry skin, and other skin conditions, such as psoriasis and eczema. Macerating aloe vera leaves in soybean oil produces aloe vera oil.

Almond, Sweet Oil
(Prunus amygdalus dulcis)
Sweet almond oil is a great emollient for softening and conditioning the skin. It is suitable for all skin types, but is especially good for dry, inflamed and irritated skin.

Amla Oil
(Emblica officinalis)
Amla oil is made from amla fruits, and is known to have one of the highest natural sources of vitamin C. Amla oil has been used in ayurvedic medicine to treat hair loss and to promote stronger and healthier hair growth. For a hot oil treatment, use it with brahmi oil.

Apricot Kernel Oil
(Prunus armeniaca)
Apricot kernel oil is taken from the kernel of the apricot seed and is similar in texture and properties to almond oil. It is extremely nourishing to the skin, and excellent to apply around the eyes and neck. Apricot kernel oil is an emollient. It does help make the skin feel softer and smoother, reduce roughness, cracking and irritation. Apricot kernel oil may possibly retard the fine wrinkles of aging.

Argan Oil
(Argania spinosa)
Argan oil comes from Morocco and is high in vitamin E. It also contains sterols, anti-oxidant and anti-inflammatory properties. This oil is excellent to use on dry, inflamed and eczema prone skin.

Avocado Oil
(Persea gratissima)
Avocado oil is reputed to be beneficial in reducing age spots, healing scars and moisturizing the skin. Avocado oil is also known to soften the skin. It is easily absorbed into the deep tissues and is therefore excellent for mature skin. It can help relieve dryness and itching of psoriasis and eczema. The unrefined oil has a higher level of protein and vitamins A, B1, B2, Panthothenic acid, D and E than refined oil.

Baobab
(Adansonia digitata)
Baoba (Mbuyu in Swahili) oil is derived from the seeds of the baobab tree, native to eastern and southern Africa. This oil has been used in African skin care for centuries, providing moisturizing benefits to the skin and hair. It absorbs quickly, improves elasticity, encourages regeneration of skin cells and does not clog the pores. It is extremely stable against rancidity.

Black Currant Seed Oil
(Ribes nigrum)
Black currant seed oil has a very high content of gamma linolenic acid, an important ingredient for maintaining the elasticity of the skin. Excellent for dry, devitalized, damaged and aging skin, as it assists in the reconstruction of cell membranes.

Black Seed Oil
(Nigella sativa)
Black seed oil is known to "cure all illnesses, except death", according to the writings in the Koran. Black seed oil is anti-bacterial and anti-inflammatory.

Borage
(Borago officinalis)
This oil contains an abundance of gamma linolenic acid (GLA), an essential fatty acid that the body uses to manufacture prostaglandins - hormone like substances that balance and regulate cellular activity. It reduces the aging process of the skin and reverses damage from ultraviolet rays. Borage oil regulates the hydration of the skin. This oil is also used to treat PMS, endometriosis, and menopausal discomforts, as well as for psoriasis and eczema. Borage seed oil's benefit is apparent even when it is used in small quantities.

Brahmi Oil
(Bacopa monniera)
Used in ayurvedic medicine to treat hair loss, skin problems, eczema, psoriasis and more. It is said to strengthen the hair roots, relieve itchy scalp and dandruff. Purifies and tightens the skin. Combine with amla oil to make a hair conditioning oil.

Camelina Oil
(Camelina sativa)
Camelina oil is taken from the cruciferous annual camelina, known as false flax or gold-of-pleasure. It is high in omega-3 linolenic acid. Records of plant cultivation date back as far as the Iron Age as the oil was used as a source of fuel as well as a skin moisturizer. It provides a protective coating for hair follicles and is a good to add to hair care products.

Camellia Oil
(Camellia sinensis)
This oil has been used in Japan for centuries to moisturize and condition the skin, hair and nails. Good for dry and damaged skin. Add it to hair conditioners, eye creams and sun skin care products. Green tea is made from this plant.

Castor Oil
(Ricinus communis)
Castor oil relieves dry skin and improves complexion. It acts as a humectant, attracting moisture to the skin. Castor oil has healing properties and a nourishing, alkalizing effect on the body. It penetrates deeply into the protective layer under the skin. This oil has a long shelf life. It is great for blackheads and dandruff.

Castor Oil, Sulfated (see Turkey Red Oil)

Coconut Oil
(Cocos nucifera)
Coconut oil is expressed from coconut kernels and is solid at temperatures below 76 degrees. Relatively light, unctuous and cooling, suitable for people living in hot climates. Place it in a blue bottle for added cooling qualities. It is easily absorbed by the skin and improves its texture. Coconut oil makes hair healthy, shiny and long.

Coconut Oil, Fractionated
(Cocos nucifera)
Fractionated coconut oil contains the medium-chain triglycerides (MCT's) of coconut oil. It is produced through hydrolysis of coconut oil and is then fractionated by steam distillation to isolate the MCT's. It has a water-clear, light texture, odorless, tasteless, with an indefinite shelf life. An excellent replacement for mineral oil, it is used as a viscosity modifier, carrier, and base oil. The great thing about using this carrier oil is it does not stain sheets or clothing. Massage therapists love this unscented base oil. It has a nice glide, absorbs well, and is not sticky. It leaves your skin smooth as silk. Suitable for all skin types, especially dry, mature or sensitive skin.

Coconut Oil, Virgin
(Cocos nucifera)
Virgin coconut oil is made from freshly harvested coconuts. They are grated and expeller pressed to produce coconut milk. This milk is then centrifuged to separate the milk from the solids. This separation is so thorough that the oil has no moisture left in it, therefore, it does not have to be heated. This unique cold process extraction method yields the finest, creamiest, most flavorful coconut oil, conserving all of the functional components of coconut oil: squalene, tocopherols, sterol etc. Virgin coconut oil is very light, penetrating, with an excellent shelf life and stability. It is known for its moisturizing and protective properties for skin and hair. Anti-fungal, non-greasy and high in vitamin E. Virgin coconut oil is an excellent cooking oil that enhances the flavor of many foods and bakery items. It is fabulous in protein shakes, salads and popcorn.

Cottonseed Oil
(Gossyoium hirsutum, barbadense)
Cottonseed oil is taken from the seed that is embedded in the cotton fiber. The oil contains about 20 IU of vitamin E per ounce.

Cranberry Seed Oil
(Vaccinium macrocarpon)
Cranberry seed oil contains 70% essential fatty acids, making it a superb emollient, lubricant and conditioner for the skin. This oil is excellent for use in skin, hair, lip and baby care. Cranberry seed oil contributes to the lipid barrier protection to the skin and assists in moisture retention.

Evening Primrose Oil
(Oenothera biennis)
Evening Primrose oil is a rich source of GLA (an essential fatty acid) and is useful for the relief of many skin conditions, PMS and tender breasts. Since the body does not produce EFA's it is important to get these nutrients through diet and topical applications. EFA's inhibit bacterial growth and allow our systems to defend against infection and inflammation. Internally, you may take one teaspoon daily. For external use, mix 20 % evening primrose oil with another carrier oil. Helps in making the skin feel softer and smoother, reduce roughness, cracking and irritation, and may possibly retard the fine wrinkles of aging.

Flaxseed Oil
(Linum usitatissimum)
This oil is rich in essential fatty acids, lecithin and contains all of the essential amino acids and almost every known trace minerals. Topical use of flaxseed oil allows the body to absorb some of the essential fatty acids necessary for healthy cellular activity. It softens and heals skin abrasions, reduces the swelling and redness of lesions due to skin disease and improves the overall health of the skin. This oil is commonly used for eczema, psoriasis, burns, inflammatory skin and other skin conditions.

Foraha Oil/Tamanu
(Calophyllum inophyllum)
This oil is obtained by crushing the dried nuts of the tamanu tree, which is native to Tahiti. This rich oil stimulates cell regeneration and is good for fragile or broken capillaries. Foraha is used in the South Pacific as a medicine, as an analgesic, anti-inflammatory and cicatrisant. Long ago, foraha was used to treat leprosy. It is wound healing, soothing for eczema and other skin problems, such as burns and rashes, as well as for insect bites. It is used as an aid for relieving pain, healing wounds, herpes lesions and post-surgical scars. A combination of foraha and ravensara aromatica essential oil has been used successfully as a treatment for shingles. Use no more than 25 percent of foraha oil in your base blend.

Grape Seed Oil
(Vitis vinifera)
Grape seed oil is non-greasy and suits all skin types. As its name suggests, it is produced from the grape seed. Grape seed oil's very fine texture quickly penetrates into the skin, wonderful to use around the eyes and neck. It helps preserve the natural moisture of the skin. Widely used in hypoallergenic natural products because it does not often cause allergic reactions in the highly allergic people.

Hazelnut Oil
(Corylus americana)
Hazelnut oil has unusual astringent qualities that are particularly valuable for oily, acne prone and combinations skins. Moisturizes, softens and repairs dry and damaged skin. Studies have shown that it can filter sunrays and is commonly used in sun care products.

Hemp Oil
(Cannabis sativa)
Hemp oil is a rich source of GLA and is useful for the relief of many skin conditions. It is wonderful for dry or mature skin, since it helps stimulate cell growth. Hemp oil has the lowest amount of saturated fatty acids and the highest amount of the polyunsaturated essential fatty acids, making it a key nutritive ingredient in anti-inflammatory skin care formulations.

Jojoba Oil
(Simmondsia chinensis)
Jojoba oil is not actually an oil, it is a liquid wax. Jojoba oil is an excellent lubricant and hair conditioner, good for all skin types. It penetrates more easily then other oils. It is rich in vitamin E and is excellent for massaging faces with sensitive or oily complexions. It also contains anti-bacterial properties, useful for the treatment of acne. Use in sun tanning oil for those who burn easily in the sun. Jojoba oil is similar to sperm whale oil and has been used as a substitute for it. Jojoba is actually a liquid wax and properly stored can last for many years without spoiling. It also closely resembles the natural moisturizing oil, sebum, which is secreted by human skin. Jojoba helps to heal inflamed skin conditions such as psoriasis or any form of dermatitis, helps control acne and oily scalps. Since it has antioxidant properties, it can keep other oils from going rancid.

Kukui Nut Oil
(Aleurites moluccana)
Kukui nut oil is pressed from the nut of the tropical kukui tree, which comes mainly from Hawaii. Kukui oil is high in essential fatty acids, helpful for softening and restructuring the skin. It is excellent for sensitive, mature, damaged, sunburned, burned or wrinkled skin.

Macademia Oil
(Macademia ternifolia)
Macademia oil has a fine texture with very little aroma. Macademia nut oil is similar to sebum, the oil naturally produced by human skin to protect it. It is a good emollient, making it especially beneficial for dry and aging skin. This oil has a long shelf life and has good resistance to rancidity. It has a mild laxative action and thus, some have said, to be effective in reducing weight.

Marula Oil
(Sclerocarya birrea)
Marula is Africa's greatest skin care oil. It is rich in anti-oxidants and an extremely stable oil. It creates a protective coating on the surface of the skin making it great for dry skin sufferers. It absorbs quickly, hydrates the skin, heals tissues, reduces trans-epidermal water loss and increases smoothness of the skin.

Meadowfoam Oil
(Limnanthes alba)
Meadowfoam oil is a winter annual plant native to the pacific northwest of the United States. This oil was developed in the 70's to replace sperm whale oil in an effort to protect this species. Meadowfoam is known to moisturize the skin and hair better than any oils and prevents moisture loss. Makes hair shiny, revitalizes dry, cracked lips, keeping them moist longer.

Mustard Oil
(Brassica alba)
Mustard oil is an excellent oil for kapha. It loosens lung mucus, relieves respiratory congestion, colds, joint pain, arthritis and abdominal pain.

Neem Oil
(Azadirachtin indica)
Neem is used widely in India and Africa as an anti-bacterial, anti-viral, anti-fungal, anti-septic, and anti-parasitic agent in toiletries, soap, toothpaste, and skin/hair care products. It is used to treat skin disorders such as eczema, psoriasis ringworm, scabies and chicken pox. Neem oil can be used to get rid of lice and control dandruff. Use it for pets to kill and repel fleas and to treat hot spots.

Olive Oil
(Olea europaea)
The highest quality of olive oil available is expeller expressed from the olive fruit. You can purchase different grades of this oil. The first pressing is dark green, has the highest amount of vitamins and minerals and is called "extra virgin". The second pressing is referred to as "classico" or "virgin" olive oil and is golden in color. Olive oil has the properties of being calming, demulcent and emollient and can be used pure or in blends for burns, sprains, bruises, insect bites, to relieve itchy skin and to massage the gums of people suffering from pyorrhea.

Palm Oil
(Elaeis guineensis)
Palm oil is produced from the pulp or flesh of the fruit of the oil palm. It is a natural source of vitamin E and is also a rich source of beta-carotene. Palm oil can be used in balms, body butters and stick formulations, where rigidity is required. Good for soap making, it makes a nice hard bar.

Palm Kernel Oil
(Elaeis guineensis)
This oil is obtained from the kernels, taken from the cracked nuts of the palm. Soaps made with palm kernel oil are white, very hard and lather beautifully. It is a good substitute for beeswax.

Passion Fruit Seed Oil
(Passiflora edulis)
Also known as maracuya, this oil is extracted from the seed of the passion fruit and is rich in essential fatty acids. It has great spreading properties, yet it leaves the skin feeling less greasy than some other oils. Passion fruit seed oil has anti-bacterial (for acne), anti-itching and anti-inflammatory properties.

Peach Kernel Oil
(Prunus persica)
Peach kernel oil is very similar to apricot oil. It is a light, penetrating oil that is good for mature or sensitive skin. Use it to make light creams and lotions. Great for lip balms, as it absorbs quickly and does not leave a greasy feeling.

Peanut Oil
(Arachis hypogaea)
Peanut oil is heavy, scented, penetrates the skin well, and is often used to increase a products nutritive value. Peanut oil is excellent for oily skin or for use in facials.
Caution: Many people are allergic to peanut oil.

Pecan Oil
(Algooquian paccan.)
Pecan oil is an excellent source of monounsaturated fatty acid - similar to olive oil. It is moisturizing, emollient and healing.

Pistachio Oil
(Pistacia vera)
Pistachio oil is a great skin moisturizer. It is rapidly absorbed into the skin and does not leave a greasy feel to the skin. Pistachio oil softens and nourishes the skin. Some of the documented properties are: analgesic, anticoagulant, aphrodisiac, digestive and hepatic. Pistachio oil contains phytosterols, which may have anti-cancer properties.

Pomegranate Seed Oil
(Punica granatum linn.)
Pomegranate Seed oil is known for its anti-bacterial (acne) properties, hydrates, moisturizes and nourishes the skin. It also restores the pH balance of the skin. Has anti-wrinkle properties and smoothes fines lines.

Pumpkin Seed Oil
(Cucurbita pepo)
Pumpkin seed oil is highly emollient, rich in vitamins A, C, E and K and Zinc. Pumpkin seed oil is high in unsaturated fatty acids (about 60%). Use this oil to add nutrients to your cosmetics and massage oils. Native Americans used pumpkin seeds to treat enlarged prostate. Herbalists use it as a non-irritating diuretic.

Red Raspberry Seed Oil
(Rubus idaeus)
Raspberry seed oil is emollient, lubricating, conditioning, a lipid barrier, providing protection and moisture retention for the skin. It is a superior radical scavenger oil. Raspberry seed oil has UV absorptive properties, beneficial for photo sensitivity protection. It contains high concentrations of mixed tocopherol, tocotrienols and carotenoid. The oil reveals mild raspberry flavor and aroma, excellent to add to salad dressings.

Rice Bran Oil
(Oryza sativa)
Rice bran oil is derived from rice and makes a soothing oil for sunburns. Use rice bran oil where softening and moisturizing properties are needed. Good for mature, delicate or sensitive skin.

Rosehip Oil
(Rosa canina, Rosa mosqueta)
Rosa mosqueta grows wild in the southern Andes as well as other parts of the world. High in essential fatty acids and vitamin C, valuable in treating skin problems such as eczema and psoriasis. This oil is the best anti-aging oil to use. It is known to reduce scarring and to heal burns. Rosehip oil can diminish broken capillaries. It may turn rancid quickly and should be stored in a cool place or refrigerated.

Safflower Oil
(Carthamus tinctorius)
Safflower oil helps moisturize, nourish and restructure the skin and is nice to use in balms, creams and lip balm. Safflower oil has one of the highest linoleic acid (70%) contents of all oils. The moisture content of human skin is proportional to the content of essential unsaturated fatty acids. It is wonderfully moisturizing.

Sea Buckthorn Berry Oil/Sanddorn

(Hippophae rhamnoides)

Sea buckthorn was known for centuries as a skin care remedy and cosmetic aid with nourishing, revitalizing, and restorative action. Sea buckthorn oil is used to promote the healing of skin injuries, such as burns, sunburns, wounds, eczema and help improve conditions of mucous membranes, including ulcers, lesions. Since sea buckthorn is rich in nutrients required for healthy skin metabolism, it is known to combat wrinkles, dryness and other symptoms of malnourished or prematurely aging skin. It is also taken internally to improve the condition of the mucous membranes in the gastro-intestinal tract and as a natural dietary supplement. Use up to 30 % in a base oil.

Sesame Seed Oil

(Sesamum indicum)

Sesame seed oil is used in ayurveda when a warming effect is needed. It grounds Vata, tonifies the female reproductive system and is used for a wide variety of other conditions. It penetrates deep into the skin, nourishing and detoxifying the deepest tissue layers. Sesame seed oil aggravates Pita skin and eye conditions, as it is heating. Since it contains tryptophane, it can be massaged into the feet before bed, for a good night's sleep.

Shea Oil

(Butyrospermum parkii)

Shea oil is made from the nuts of the shea nut tree in South Africa. High in vitamin E, it softens the skin and has a slight sunscreen effect. Useful in baby formulations, sun protection products, lip care products, hair care products, and more, for healing and protecting the skin. Use 3% to 20% in creams and lotions, soaps and balms, or 100% pure as a moisturizing serum.

Soybean Oil

(Glycine soja)

Soybean oil is made form the soybean. It has very little color and is high in polyunsaturated fatty acids, vitamin E and lecithin. Unsaponifiables are a large group of compounds called plant steroids or sterolins. They soften the skin, have superior moisturizing effect on the upper layer of the skin and reduce scars. The sterolins in avocado oil have been found to diminish age sports. Oils with the highest unsaponifiables are shea butter, avocado oil, sesame seed oil, soybean oil and olive oil.

Sunflower Oil
(Helianthus annuus)
Sunflower oil is pressed from the sunflower seeds and is rich in vitamins A, E and minerals. This light oil leaves a protective layer on the skin after drying. Sunflower oil is particularly useful in the winter when extra protection is desirable.

Tamanu Oil *(see Foraha Oil)*

Turkey Red Oil
(Sulphated Ricinus communis)
Adding sulfuric acid to castor oil creates turkey red oil or sulfonated castor oil. This oil is water-soluble and emulsifies other oils in water. When making bath oils, use 3 parts of turkey red oil and 1 part essential oils.

Vitamin E Oil
(Tocopherol)
Vitamin E oil is produced by vacuum distillation of various vegetable oils. The potency of vitamin E is measured by its alpha tocopherol content. It is important to know the IU of the vitamin E oil you are using. A 200 IU/g vitamin E contains 200 units of alpha tocopherol per gram of oil and the rest is unspecified amounts of other components. Since the alpha tocopherol is responsible for repairing, healing and protecting the skin, use the high alpha tocopherol natural vitamin E oil. The most important and well-known biological function of vitamin E is related to its anti-oxidant properties. It protects the cellular structure against damage from free radicals. It acts as a free radical scavenger to prevent cell damage. Vitamin E may help decrease the toxicity of certain chemotherapy drugs, the harmful effects of solar radiation, and burns from radiation therapy on the skin.. Vitamin E moisturizes the skin, reduces UV induced damage and is appropriate to use in sun care products including lip balms. Helps heal scar tissues, prevents aging by rejuvenating skin cellular activity.

Walnut Oil
(Juglans regia)
Walnut oil is high in linoleic acid and helps to regenerate, tone and moisturize damaged dry skin. Walnut oil strengthens the liver and gallbladder. It is known to help balance the nervous system. Topically, it is applied to the eyes to strengthen dim vision.

Watermelon Seed Oil
(Citrullus vulgaris)
Watermelon oil (Ootanga or Kalahari oil) is a light, penetrating and emollient oil, and rich in Omega 6. It absorbs into the skin rapidly, dissolving sebum build up. It has a non-greasy feel to it. Its moisturizing properties make it ideal for mature skin as it restores elasticity. It can be used as a natural baby oil.

Wheat Germ Oil
(Triticum vulgare)
Wheat germ oil is rich in vitamin E and is useful for dry, mature skin. It is well known for its ability to heal scar tissue, smooth stretch marks, and soothe burns. As it is too sticky to use on it's own for massage oil, add small amounts to a lighter oil, in 10% dilution. Do not use on people with wheat intolerance.

VEGETABLE, NUT & SEED BUTTERS

Vegetable butters are fats that are solid at room temperature. Today, vegetable butters are being used more and more in cosmetics and skin care products. They are rich in nutrients that are beneficial to the skin. Vegetable butters give viscosity and stability to lotions, creams and balms.

Basic Body Butter Bar

2 parts cocoa butter
1 part shea butter
1 part mango butter
2 parts virgin coconut oil
Essential oils
Vibrational Essences

Melt butters and oil in a double boiler. Add essential oils and Vibrational Essences. Add mica for coloring, if desired. Pour into deodorant containers.

Exfoliating Body Wash

3 parts castile soap
1 part shea butter
1 part apricot meal
½ part walnut hulls, ground
¼ part grapefruit essential oil
¼ part cypress essential oil

Melt shea butter. When the butter has melted, add warmed castile soap. Add the rest of the ingredients and pour into a container.

Rich Body Butter Bar

2 parts almond butter
1 part shea butter
1 part avocado butter
½ oz rosehip oil
8 drops rose essential oil
10 drops jasmine essential oil
12 drops neroli essential oil

Melt butters in a double boiler. Let it cool for a while then add rosehip oil and essential oils. Pour into desired forms.

Aloe Butter
(Cocos nucifera and Aloe barbadensis)
Aloe butter is an extract of aloe vera using a fatty coconut fraction, which produces a soft and solid butter. Aloe butter is solid at room temperature, but melts on the skin. Aloe butter can be used for dry skin and to moisturize after exposure to sun, wind and cold. To enhance moisture in the skin add a small amount to your cosmetics.

Apricot Kernel Butter
(Prunus armeniacae)
Apricot butter is obtained from apricot kernel oil, and possesses all the natural qualities of the oil. It moisturizes and soothes the skin and is suitable for mature or sensitive skin.

Avocado Butter
(Persea gratissima)
Avocado butter is made from the fresh of the avocado fruit. Avocado butter is very rich in nutrients, proteins and minerals. It is a much softer butter than any other butter. It has some natural sunscreen properties, which makes it an ideal butter in lip balms, creams (under the eyes creams), hair conditioners and lotions.

Borneo Tallow *(see Illipe Butter)*

Cocoa Butter
(Theobroma cacao)
Cocoa butter is the solid fat from the roasted seed of the cacao plant. Cocoa butter is solid at room temperature. It's the perfect stuff for massaging daily into fast-growing pregnant bellies to prevent stretch marks from developing.

Illipe Butter
(Shorea stenoptera)
Illipe butter is also called Borneo tallow. It is taken from the nuts of the illipe tree, which grows in Africa, South America and Asia. Illipe butter is similar to cocoa butter in its texture. It moisturizes the skin and restores elasticity, and has skin-soothing properties.

Kokum Butter
(Garcinia indica)
Kokum butter is obtained from the Indian tree garcinia indica. It is used in skin care products, because of its ability to soften the skin and heal ulcerations and fissures of lips, hands and soles of feet. Kokum butter helps reduce degeneration of the skin cells and restores elasticity.

Mango Butter
(Magnifera indica)
Mango butter is taken from the seed kernels of the fruit of the mango tree. It is similar in texture to shea butter and is much softer than cocoa butter. Mango butter has good emolliency and lends protection against the sun. It is said to prevent drying of the skin and formation of wrinkles. Mango also reduces degeneration of skin cells and restores elasticity. It has a very light yellow/mango color.

Olive Butter
(Olea europea)
Olive butter is taken from very ripe and cold-pressed Olives. Olive butter possesses all of the natural qualities of olive oil and is similar to shea butter. Olive butter has excellent spread-ability and can be used as massage butter.

Sal Butter
(Shorea robusta)
Sal butter comes from the fruit kernels of the sal tree, native to Indian. It has similar properties to cocoa butter but differing slightly in scent and color. It is wonderful for the skin because of its high emollient properties and its exceptional oxidative stability. This is valuable for those who enjoy keeping their skin moist and protected from harsh elements.

Shea Butter
(Butyrospermum parkii)
Shea butter is actually a wax in semi solid form. It is made from the nuts of the South African shea nut tree and has been extensively used by African healers as the ideal treatment for dry or aging skin. High in vitamin E, it softens the skin and has a slight sunscreen effect. It is useful for healing and protecting the skin. Melt and heat Shea butter for at least 20 minutes at about 175 degrees to avoid crystallization.

WAXES

Waxes are organic compounds that are solid at room temperature, melt at low temperature, are water-repellant, and give solidity and smoothness to creams and lotions. Waxes also facilitate the emulsion of water and oil when making creams, lotions or other emulsions.

Bees Wax

(Apis)

Bees wax has many uses, firstly in the cosmetic industry for creams, ointments, lotions, pomades, lipstick, rouges, and much more. Secondly, bees wax is used in the candle making industry. Bees wax candles are drip less and smokeless, and most of all have a wonderful fragrance. Thirdly, bees wax is being used in the pharmaceutical and many other industries. Bees wax has therapeutic benefits and has been used to treat Lupus, respiratory diseases, hay fever, asthma, and sinus problems. Eating honeycomb is delicious and can desensitize someone to pollen, prevent hay fever and allergies. You can also simply chew and swallow (if desired) ½ teaspoon of bees wax. Please, only use pure and unbleached bees wax. When using bees wax for making salves, use one ounce bees wax to three to four ounces of oil. Modify the amount of wax you use depending on what you are making, and what consistency you like it. Bees wax has antiseptic properties, which help preserve your homemade products.

Bees Wax Candles

1 lb bees Wax
1 oz comfrey leaf
1 oz sweetgrass
1 oz white Sage

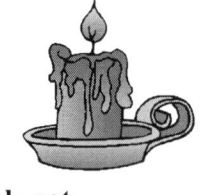

Melt bees wax in a crock-pot. Add finely crushed herbs and macerate for 2 hours, keeping the crock-pot on low. Strain, if desired, while the wax is still warm and liquid. Pour into desired forms.

Candelilla Wax
(Euphorbia cerifera, E. antisyphilitica and Pedilanthus pavonis)
Candelilla wax is a natural vegetable wax found on the outer coating of the candelilla shrubs. Candelilla is the plasticizer used in making chewing gum. The wax gives the gum its "chew". Candelilla wax holds fragrances and flavors very well. Candelilla wax can be used in place of beeswax for vegan formulations. It is also a good additive in candle making since it adds strength to wax blends.

Carnauba Wax
(Copernicia prunifera)
Carnauba is a vegetable wax exuded by the leaves of the Brazilian "tree of life". Carnauba palm grows in the northern and northeastern part of Brazil along riverbanks, valleys, and lagoons where soil is dark and fertile. This is a very, very hard wax for making cosmetics.

Emulsifying Wax
(Vegetable based)
When using emulsifying wax make sure that it is vegetable based. Emulsifying wax can be added to the oil phase in making cosmetics. Vegetable emulsifying wax helps keep the oil and water from separating in creams and lotions.

Floral Waxes

Floral waxes are extracted from plant materials via solvents. Floral waxes can be added to the oil phase when making creams and lotions, to create a thicker texture and add a pleasant fragrance.

Jasmine Wax

Jasmine wax retains the highly aromatic properties of jasmine. It is used as a thickening agent in making cosmetics for dry, greasy, irritated and sensitive skin. The aromatic benefits of jasmine are euphoric, inspiring, and aphrodisiac.

Mimosa Wax

Mimosa wax retains the highly aromatic properties of mimosa. It is used as a thickening agent in making cosmetics for sensitive or oily skin, and for skin problems caused by stress. The aromatic benefits of mimosa are calming, uplifting and bringer of joy.

Rose Wax

Rose wax retains the highly aromatic properties of rose. It is used as a thickening agent in making cosmetics to regenerate skin cells, especially for dry, wrinkles and aging skin. The aromatic benefits of rose are aphrodisiac, mood elevating, and calming/energizing.

Tuberose Wax

Tuberose wax retains the highly aromatic properties of tuberose. It is used as a thickening agent in making cosmetics and high-class perfumes. The aromatic benefits of tuberose are aphrodisiac, euphoric, and center the emotions.

Index

acid/alkaline 4, 5, 9, 11, 35, 124, 133, 178, 227, 248
see also blood
acne 26, 44, 47, 55, 56, 81, 85, 88, 89, 90, 91, 93, 100, 101,
107, 108, 127, 149, 170, 177, 180, 188, 205, 207, 208, 210,
213, 222, 224, 238, 251, 253, 254
adaptogens 127, 162, 164, 177, 180, 183, 207
adrenal glands 81, 86, 101, 102, 126, 141, 147, 151, 159, 162,
164, 180, 213
stimulant 10, 83, 101, 132, 134, 151
aging 6, 23, 31, 48, 55, 113, 122, 138, 145, 147, 177, 189,
206, 212, 223, 224, 246, 247, 248, 250, 252, 255, 256, 257,
261, 264
AIDS 22, 27, 150, 164, 197
alcoholism 91, 160
alfalfa 13, 15, 227, 228
allergies 3, 41, 47, 59, 70, 117, 124, 136, 146, 148, 149, 150,
152, 164, 168, 171, 172, 173, 177, 189, 233, 262

aloe vera 2, 14, 27, 68, 123, 175, 191, 192, 246, 260
aluminum 237
amenorrhea see menstruation
anemia 22, 41, 44, 47, 50, 128, 130, 141, 146, 152, 171, 243
aneurysm 134
animals 3, 58, 69, 121, 136, 138, 204, 207, 210
pets 79, 253, 204
anorexia 11, 45, 79, 106, 134
antibiotics 2, 7, 11, 27, 42, 44, 58, 71, 97, 106, 118, 150, 158,
184, 191
anti-aging see aging
anti-fungal 26, 61, 83, 94, 95, 97, 103, 104, 105, 130, 134,
142, 150, 156, 164, 170, 172, 188, 189, 222, 224, 249, 253
anti-histamine 81, 152, 164, 168, 171, 172
anti-oxidant 5, 11, 27, 60, 91, 113, 122, 125, 126, 132, 134,
137, 138, 150, 151, 153, 155, 164, 171, 176, 177, 178, 180,
183, 185, 191, 209, 212, 236, 247, 251, 252, 257
anxiety 16, 18, 40, 44, 49, 50, 52, 74, 75, 77, 81, 82, 83, 87,
89, 92, 93, 94, 95, 99, 100, 102, 103, 104, 107, 109, 117,
131, 153, 156, 160, 161, 165, 169, 174, 177, 179, 185, 186,
187, 191, 197, 205, 209, 213, 215, 233
aphrodisiac 23, 27, 76, 81, 88, 89, 91, 95, 97, 100, 101, 106,
107, 108, 109, 111, 137, 144, 147, 154, 179, 189, 206, 210,
213, 244, 254, 264
appendicitis 161, 189
appetite depressant 12, 148, 150, 154, 164, 189
appetite stimulant 22, 41, 44, 45, 46, 50, 51, 77, 78, 79, 91,
92, 127, 135, 136, 138, 140, 141, 144, 148, 151, 163, 167,
174, 177, 184, 185, 194, 205
arteriosclerosis 92, 147, 162, 166, 178

266

arthritis 6, 10, 25, 27, 31, 32, 42, 45, 47, 49, 59, 60, 75, 78, 80, 88, 95, 99, 106, 108, 122, 130, 136, 138, 140, 145, 147, 148, 150, 154, 157, 158, 164, 165, 173, 175, 180, 186, 188, 189, 190, 224, 252

aspirin 78, 108, 126, 165, 171, 186

asthma 4, 38, 44, 46, 47, 52, 91, 92, 96, 97, 101, 102, 125, 134, 141, 142, 147, 154, 156, 157, 159, 163, 164, 166, 167, 177, 179, 180, 184, 186, 189, 215, 225, 262

astragalus 126, 164, 191

astringent 7, 21, 56, 59, 60, 61, 62, 64, 81, 92, 122, 128, 129, 130, 133, 148, 168, 172, 176, 179, 181, 183, 184, 186, 187, 206, 207, 209, 210, 212, 213, 223, 251

atherosclerosis 41, 154, 173, 179

athlete's foot 85, 93, 94, 103, 134, 222

auto-immune disorders 162, 164
   see also lupus, rheumatoid arthritis

azulene 81, 82, 108

backache 34, 143

bacteria 2, 11, 32, 41, 42, 88, 93, 95, 105, 117, 127, 138, 141, 142, 149, 176, 189, 191, 204, 217, 222, 236, 242, 250

baths 4, 5, 9, 57, 60, 67, 74, 80, 83, 98, 102, 107, 125, 142, 157, 205, 207, 210, 224, 239, 240, 257

bedwetting 142, 171

Bell's palsy 158

beneficial bacteria *see* intestinal flora

bipolar disorder 40

birth control 139, 148, 187, 194

bladder 1, 15, 37, 52, 64, 125, 133, 138, 140, 142, 152, 157, 158, 159, 165, 173, 178, 182, 186, 205
   infection 42, 63, 212
   prolapsed 41

bleeding 18, 22, 45, 50, 51, 84, 122, 129, 130, 133, 136, 146, 152, 155, 167, 168, 176, 179, 181, 183, 186, 187, 188, 189, 213

blood 11, 16, 20, 22, 31, 33, 34, 35, 40, 41, 42, 43, 47, 48, 63, 123, 127, 128, 130, 131, 134, 138, 139, 149, 151, 152, 153, 162, 165, 167, 168, 172, 174, 176, 179, 180, 182, 183, 185, 187, 189, 198, 221, 227, 228, 230, 237, 243
   alkalizing 11, 35
   building/strengthening 7, 22, 41, 48, 49, 50, 124, 130, 142, 146, 152, 154, 155, 168, 172, 176, 242
   circulation 9, 30, 42, 47, 55, 56, 127, 128, 131, 136, 143, 151, 153, 155, 162, 166, 174, 178, 179, 180, 182, 185, 189, 223, 230
   cleansing 7, 26, 27, 34, 60, 126, 128, 133, 138, 140, 145, 146, 161, 164, 168, 176, 178, 180, 189

blood clots 49, 50, 130, 134, 179, 221

blood pressure 10, 11, 31, 38, 41, 45, 51, 89, 93, 94, 108, 127, 130, 133, 134, 138, 140, 142, 144, 145, 146, 147, 150, 154, 155, 160, 162, 163, 166, 169, 172, 177, 178, 180, 181, 187, 189, 194, 195, 197, 207, 208, 214, 225, 231, 232, 237
   see also hypertension

blood sugar 22, 24, 26, 127, 129, 145, 147, 152, 153, 155, 158, 160, 165, 169, 179, 183, 242, 243
   see also diabetes, hypoglycemia

blood thinners 176, 180, 186, 198

boils 44, 61, 130, 146, 182

bones 16, 20, 42, 52, 71, 104, 132, 225, 228, 241
   disorders 34, 42, 130
   healing 45, 132, 142, 157, 223
   strengthening 23, 45, 142
   osteoporosis(penia) 22, 34, 122, 142, 156, 157
   spurs 138

bowels 52, 61, 63, 122, 126, 133, 136, 139, 144, 155, 159, 160, 167, 168, 178, 195, 210, 227, 238
  see also colon, constipation, laxative
breastfeeding 27, 76, 79, 102, 135, 171, 176

breasts 146, 148
  cancer 11, 155, 164
  cystic/fibroids 10, 149, 174
  disorder 147
  inflammation 139
  tender 114, 250
bruises 3, 32, 43, 45, 50, 51, 52, 61, 67, 89, 100, 104, 125, 127, 128, 134, 150, 179, 206, 208, 221, 222, 246, 253
burns 67, 90, 95, 99, 105, 123, 128, 134, 143, 146, 155, 165, 191, 204, 205, 207, 208, 212, 221, 222, 223, 225, 246, 250, 253, 255, 256, 257, 258
caffeine 134, 142, 153, 154, 155, 159, 169, 177, 187, 210
calcium 7, 11, 12, 33, 56, 143, 157, 158, 168, 169, 174, 175, 185, 227, 237, 240, 241, 242
cancer 27, 60, 105, 125, 132, 133, 136, 138, 139, 140, 146, 149, 150, 153, 164, 171, 172, 179, 181, 183, 191, 223, 224, 254
  breast 11, 155, 164
  colon 150
  liver 164
  leukemia 151, 164, 183
  prostate 155
  skin 131, 221, 224, 225
  uterine 155
  see also chemotherapy
candida 85, 130, 134, 138, 140, 143, 172, 182, 205, 210
canker sores 130, 169, 176, 179, 189, 210

castor oil 32, 99, 131, 248, 257
cayenne 13, 30, 37, 137, 194, 200-203
cellulite 9, 58, 75, 76, 78, 81, 83, 84, 86, 87, 88, 89, 91, 92, 98, 100, 104, 106
chakras 36-39, 97, 212, 215, 217
chamomile 14, 37, 81, 82, 97, 138, 194, 205, 210, 222
chemotherapy 27, 122, 126, 136, 148, 151, 162, 257
chicken pox 77, 134, 160, 222, 253
childbirth 27, 46, 90, 95, 97, 131, 146, 160, 161, 171, 176, 183, 185, 225, 230
cholesterol 10, 11, 24, 25, 28, 31, 45, 125, 134, 144, 150, 154, 155, 156, 175, 177, 179, 181, 183, 187, 225, 231, 232, 243
  see also arteriosclerosis, atherosclerosis
cholelithiasis *see* gallstones
chronic fatigue syndrome (CFS) 150, 183
cinnamon 4, 14, 24, 28, 31, 37, 42, 44, 80, 82, 135, 136, 140, 141
cirrhosis 91, 144, 165, 196
coffee 46, 53, 61, 63, 80, 83, 119, 135, 139, 142, 143, 144, 159, 172, 210
colds 24, 31, 34, 38, 43, 47, 48, 50, 52, 59, 74, 76, 78, 79, 79, 80, 85, 89, 90, 92, 94, 95, 97, 98, 100, 101, 105, 124, 126, 127, 128, 130, 134, 140, 146, 148, 149, 153, 156, 157, 160, 161, 162, 163, 164, 171, 173, 176, 177, 182, 186, 188, 213, 233, 239, 252
cold sores 77, 94, 95, 100, 239
colitis 22, 32, 61, 143, 167, 173, 180, 188, 210
colon 20, 22, 32, 122, 123, 125, 136, 150, 154, 162, 165, 167, 175, 184, 189
  see also bowels, constipation, laxative
comfrey 16, 142, 194, 216, 223

268

constipation   10, 20, 22, 31, 35, 36, 42, 45, 46, 48, 49, 52, 59,
    122, 125, 127, 134, 136, 143, 144, 154, 162, 173, 176, 177,
    185, 188, 189, 197, 227, 228
coughs   11, 45, 52, 59, 79, 85, 91, 94, 95, 97, 98, 101, 102,
    105, 108, 124, 131, 134, 135, 148, 154, 156, 162, 163, 165,
    167, 170, 171, 174, 178, 180, 182, 186, 189, 225
cramps   16, 35, 41, 59, 87, 91, 92, 134, 135, 136, 143, 144,
    148, 152, 161, 164, 172, 177, 182, 184, 187, 205, 211, 225
    menstrual   34, 35, 50, 76, 79, 82, 83, 89, 93, 124, 129, 164,
        187, 206, 211, 225, 230
Crohn's disease   136, 150, 210
cuts   3, 45, 67, 85, 95, 99, 104, 127, 146, 208, 222, 223, 246
cystitis   62, 81, 128, 142, 157, 180, 184, 189, 212
cysts   60, 63, 146, 227
    breasts   149, 174
    ovarian   44
dandelion   16, 23, 134, 140, 144-145, 223, 228, 241
depression   17, 20, 32, 39, 40, 52, 74, 76, 77, 80, 82, 83, 86,
    87, 88, 89, 90, 91, 95, 97, 98, 100, 107, 109, 127, 144, 147,
    152, 153, 156, 161, 164, 171, 177, 178, 179, 184, 185, 195,
    215, 233
dermatitis   44, 78, 80, 81, 136, 154, 192, 222, 251
detoxification & cleansing
    blood   26, 60, 63, 126, 128, 133, 140, 161, 176, 178
    cleansing   13, 15, 22, 23, 25, 31, 54, 55, 56, 83, 84, 86,
        102, 128, 136, 145, 148, 153, 156, 159, 160, 161, 172,
        175, 178, 181, 187, 189, 191, 207, 210, 211
    detoxification   12, 25, 32, 54, 58, 86, 88, 91, 98, 126, 146,
        164, 185, 207, 216, 223, 239, 240, 256
    liver   26, 30, 144, 156, 180, 208
    lymphatic   138, 141, 146, 188
    skin   56, 57, 68, 83, 131, 146, 175, 222, 225, 239, 240

diabetes   22, 37, 62, 63, 125, 128, 129, 131, 141, 152, 154,
    165, 169, 171, 183, 194, 196, 231
    see also blood sugar
diaper rash   5, 67, 108, 139, 171, 204, 205, 222, 226
digestion   2, 7, 10, 12, 19, 20, 22, 24, 25, 26, 27, 30, 31, 34,
    37, 40, 41, 42, 43, 44, 45, 46, 47, 48, 50, 51, 52, 59, 64, 75,
    76, 80, 81, 84, 85, 86, 87, 88, 89, 91, 92, 94, 95, 96, 97, 98,
    99, 103, 104, 106, 107, 123, 124, 126, 128, 130, 131, 132,
    133, 135, 136, 137, 138, 139, 140, 141, 142, 143, 144, 146,
    148, 151, 152, 153, 156, 159, 161, 162, 163, 165, 166, 167,
    169, 170, 171, 172, 174, 175, 177, 178, 179, 180, 184, 185,
    186, 188, 189, 198, 199, 205, 207, 208, 209, 210, 211, 213,
    227, 237, 238, 241, 254
disinfectant   60, 64, 74, 80, 83, 88, 99, 133, 236
diuretics   78, 86, 88, 97, 108, 128, 131, 134, 138, 140, 141,
    142, 143, 146, 154, 156, 159, 165, 166, 168, 169, 172, 173,
    181, 182, 184, 186, 189, 206, 207, 213, 254
diverticulitis(osis)   134, 136
dizziness   20, 29, 40, 43, 44, 47, 50, 51, 79, 89, 134, 138, 140,
    161, 162, 176, 178, 181, 197
douches   128, 205, 210, 221
dreams   17, 18, 23, 40, 49, 52, 76, 94, 102, 134, 209
drug withdrawal   181
dysmennorhea   *see* menstruation
earaches   78, 89, 167, 170
ears   20, 38, 43, 52, 70-73, 167
    infections   3, 32, 42, 44, 97, 223
eczema   44, 77, 78, 80, 81, 93, 99, 107, 125, 127, 131, 146,
    147, 149, 155, 171, 177, 180, 188, 205, 221, 222, 224, 226,
    238, 246, 247, 248, 250, 253, 255, 256
edema   78, 80, 144, 150, 165, 171, 196
endocrine system   15, 36, 141, 142, 147, 162, 163, 169, 211

endometriosis 44, 139, 225, 248

enzymes 2, 7, 28, 31, 58, 124, 132, 144, 175, 188, 227, 235, 237, 243

epilepsy 79, 88, 134

Epstein-Barr virus 27, 183

equilibrium *see* dizziness

estrogen 25, 88, 122, 124, 129, 162, 183, 185, 187, 225
  see also hormones

eyes 14, 20, 22, 23, 32, 37, 39, 40, 44, 47, 48, 49, 52, 62, 67, 91, 124, 127, 128, 131 ,132, 138, 139, 140, 148, 151, 152, 153, 157, 162, 163, 166, 168, 181, 189, 194, 205, 206, 211, 228, 233, 246, 248, 251,256, 257, 260

fatigue 23, 32, 40, 41, 42, 43, 44, 45, 48, 50, 63, 76, 83, 87, 89, 91, 93, 95, 97, 98, 99, 101, 106, 124, 137, 141, 142, 150, 151, 159, 162, 164, 178, 180, 184, 189, 194, 208

fever blisters 89

fevers 7, 16, 17, 42, 43, 44, 50, 51, 64, 67, 76, 77, 79, 85, 89, 92, 124, 126, 129, 130, 131, 132, 134, 140, 146, 148, 149, 150, 160, 162, 163, 164, 165, 169, 171, 172, 174, 176, 186, 187, 188, 194, 212, 213, 243

fibroids 10, 44, 227

fibromyalgia 125, 159, 184, 187

flatulence 79, 80, 86, 91, 95, 124, 157, 187, 238
  see also gas

flu *see* influenza

food poisoning 42, 139

frigidity 37, 95, 107

gallbladder 1, 16, 32, 46, 48, 52, 101, 127, 132, 133, 134, 135, 143, 145, 150, 179, 186, 188, 225, 257

gallstones 46, 52, 90, 101, 136, 137, 138, 150, 183, 187, 193, 195

gas 11, 22, 24, 41, 42, 51, 59, 77, 80, 85, 86, 87, 103, 105, 123, 124, 126, 135, 139, 140, 141, 143, 144, 148, 151, 152, 170, 171, 172, 178, 186, 187
  see also flatulence

gastritis 11, 79, 88, 131, 134, 136, 139, 173, 177, 189

ginger 13, 24, 30, 31, 67, 86, 87, 151, 160, 181, 195, 207

gingivitis 142, 208

ginseng
  panax 14, 151, 152, 191
  pseudo 23, 141, 146, 147, 152, 183, 191

glaucoma 128

gout 4, 22, 25, 75, 80, 88, 95, 105, 128, 138, 140, 143, 145, 148, 151, 159, 173, 176, 178, 180, 186, 205

HIV 164

hair 2, 3, 6, 10, 12, 18, 23, 48, 49, 52, 55, 60, 61, 77, 78, 81, 90, 101, 119, 120, 125, 145, 146, 157, 168, 178, 208, 211, 228, 238, 247, 248, 249, 250, 251, 252, 253, 256, 260
  growth 12, 23, 91, 102, 111, 163, 221, 224, 246
  loss 10, 22, 77, 78, 81, 106, 146, 246, 248

hay fever 47, 152, 164, 177, 189, 262

headaches 4, 39, 41, 47, 76, 79, 89, 90, 92, 98, 101, 129, 131, 134, 138, 140, 141, 143, 160, 161, 162, 165, 170, 177, 178, 181, 185, 186, 233
  migraine 46, 84, 88, 141, 148, 160, 233
  nervous 26, 107, 186
  sinus 4
  stress 128, 185, 187
  tension 81, 106
  see also migraines

hearing 23, 38, 52, 70, 71, 88

heart 1, 10, 14, 22, 23, 26, 40, 42, 49, 52, 82, 87, 111,130, 133, 134, 136, 137, 146, 147, 150, 151, 152, 153, 154-155,

270

157, 159, 160, 161, 162, 166, 178, 178, 179, 181, 183, 188, 242
   conditions   22, 31, 63, 152, 162, 166, 189
   congestive heart failure (CHF)   147, 150, 157, 160
   disease   10, 38, 41, 132, 194
   emotional heart   38, 82, 92, 100, 111, 161, 206, 207, 208, 211, 217
   heartbeat   108, 133, 142, 145, 154, 185, 214
   mitral valve   155
   palpitations   26, 91, 161, 166, 224
heartburn   41, 80, 130, 131, 139, 177, 213
heavy (toxic) metals   10, 138, 140, 159, 176, 237
   see also   aluminum
hemoglobin   10, 20, 122
hemorrhoids   34, 36, 41, 44, 61, 67, 84, 134, 139, 149, 155, 183, 187, 189, 205, 212, 222, 224
hepatitis   22, 46, 124, 131, 133, 140, 150, 164, 166, 184
hiatal hernia   11, 131, 165
hives   44, 47, 50
hoarseness   11, 45, 141, 156
hormones   26, 43, 58, 74, 102, 128, 139, 146, 163, 183, 224
   see also   estrogen, progesterone, testosterone
hot flashes   42, 51, 83, 102, 129, 147, 179, 204, 206, 225
hydrochloric acid   124, 137, 144, 159, 170, 175, 186, 188
hypertension   45, 63, 92, 125, 137, 144, 155, 162, 164, 169, 177, 196, 205
   see also   blood pressure
hypoglycemia   37, 126, 158, 162
   see also   blood sugar
immune system   2, 10, 18, 27, 30, 48, 75, 77, 87, 93, 96, 100, 101, 105, 107, 117, 123, 124, 126, 132, 136, 141, 146, 147, 149, 150, 151, 153, 155, 159, 162, 164, 168, 171, 172, 176, 177, 179, 180, 182, 183, 185, 191, 204, 206, 207, 210, 215, 216, 231, 232
impotence   27, 37, 45, 50, 95, 137, 144, 147, 148, 153, 164
indigestion   *see* digestion
infections   18, 85, 91, 92, 96, 98, 123, 124, 127, 146, 153, 168, 170, 183, 184, 185, 197, 210, 250
   bacterial   88, 95, 105
   fungal   44, 81, 85, 93, 97, 105, 155, 184
   gastro-intestinal   87, 156
   lung   42, 75, 76, 79, 81, 84, 85, 99, 126, 147 ,153, 178
   sinus   74, 85
   skin & nail   44, 85, 91, 93, 101, 102, 153
   throat   79
   urinary tract   25, 42, 46, 62, 63, 87, 122, 128, 143, 170, 173, 178, 181, 183, 189, 195, 205 ,212
   vaginal   81, 205
   viral   42, 124, 147
infertility   27, 45, 139, 144, 148, 225
influenza   43, 48, 50, 64, 74, 78, 79, 85, 92, 95, 97, 98, 101, 105, 124, 127, 130, 131, 132, 140, 146, 147, 149 ,153, 156, 157, 163, 164, 173, 177, 182, 186, 188, 209, 213, 239
insects
   bites   27, 67, 76, 85, 90, 95, 98, 127, 139, 155, 160, 173, 179, 207, 250, 253
   repellants   3, 79, 80, 81, 83, 85, 91, 92, 94, 98, 127
insomnia   16, 20, 34, 40, 41, 44, 47, 49, 51, 52, 88, 90, 91, 92, 93, 94, 103, 107, 109, 128, 135, 137, 143, 150, 159, 160, 161, 162, 164, 165, 166, 171, 174, 176, 177, 179, 185, 186, 209, 214
intestinal flora   7, 10, 123, 190
iron   11, 17, 34, 56, 57, 135, 144, 168, 171, 175, 176, 177, 188, 228, 239, 240, 242

iodine 11, 17, 130, 229, 240

itching 4, 26, 44, 47, 50, 51, 93, 98, 99, 103, 125, 133, 154, 155, 162, 180, 188, 205, 210, 212, 222, 223, 247, 248, 253

Jerusalem artichoke 158

joints 3, 6, 7, 10, 19, 23, 25, 27, 45, 49, 59, 78, 79, 87, 88, 91, 93, 94, 95, 97, 98, 99, 106, 108, 132, 133, 138, 140, 145, 151, 158, 164, 182, 184, 187, 189, 190, 207, 213, 223, 227, 237, 238, 252

kelp 9, 11, 159, 191, 225, 227, 229

kidneys 1, 10, 15, 17, 24, 41, 42, 43, 45, 48, 51, 52, 100, 122, 128, 130, 132, 133, 134, 135, 138, 141, 146, 150, 152, 154, 155, 162, 168, 173, 176, 178, 180, 181, 183, 185, 198, 231, 232

    infection 25, 46, 195

    inflammation 133, 142, 196, 197

    disorders 32, 37, 80, 148, 151, 157, 159, 171, 196, 199, 237

    stones 128, 138, 143, 152, 153, 172, 178, 179, 183, 198, 199, 205, 207

labor 95, 129, 131, 176, 182

lactation 76, 104, 125, 139

    see also breastfeeding

lavender 5, 14, 15, 39, 78, 90, 101, 103, 107, 141, 161, 208

laxatives 46, 49, 123, 125, 127, 131, 134, 135, 136, 140, 143, 148, 149, 154, 177, 181, 227, 252

leaky gut syndrome 136, 175

libido 89, 101, 142, 147, 167, 169,

    see also aphrodisiac

lice 62, 78, 79, 85, 99, 105, 184, 253

ligaments 16, 34

liver 1, 9, 15, 16, 22, 37, 40, 41, 42, 46, 48, 49, 50, 52, 53, 63, 80, 81, 91, 92, 97, 106, 107, 122, 125, 126, 127, 128, 131,

132, 133, 136, 137, 138, 140, 143, 144, 146, 150, 151, 155, 156, 162, 163, 164, 165, 171, 178, 179, 180, 181, 183, 186, 187, 188, 207, 211, 241, 257

    detoxification 26, 30, 144, 156, 180, 207, 208

    disorders 32, 92, 136, 144, 145, 148, 150, 165-166, 184, 193, 194, 196, 197, 199, 208

    tonic 60, 122, 138, 144, 155, 170, 188, 231, 232

longevity 22, 28, 147, 151, 163, 177, 185

    see also aging

lungs 1, 22, 23, 24, 38, 40, 42, 43, 45, 46, 47, 48, 52, 61, 68, 77, 99, 100, 103, 130, 132, 133, 135, 139, 141, 144, 154, 156, 163, 165, 167, 174, 180, 181, 182, 184, 186, 187, 189, 225, 231, 232, 252

lupus 150, 184, 262

Lyme's disease 154, 163, 182, 184

lymphatic system 20, 32, 42, 50, 56, 63, 70, 75, 77, 81, 83, 84, 86, 87, 88, 91, 104, 131, 133, 138, 141, 146, 148, 149, 150, 153, 157, 164, 168, 174, 176, 181, 182, 183, 186, 188, 207, 210, 222

massage 67, 74, 75, 76, 77, 79, 82, 85, 86, 87, 88, 89, 90, 94, 97, 98, 99, 100, 101, 103, 104, 105, 107, 126, 174, 221, 225, 249, 253, 254, 256, 258, 261

memory 18, 23, 27, 28, 30, 40, 42, 52, 76, 79, 84, 89, 98, 101, 117, 126, 127, 134, 137, 153, 164, 172, 177, 178, 179, 222

menopause 51, 84, 87, 88, 101, 129, 147, 225

    see also estrogen, hot flashes, hormones, progesterone, testosterone

menorrhagia *see* menstruation

menstruation

    amenorrhea 94, 162,

    cramps 34, 35, 50, 76, 79, 82, 83, 89, 93, 124, 129, 164, 187, 206, 211, 225, 230

dysmenorrhea 44, 143, 158, 162
irregular 41, 50, 139, 176
menorrhagia 176
pain 50, 61, 94, 105, 130, 133, 134, 136, 143, 144, 145, 158, 162, 172, 225
mental alertness 77, 85, 92, 96, 99, 105, 147
mental disorders 22
metabolism 9, 12, 24, 27, 30, 31, 58, 126, 131, 133, 138, 139, 140, 143, 151, 157, 164, 165, 173, 179, 180, 185, 227, 256
migraines 29, 46, 76, 84, 88, 92, 103, 134, 141, 148, 160, 161, 166, 172, 205, 233
see also headaches
milk thistle 133, 165, 176, 191, 208
minerals 9, 10, 11, 12, 33-35, 55, 56, 57, 58, 66, 114, 117, 122, 130, 139, 144, 146, 157, 159, 168, 176, 177, 179, 185, 224, 227-229, 237, 238, 239, 240, 242, 243, 244, 245, 250, 253, 257, 260
see also calcium, iodine, iron, potassium
miscarriage 27, 130, 143, 148, 176, 184, 187, 225
mononucleosis 100
mood swings 41, 52, 101, 152
morning sickness 46, 48, 176, 182
motion sickness 24, 41, 98, 151
mucous membranes 11, 34, 122, 132, 139, 148, 153, 155, 159, 165, 166, 167, 168, 173, 182, 183, 185, 189, 236, 256
mucus 11, 18, 108, 127, 132, 161, 163
mullein 16, 36, 167, 223
muscles 3, 16, 20, 27, 29, 34, 43, 45, 52, 53, 59, 61, 75, 76, 77, 78, 79, 81, 86, 87, 88, 89, 91, 93, 94, 95, 98, 99, 100, 104, 106, 107, 122, 125, 126, 128, 130, 132, 134, 135, 137, 138, 142, 143, 147, 154, 156, 158, 159, 160, 163, 164, 165, 166, 167, 171, 172, 174, 176, 179, 181, 186, 187, 188, 207, 210, 214, 237, 238, 239, 242
nausea 24, 41, 42, 43, 46, 50, 51, 78, 80, 84, 86, 87, 89, 91, 95, 97, 98, 124, 132, 140, 141, 142, 143, 144, 148, 151, 157, 163, 165, 170, 172, 177, 178, 182, 186, 193, 194, 196, 197, 209
nervous system 6, 14, 15, 16, 17, 18, 20, 23, 25, 26, 27, 32, 34, 60, 71, 73, 74, 75, 76, 77, 79, 81, 82, 87, 88, 89, 90, 91, 92, 94, 95, 97, 98, 99, 100, 102, 104, 107, 109, 124, 126, 127, 129, 131, 133, 134, 137, 138, 140, 142, 144, 145, 147, 150, 152, 153, 154, 156, 157, 158, 159, 161, 162, 164, 165, 166, 167, 169, 171, 172, 177, 178, 179, 180, 181, 184, 185, 186, 187, 189, 194, 205, 211, 213, 214, 215, 217, 224, 225, 227, 228, 229, 231, 241, 257
neuralgia 47, 84, 99
nicotine 163, 169
see also smoking
nosebleed 41, 129, 146, 155, 183
oats 169, 227
osteoporosis(penia) *see* bones
ovaries 44, 148, 162, 165, 225
pancreas 20, 37, 86, 136, 137, 147
parasites 78, 87, 92, 94, 103, 106, 126, 130, 138, 156, 163, 166, 182, 184
peppermint 3, 6, 13, 14, 15, 98, 103, 161, 172, 174, 182, 210
pineal gland 39, 188
pituitary gland 81
poisoning 23, 42, 90, 92, 138, 139, 163, 180, 191
potassium 2, 11, 12, 56, 58, 144, 175, 184, 196, 227-228, 238, 240, 242
pregnancy 27, 128, 129, 140, 142, 148, 160, 171, 176, 182, 187, 192, 193, 194, 195, 196, 197, 198, 199, 242

premenstrual syndrome (PMS)   44, 48, 50, 83, 84, 87, 101, 114, 131, 139, 144, 206, 207, 211, 215, 248, 250

probiotics   *see* intestinal flora

progesterone   180, 187, 225

prostate   25, 31, 41, 45, 63, 64, 98, 133, 142, 148, 155, 157, 168, 175, 182, 194, 199, 254

protein   7, 9, 10, 11, 12, 27, 36, 62, 117, 122, 130, 132, 135, 137, 139, 143, 148, 159, 164, 171, 175, 177, 197, 235, 247, 249, 260

psoriasis   2, 58, 75, 78, 80, 92, 125, 127, 142, 149, 163, 166, 170, 180, 188, 224, 238, 246, 247, 248, 250, 251, 253, 255

radiation   2, 105, 123, 126, 138, 148, 162, 191, 257

rashes   25, 44, 47, 66, 80, 93, 97, 107, 108, 158, 160, 162, 163, 173, 183, 195, 196, 205, 207, 210, 212, 222, 223, 224, 250

red clover   36, 146, 176, 198, 224, 228

respiratory system   4, 6, 11, 12, 14, 17, 24, 26, 35, 68, 75, 76, 79, 87, 90, 97, 99, 100, 101, 103, 108, 126, 127, 132, 147, 148, 151, 153, 157, 162, 163, 167, 170, 173, 174, 175, 176, 178, 184, 186, 189, 205, 208, 211, 215, 219, 225, 231, 232, 233, 252, 262

rheumatoid arthritis   10, 88, 147, 150, 154, 180, 189

ringworm   32, 93, 99, 105, 130, 131, 253

rosehips   54, 114, 177-178, 191, 255, 259

sedatives   26, 29, 49, 82, 83, 84, 88, 92, 95, 104, 109, 128, 129, 135, 136, 141, 142, 143, 156, 159, 160, 166, 171, 174, 175, 185, 186, 187, 205, 210

seizures   79, 134

shingles   77, 100, 179, 209, 250

sinus   4, 68, 70, 74, 85, 91, 104, 105, 125, 127, 128, 147, 148, 156, 160, 164, 167, 225, 233, 233- 234, 262

sinusitis   34, 89, 97, 100, 142, 233

skin   2, 3, 5, 6, 9, 11, 12, 16, 18, 20, 26, 34, 48, 49, 52, 58, 60, 61, 67, 75, 76, 78, 80, 83, 84, 85, 87, 88, 93, 94, 97, 101, 102, 103, 106, 109, 113, 117, 123, 130, 134, 142, 155, 157, 162, 168, 170, 171, 189, 204-205, 206, 209, 211, 212, 221, 222, 223, 224, 225, 228, 230, 236, 238, 239, 247, 249, 250, 251, 252, 253, 254, 255, 256, 257, 258, 259, 260, 261

cleansing   55-57, 68, 74, 116, 123, 125, 131, 146, 175, 176, 211, 222

conditions   4, 31, 44, 46, 75, 78, 80, 81, 85, 87, 90, 94, 95, 96, 99, 100, 101, 102, 106, 108, 114, 122, 131, 133, 136, 138, 139, 143, 146, 148, 149, 153, 161, 171, 172, 177, 179, 180, 188, 189, 205, 207, 208, 212, 213, 221, 222, 224, 225, 226, 238, 246, 248, 250, 251, 253, 255, 256, 257

dry   2, 5, 6, 32, 34, 46, 66, 77, 86, 95, 97, 99, 100, 113, 188, 207, 212, 224, 246, 248, 249, 252, 257, 260, 264

irritated   67, 89, 99, 104, 108, 113, 146, 208, 209, 212, 222, 224, 246

moisturizing   2, 17, 114, 122, 131, 178, 206, 246, 247, 248, 250, 254, 255, 257, 260

oily   55, 56, 84, 87, 88, 89, 91, 94, 95, 100, 102, 107, 108, 208, 209, 254, 264

sensitive   89, 95, 100, 113, 125, 127, 207, 208, 249, 254, 255, 260, 264

wrinkles   6, 10, 80, 85,87, 90, 94, 95, 97, 98, 100, 101, 102, 103, 107, 113, 115, 142, 175, 206, 208, 246, 247, 248, 249, 250, 251, 252, 256, 258, 261

skin tags   26

sleep   18, 20, 23, 40, 41, 49, 51, 52, 75, 80, 81, 85, 95, 96, 104, 107, 117, 125, 135, 138, 139, 142, 156, 157, 158, 165, 167, 169, 172, 175, 177, 189, 194, 208, 210, 212, 225, 255, 256

see also insomnia
slippery elm 16, 182
smoking 46, 60, 136, 141, 163, 185, 210
   see also nicotine
sore throat 34, 38, 40, 42, 43, 44, 45, 50, 59, 60, 61, 63, 64, 66, 70, 77, 89, 94, 102, 105, 106, 124, 127, 129, 146, 148, 151, 156, 158, 170, 210, 212, 239
splinters 67, 182
sprains 32, 45, 54, 67, 78, 85, 134, 150, 179, 187, 210, 221, 239, 253
stomach 1, 7, 14, 20, 22, 37, 41, 42, 44, 45, 52, 67, 77, 84, 86, 89, 91, 94, 101, 103, 122, 126, 130, 131, 136, 137, 138, 139, 140, 142, 146, 150, 151, 156, 159, 160, 161, 164, 165, 167, 168, 172, 173, 174, 176, 177, 178, 180, 182, 184, 186, 187, 197, 209, 210, 227, 237, 238
stool softener 125, 149
stress 6, 16, 17, 23, 30, 44, 46, 48, 49, 50, 69, 76, 77, 81, 82, 88, 89, 92, 94, 96, 99, 100, 101, 103, 104, 107, 109, 122, 127, 128, 142, 147, 152, 153, 159, 160, 161, 162, 164, 177, 180, 183, 185, 187, 189, 191, 205, 207, 208, 209, 210, 214, 215, 224, 227, 231, 232, 239, 264
stretch marks 104, 258, 260
sugar cravings 141, 158
TMJ 158
tendonitis 207, 230
testosterone 25, 147, 180, 189
thrush 34, 130, 134, 205, 208, 236
thyroid gland 10, 11, 38, 94, 133, 145, 146, 159, 168, 171, 188, 193, 194, 229
tinnitus 29, 43, 130, 146, 151, 162
tonsillitis 34, 42, 44, 89, 106, 127, 155, 176

tumors 11, 60, 63, 126, 129, 136, 138, 153, 164, 176, 177, 183, 185, 186, 231, 232
ulcers 2, 11, 16, 37, 41, 49, 61, 79, 96, 127, 131, 134, 136, 139, 152, 155, 162, 168, 173, 177, 182, 185, 189, 194, 195, 196, 198, 222, 256, 261
urinary system 17, 25, 31, 36, 37, 46, 61, 62, 80, 81, 87, 98, 122, 128, 129, 130, 131, 134, 138, 139, 141, 143, 144, 146, 148, 153, 156, 157, 159, 163, 166, 167, 170, 172, 173, 176, 178, 180, 181, 183, 184, 185, 189, 205, 206
   incontinence 45, 138, 143, 185
   infections *see* infections
   see also bladder and kidneys
uterus 14, 41, 63, 122, 128, 129, 133, 153, 160, 171, 176, 187, 188
vagina 27, 41, 42, 46, 51, 67, 81, 107, 122, 153, 158, 165, 173, 205
   infections *see* infections
vaginitis 61, 85, 208, 210
valley fever 130
varicose veins 34, 52, 84, 128, 155, 156, 163, 165, 174, 183, 186, 187, 188, 212, 222, 223, 225
viruses 4, 11, 32, 77, 93, 94, 117, 129, 136, 146, 157, 170, 191, 209, 217
vision 28, 29, 39, 47, 50, 51, 70, 146, 169, 197, 257
   see also eyes
vitamins 10, 58, 122, 139, 144, 159, 222, 235, 242, 243, 244, 245, 253
   A 11, 144, 185, 247, 254, 257
   B 6, 11, 12, 117, 177, 222, 243, 247
   C 11, 22, 100, 122, 124, 135, 140, 173, 174, 175, 177, 185, 191, 199, 246, 254, 255
   D 11, 113, 247

E 11, 113, 146, 177, 236, 247, 249, 251, 253, 254, 256, 257, 258, 261

K 10, 168, 177, 254

warts 32, 94, 105, 131, 137, 221

water retention 54, 75, 86, 87, 92, 133, 134, 156, 162, 163, 184, 206, 239

weight 2, 10, 18, 19, 24, 28, 31, 41, 45, 117, 138, 142, 150, 154, 158, 165, 167, 173, 178, 180, 252

wounds 3, 51, 66, 67, 84, 85, 87, 99, 100, 105, 106, 108, 123, 138, 142, 148, 152, 155, 173, 179, 180, 184, 185, 187, 192, 194, 208, 210, 213, 217, 221, 222, 223, 239, 250, 256

wrinkles *see* skin

yeast infection 3, 52, 134

Made in the USA
San Bernardino, CA
11 May 2014